MW01681011

CACHEXIA

A Medical Dictionary, Bibliography, and Annotated Research Guide to Internet References

James N. Parker, M.D.
and Philip M. Parker, Ph.D., Editors

ICON Health Publications
ICON Group International, Inc.
4370 La Jolla Village Drive, 4th Floor
San Diego, CA 92122 USA

Printed in the United States of America.

Last digit indicates print number: 10 9 8 7 6 4 5 3 2 1

Publisher, Health Care: Philip Parker, Ph.D.
Editor(s): James Parker, M.D., Philip Parker, Ph.D.

Publisher's note: The ideas, procedures, and suggestions contained in this book are not intended for the diagnosis or treatment of a health problem. As new medical or scientific information becomes available from academic and clinical research, recommended treatments and drug therapies may undergo changes. The authors, editors, and publisher have attempted to make the information in this book up to date and accurate in accord with accepted standards at the time of publication. The authors, editors, and publisher are not responsible for errors or omissions or for consequences from application of the book, and make no warranty, expressed or implied, in regard to the contents of this book. Any practice described in this book should be applied by the reader in accordance with professional standards of care used in regard to the unique circumstances that may apply in each situation. The reader is advised to always check product information (package inserts) for changes and new information regarding dosage and contraindications before prescribing any drug or pharmacological product. Caution is especially urged when using new or infrequently ordered drugs, herbal remedies, vitamins and supplements, alternative therapies, complementary therapies and medicines, and integrative medical treatments.

Cataloging-in-Publication Data

Parker, James N., 1961-
Parker, Philip M., 1960-

Cachexia: A Medical Dictionary, Bibliography, and Annotated Research Guide to Internet References / James N. Parker and Philip M. Parker, editors
p. cm.
Includes bibliographical references, glossary, and index.
ISBN: 0-497-00195-0
1. Cachexia-Popular works. I. Title.

Disclaimer

This publication is not intended to be used for the diagnosis or treatment of a health problem. It is sold with the understanding that the publisher, editors, and authors are not engaging in the rendering of medical, psychological, financial, legal, or other professional services.

References to any entity, product, service, or source of information that may be contained in this publication should not be considered an endorsement, either direct or implied, by the publisher, editors, or authors. ICON Group International, Inc., the editors, and the authors are not responsible for the content of any Web pages or publications referenced in this publication.

Copyright Notice

Acknowledgements

The collective knowledge generated from academic and applied research summarized in various references has been critical in the creation of this book which is best viewed as a comprehensive compilation and collection of information prepared by various official agencies which produce publications on cachexia. Books in this series draw from various agencies and institutions associated with the United States Department of Health and Human Services, and in particular, the Office of the Secretary of Health and Human Services (OS), the Administration for Children and Families (ACF), the Administration on Aging (AOA), the Agency for Healthcare Research and Quality (AHRQ), the Agency for Toxic Substances and Disease Registry (ATSDR), the Centers for Disease Control and Prevention (CDC), the Food and Drug Administration (FDA), the Healthcare Financing Administration (HCFA), the Health Resources and Services Administration (HRSA), the Indian Health Service (IHS), the institutions of the National Institutes of Health (NIH), the Program Support Center (PSC), and the Substance Abuse and Mental Health Services Administration (SAMHSA). In addition to these sources, information gathered from the National Library of Medicine, the United States Patent Office, the European Union, and their related organizations has been invaluable in the creation of this book. Some of the work represented was financially supported by the Research and Development Committee at INSEAD. This support is gratefully acknowledged. Finally, special thanks are owed to Tiffany Freeman for her excellent editorial support.

About the Editors

James N. Parker, M.D.

Dr. James N. Parker received his Bachelor of Science degree in Psychobiology from the University of California, Riverside and his M.D. from the University of California, San Diego. In addition to authoring numerous research publications, he has lectured at various academic institutions. Dr. Parker is the medical editor for health books by ICON Health Publications.

Philip M. Parker, Ph.D.

Philip M. Parker is the Eli Lilly Chair Professor of Innovation, Business and Society at INSEAD (Fontainebleau, France and Singapore). Dr. Parker has also been Professor at the University of California, San Diego and has taught courses at Harvard University, the Hong Kong University of Science and Technology, the Massachusetts Institute of Technology, Stanford University, and UCLA. Dr. Parker is the associate editor for ICON Health Publications.

About ICON Health Publications

To discover more about ICON Health Publications, simply check with your preferred online booksellers, including Barnes&Noble.com and Amazon.com which currently carry all of our titles. Or, feel free to contact us directly for bulk purchases or institutional discounts:

ICON Group International, Inc.
4370 La Jolla Village Drive, Fourth Floor
San Diego, CA 92122 USA
Fax: 858-546-4341
Web site: **www.icongrouponline.com/health**

Table of Contents

FORWARD 1
CHAPTER 1. STUDIES ON CACHEXIA 3
Overview 3
The Combined Health Information Database 3
Federally Funded Research on Cachexia 4
E-Journals: PubMed Central 50
The National Library of Medicine: PubMed 50
CHAPTER 2. NUTRITION AND CACHEXIA 93
Overview 93
Finding Nutrition Studies on Cachexia 93
Federal Resources on Nutrition 95
Additional Web Resources 95
CHAPTER 3. ALTERNATIVE MEDICINE AND CACHEXIA 97
Overview 97
National Center for Complementary and Alternative Medicine 97
Additional Web Resources 105
General References 106
CHAPTER 4. PATENTS ON CACHEXIA 107
Overview 107
Patents on Cachexia 107
Patent Applications on Cachexia 118
Keeping Current 133
CHAPTER 5. BOOKS ON CACHEXIA 135
Overview 135
Book Summaries: Online Booksellers 135
CHAPTER 6. PERIODICALS AND NEWS ON CACHEXIA 137
Overview 137
News Services and Press Releases 137
Academic Periodicals covering Cachexia 138
CHAPTER 7. RESEARCHING MEDICATIONS 141
Overview 141
U.S. Pharmacopeia 141
Commercial Databases 142
Researching Orphan Drugs 142
APPENDIX A. PHYSICIAN RESOURCES 147
Overview 147
NIH Guidelines 147
NIH Databases 149
Other Commercial Databases 151
APPENDIX B. PATIENT RESOURCES 153
Overview 153
Patient Guideline Sources 153
Finding Associations 156
APPENDIX C. FINDING MEDICAL LIBRARIES 159
Overview 159
Preparation 159
Finding a Local Medical Library 159
Medical Libraries in the U.S. and Canada 159

ONLINE GLOSSARIES 165

Online Dictionary Directories 165

CACHEXIA DICTIONARY 167

INDEX 245

FORWARD

In March 2001, the National Institutes of Health issued the following warning: "The number of Web sites offering health-related resources grows every day. Many sites provide valuable information, while others may have information that is unreliable or misleading."[1] Furthermore, because of the rapid increase in Internet-based information, many hours can be wasted searching, selecting, and printing. Since only the smallest fraction of information dealing with cachexia is indexed in search engines, such as **www.google.com** or others, a non-systematic approach to Internet research can be not only time consuming, but also incomplete. This book was created for medical professionals, students, and members of the general public who want to know as much as possible about cachexia, using the most advanced research tools available and spending the least amount of time doing so.

In addition to offering a structured and comprehensive bibliography, the pages that follow will tell you where and how to find reliable information covering virtually all topics related to cachexia, from the essentials to the most advanced areas of research. Public, academic, government, and peer-reviewed research studies are emphasized. Various abstracts are reproduced to give you some of the latest official information available to date on cachexia. Abundant guidance is given on how to obtain free-of-charge primary research results via the Internet. **While this book focuses on the field of medicine, when some sources provide access to non-medical information relating to cachexia, these are noted in the text.**

E-book and electronic versions of this book are fully interactive with each of the Internet sites mentioned (clicking on a hyperlink automatically opens your browser to the site indicated). If you are using the hard copy version of this book, you can access a cited Web site by typing the provided Web address directly into your Internet browser. You may find it useful to refer to synonyms or related terms when accessing these Internet databases. **NOTE:** At the time of publication, the Web addresses were functional. However, some links may fail due to URL address changes, which is a common occurrence on the Internet.

For readers unfamiliar with the Internet, detailed instructions are offered on how to access electronic resources. For readers unfamiliar with medical terminology, a comprehensive glossary is provided. For readers without access to Internet resources, a directory of medical libraries, that have or can locate references cited here, is given. We hope these resources will prove useful to the widest possible audience seeking information on cachexia.

The Editors

---

[1] From the NIH, National Cancer Institute (NCI): **http://www.cancer.gov/cancerinfo/ten-things-to-know.**

Chapter 1. Studies on Cachexia

Overview

In this chapter, we will show you how to locate peer-reviewed references and studies on cachexia.

The Combined Health Information Database

The Combined Health Information Database summarizes studies across numerous federal agencies. To limit your investigation to research studies and cachexia, you will need to use the advanced search options. First, go to **http://chid.nih.gov/index.html**. From there, select the "Detailed Search" option (or go directly to that page with the following hyperlink: **http://chid.nih.gov/detail/detail.html**). The trick in extracting studies is found in the drop boxes at the bottom of the search page where "You may refine your search by." Select the dates and language you prefer, and the format option "Journal Article." At the top of the search form, select the number of records you would like to see (we recommend 100) and check the box to display "whole records." We recommend that you type "cachexia" (or synonyms) into the "For these words:" box. Consider using the option "anywhere in record" to make your search as broad as possible. If you want to limit the search to only a particular field, such as the title of the journal, then select this option in the "Search in these fields" drop box. The following is what you can expect from this type of search:

- **Diabetic Neuropathic Cachexia**

  Source: Western Journal of Medicine. 165(6): 382-385. December 1996.

  Summary: This article presents a case of diabetic neuropathic **cachexia,** a rare syndrome seen predominately in patients in their sixth or seventh decade with noninsulin dependent diabetes mellitus (NIDDM). The syndrome is characterized by substantial involuntary weight loss, anorexia, depression, severe autonomic dysfunction, and peripheral neuropathy that develop over a short period of time. Generally, other specific end-organ complications of diabetes mellitus, such as retinopathy or nephropathy, are absent. Because of its highly variable and profound clinical presentation, this syndrome is often confused with neuropathic carincomatosis or an occult cancer. The overall prognosis is good, and symptoms generally resolve spontaneously over 1 to 2 years. The authors present the case of a 57-year-old man and review the related literature. Strong reassurance to patients, optimistic views about the course of the disease, and close followup are important in managing these patients. Most patients resume their normal lifestyle, with most maintaining good diabetes control with diet alone or with a low-dose oral hypoglycemic agent. Followup for longer than 5 years has shown no relapse of this symptom complex. 1 table. 16 references.

Federally Funded Research on Cachexia

The U.S. Government supports a variety of research studies relating to cachexia. These studies are tracked by the Office of Extramural Research at the National Institutes of Health.[2] CRISP (Computerized Retrieval of Information on Scientific Projects) is a searchable database of federally funded biomedical research projects conducted at universities, hospitals, and other institutions.

Search the CRISP Web site at **http://crisp.cit.nih.gov/crisp/crisp_query.generate_screen**. You will have the option to perform targeted searches by various criteria, including geography, date, and topics related to cachexia.

For most of the studies, the agencies reporting into CRISP provide summaries or abstracts. As opposed to clinical trial research using patients, many federally funded studies use animals or simulated models to explore cachexia. The following is typical of the type of information found when searching the CRISP database for cachexia:

- **Project Title: ACTG 313--PHASE II DOUBLE BLIND COMPARING MEGACE + TESTOSTERONE VS MEGACE**

  Principal Investigator & Institution: Bartlet, John; Johns Hopkins University 3400 N Charles St Baltimore, Md 21218

  Timing: Fiscal Year 2002

  Summary: Compare the effects of treatment with megestrol acetate alone and in combination with testosterone on lean body mass in patients with HIV- associated wasting disease.

  Website: http://crisp.cit.nih.gov/crisp/Crisp_Query.Generate_Screen

- **Project Title: ACTG 382--HI PROTEIN SUPPLEMENTS IN HIV+ WEIGHT LOSS PTS**

  Principal Investigator & Institution: Bartlett, John G.; Johns Hopkins University 3400 N Charles St Baltimore, Md 21218

  Timing: Fiscal Year 2002

  Summary: ACTG 392 is designed to determine whether use of a conventional oral supplement containing increased amounts of high biologic qualityprotein which is rich in cysteine and glutamine will result in better repletion and maintenance of lean tissue than an isocaloric supplement without whey protein or amino acid supplementation.

  Website: http://crisp.cit.nih.gov/crisp/Crisp_Query.Generate_Screen

---

2 Healthcare projects are funded by the National Institutes of Health (NIH), Substance Abuse and Mental Health Services (SAMHSA), Health Resources and Services Administration (HRSA), Food and Drug Administration (FDA), Centers for Disease Control and Prevention (CDCP), Agency for Healthcare Research and Quality (AHRQ), and Office of Assistant Secretary of Health (OASH).

- **Project Title: ACTG313--EFFECT OF MEGASE AND TESTOSTERONE IN HIV WASTING**

  Principal Investigator & Institution: Sattler, Fred R.; University of Southern California 2250 Alcazar Street, Csc-219 Los Angeles, Ca 90033

  Timing: Fiscal Year 2002

  Summary: This abstract is not available.

  Website: http://crisp.cit.nih.gov/crisp/Crisp_Query.Generate_Screen

- **Project Title: ACUTE AND CHRONIC MICRODIALYSIS IN THE GUSTATORY SYSTEM**

  Principal Investigator & Institution: Travers, Joseph B.; Associate Professor; Oral Biology; Ohio State University 1960 Kenny Road Columbus, Oh 43210

  Timing: Fiscal Year 2002; Project Start 01-APR-2001; Project End 30-SEP-2004

  Summary: (provided by applicant): We propose to establish microdialysis in the awake, behaving preparation as a technique for investigating amino acid transmitters and neuropeptides in the gustatory-responsive (rostral) nucleus of the solitary tract (rNST). Although microdialysis has been used in many regions of the CNS with great success, the potential of this technique has remained unexploited in the gustatory system. Salt deprivation, hunger, satiety and conditioned aversions have all been demonstrated to impact neural responsiveness in the gustatory system. The neural basis for these state-dependent changes is unknown, but, based on their role in other sensory systems, a predominant role for peptide neuromodulators, perhaps acting via interneurons utilizing excitatory or inhibitory amino acids, is a compelling hypothesis. Understanding the functional neurochemistry of gustatory processing would be greatly facilitated by the ability to monitor the release of multiple neuroactive agents in an animal actively engaged in gustatory-driven behavior. Microdialysis can meet these requirements. The present studies will provide a foundation for assessing this hypothesis by establishing the capabilities of microdialysis followed by HPLC and electrochemical detection in the first-order gustatory relay. The first experiments will monitor amino acid release in an anesthetized preparation, in which precisely controlled taste stimulation is possible. The results of these experiments will be critical in interpreting data obtained in a second series of studies which will apply microdialysis to monitor amino acid release in an awake preparation. A third series of studies will develop microdialysis for assessing the release of multiple neuropeptides, by adapting electrochemical detection techniques to this purpose. When the proposed studies are brought to fruition, future work will be directed at examining the neurochemical basis for fluctuations in gustatory sensitivity as a function of metabolic or nutritional status, and as a function of learning or task demands. The characterization of the dynamic neurochemistry associated with gustatory processing under varying homeostatic conditions offers therapeutic avenues to either increase food intake in response to **cachexia** or to limit intake for obesity.

  Website: http://crisp.cit.nih.gov/crisp/Crisp_Query.Generate_Screen

- **Project Title: ACUTE WT LOSS NUTRITIONAL ASSESSMENT FOR HIV POSITIVE PERSONS**

  Principal Investigator & Institution: Gorbach, Sherwood L.; Professor; New England Medical Center Hospitals 750 Washington St Boston, Ma 021111533

  Timing: Fiscal Year 2002; Project Start 01-MAR-2002; Project End 28-FEB-2003

Summary: This abstract is not available.

Website: http://crisp.cit.nih.gov/crisp/Crisp_Query.Generate_Screen

- **Project Title: ADJUVANT GINSENG USE DURING BREAST CANCER DRUG THERAPY**

  Principal Investigator & Institution: Murphy, Laura L.; Associate Professor; Physiology; Southern Illinois University Carbondale 900 S. Normal Carbondale, Il 629014709

  Timing: Fiscal Year 2004; Project Start 01-APR-2004; Project End 31-MAR-2006

  Summary: (provided by applicant): Ginseng is an herb widely used by humans to treat lack of stamina, loss of appetite and **cachexia,** and impotence. In Asian medicine, ginseng is a common component in herbals used in treatment of cancer, including breast cancer. There is recent scientific evidence that ginseng and its ginsenoside components are effective in inhibiting breast cancer cell proliferation in vitro and tumor growth in vivo. Consequently, many patients may be taking ginseng supplements during treatment with standard chemotherapy and hormonal therapy regimens in an effort to enhance therapeutic results as well as ameliorate side effects of the cancer chemotherapeutic drugs. However, there is no information on how adjuvant ginseng use could influence the efficacy of the cancer therapeutic drugs. This R21 proposal will address the following questions. Will the adjuvant use of ginseng aid in or interfere with standard breast cancer chemo- or hormonal therapy? Will adjuvant ginseng use produce palliative effects in the breast cancer patient undergoing chemotherapy? To answer these questions, we will examine the effects of a wide dose-range of individual chemotherapy (doxorubicin, cyclophosphamide, paclitaxel) or hormonal (tamoxifen) therapy drugs, alone and in combinations with an extract of American ginseng, on the proliferation of human breast cancer cells (MCF-7, MDA-MB-231) in vitro. The results of this study will allow us to determine if adjuvant ginseng treatment alters the efficacy of standard cancer therapeutic drugs. From these results, we will determine the treatment regimens to be tested in vivo in female athymic nude mice inoculated with either MCF-7 or MDA-MB- 231 cells, monitoring tumor growth as well as general well-being and systemic toxicity. These preclinical studies will allow us to determine the potential palliative effects concomitant ginseng treatment may have in animals receiving the potent cancer therapeutic drugs. Thirdly, we will examine potential additive, synergistic or sub-additive effects of combination ginseng/chemotherapy treatment on pathway-specific genes/proteins involved in cell cycle regulation, apoptosis and cytotoxicity. Together, the results of these studies will provide us with a better understanding of American ginseng and will allow evidence-based decisions to be made by breast cancer patients and their physicians regarding complementary ginseng use during standard chemotherapy.

  Website: http://crisp.cit.nih.gov/crisp/Crisp_Query.Generate_Screen

- **Project Title: AIDS AND THE GASTROINTESTINAL TRACT**

  Principal Investigator & Institution: Mansfield, Keith G.; Associate Professor of Pathology; Pathology; Harvard University (Medical School) Medical School Campus Boston, Ma 02115

  Timing: Fiscal Year 2002; Project Start 30-SEP-2000; Project End 28-FEB-2005

  Summary: Human immunodeficiency virus (HIV)-infected patients commonly have unintentional weight loss and low serum micronutrient levels that have been correlated with disease progression. However, the relationship among these nutritional parameters, direct effects of the virus on the intestinal immune system and intestinal dysfunction and the role of opportunistic infections in progressive weight loss are not clear. These issues are extremely difficult to address in persons infected with HIV because a large percentage of HIV/AIDS patients are already taking a variety of nutritional supplements in an uncontrolled manner and dietary intake varies greatly. Furthermore, the rapid evolution of antiretroviral therapy complicates obtaining answers to these questions. To obviate these problems and also to control for additional variable such as time since inoculation and differences in viral inocula, we propose to use the simian immunodeficiency virus (SIV)-infected macaque model of AIDS. The organization of the program project involves three projects and four cores. One project will define the natural history of weight loss and micronutrient deficiency in SIV-infected macaques and conduct two interventions to try and alleviate wasting. The next project will examine direct effects of SIV infection on the intestinal immune system and intestinal function. Another project will determine the relationship between key gastrointestinal opportunists (C. parvum, E. bieneusi, and M. avium) and weight loss. Thus this program project represents a multi-disciplinary approach by a group of interactive, experienced investigators to examine the interplay between 1) nutrition, 2) direct effects of SIV infection, and 3) opportunistic infections of the gastrointestinal tract on the pathogenesis of wasting.

Website: http://crisp.cit.nih.gov/crisp/Crisp_Query.Generate_Screen

- **Project Title: ANABOLIC THERAPIES AND THEIR METABOLIC EFFECT IN AIDS**

  Principal Investigator & Institution: Schambelan, Morris; Professor; University of California San Francisco 500 Parnassus Ave San Francisco, Ca 941222747

  Timing: Fiscal Year 2002; Project Start 01-DEC-2001; Project End 30-NOV-2002

  Summary: This abstract is not available.

  Website: http://crisp.cit.nih.gov/crisp/Crisp_Query.Generate_Screen

- **Project Title: ANDROGEN EFFECTS AND INSULIN RESISTANCE IN HIV DISEASE**

  Principal Investigator & Institution: Grinspoon, Steven K.; Associate Professor of Medicine; Massachusetts General Hospital 55 Fruit St Boston, Ma 02114

  Timing: Fiscal Year 2003; Project Start 15-MAR-2003; Project End 29-FEB-2008

  Summary: (provided by applicant): The goal of this application is to support my professional development as a clinical investigator and successful mentor to junior faculty and fellows in patient-oriented research My research focus has been to investigate the effects of nutritional status on neuroendocrine function, and as such, I have used HIV disease as a relevant disease model, with two funded NIH R01 grants for which I am the PI. The three Specific Aims of this grant stem from a significant body of work accomplished over the past few years demonstrating hypogonadism in HIV-infected women and a severe insulin resistance pattern in HIV-infected patients with lipodystrophy In these funded studies, I will investigate the mechanisms of androgen deficiency and also the effects of long-term physiologic testosterone replacement in this population Furthermore, I will study the mechanisms of insulin resistance, investigating the critical role of increased lipolysis and the effects of thiazolidinediones in this population The grant for the first Specific Aim, to study the effects of androgens in HIV-infected women, will expire at the end of this year, and a follow-up proposal, recently submitted will further investigate adrenal androgen shunting and DHEA in this population Preliminary data in this regard show a novel effect of HIV on adrenal metabolism, with shunting toward cortisol and away from androgen production The grant for the third Specific Aim is funded until 2005 I have had good success as a mentor, with two recent K-23 awardees and six former or current trainees There has been significant interest in my research from Endocrine Fellows and also from Fellows in Harvard Nutrition Division The Institutional Environment at the MGH, with a strong and diverse Endocrine Division, GCRC, and Center for AIDS Research is outstanding The Department of Medicine has made a substantial commitment toward my development as a clinical researcher responsible for training a large number of fellows However, it is clearly necessary to reduce my clinical activities in order to devote sufficient time to the training and mentoring of junior faculty and fellows The Mid-career Investigator Award in Patient Oriented Research is an ideal mechanism to ensure the necessary support to reduce clinical and administrative responsibilities, and ensure my continued success as a mentor and clinical researcher.

Website: http://crisp.cit.nih.gov/crisp/Crisp_Query.Generate_Screen

- **Project Title: ANIMAL MODEL DEVELOPMENT FOR MICROSPORIDIOSIS:OPPORTUNISTIC INFECTIONS**

  Principal Investigator & Institution: Didier, Elizabeth Schmidt.; Research Scientist; Tulane University of Louisiana New Orleans, La New Orleans, La 70112

  Timing: Fiscal Year 2002

  Summary: Microsporidia cause opportunistic infections in persons with AIDS, organ transplant recipients, children, and travelers. Enterocytozoon bieneusi is the most prevalent microsporidian but attempts to establish a tissue culture system for generating organisms has been unsuccessful. The only nonhuman hosts known for E. bieneusi include pigs and nonhuman primates (eg. Macaca mulatta). Ten SIV-infected rhesus macaques were inoculated orally with E. bieneusi harvested from the stool and duodenal lavage aspirates of human AIDS patients. Spores were detected in stools one week later and continued sporadically for approximately two years or until death of the monkeys, but the inconsistency of spore shedding presently renders this model inadequate for testing antimicrosporidial compounds. However, the monkeys did become infected with E. bieneusi and parasite-associated lesions were identified in the gall bladder, liver, and small intestine. Attempts to infect small animals (eg. gerbils, at hymic mice, immunesuppressed mice) with E. bieneusi also have failed to date. Due to the difficulties in establishing a useful animal model for E. bieneusi, a surrogate microsporidian, Vittaforma corneae is presently being used to develop an animal model for testing lead compounds in vivo. Athymic mice developed wasting (**cachexia**) and ascites and died 15 - 60 days after intraperitoneal inoculation with 5 x 107 - 1 x 104 V. corneae organisms. Athymic mice infected with 1 x 107 V. corneae and treated with fumagillin survived only a few days longer than non-treated mice but there were statistically significantly fewer parasite-associated lesions in the small intestines, gall bladder, and liver of treated mice. Since fumagillin is toxic in mammals, attempts are underway to obtain fumagillin analogues and related compounds for testing against V. corneae in the murine model. If the simian model can be improved, the effective compounds will then be tested in monkeys, as well. FUNDING NIH; UO1AI0402 (J.A. Shadduck, P.I.); 05/01/96-04/31/00;$277,178 (year 3 total direct; subcontract = approx. 50% of total directs went to RPRC) NIH; NO1-AI-75327 (E.S. Didier, P.I.); 08/15/97-08/14/02; $360,781 (year 2 directs; 100% to RPRC) Venture research funding at TRPRC PUBLICATIONS Abstracts Snowden, K, E.S. Didier, and D. Phalen. 1998. What is the source of Encephalitozoon infections in immunocompromised humans? 49th Ann. Southwest Conference on Disease in Nature Transmissible to Man. College Station, TX (abstract). Snowden, K.F., J.A. Shadduck, and E.S. Didier. 1998. Evaluation of antimicrosporidial therapies using an immunedeficient mouse model. National Cooperative Drug Discovery Groups for the Treatment of Opportunistic Infections (abstract). Snowden, K., D. Phalen, and E.S. Didier. 1998 Where are the reservoirs of human microsporidial infections? Second European Congr. Trop. Med., Liverpool, U.K. (abstract 438) and Amer. J. Trop. Med. Hyg. 59:302 (abstract 554). Green, L.C., L.B. Rogers, P.J. Didier, and E.S. Didier. 1998. Enterocytozoon bieneusi infection immunocompromised rhesus monkeys. Amer. J. Trop. Med. Hyg. 59:332 (abstract 644). Reviews and book chapters Didier, P.J., E.S. Didier, K. Snowden, and J.A. Shadduck. 1998. Encephalitozoonosis. In Infectious Diseases of the Dog and Cat. C.E. Greene (ed.). W.B. Saunders, Philadelphia, PA. pp. 465-469. Didier, E.S., K.A. Snowden, J.A. Shadduck. 1998. The biology of Microsporidian species infecting mammals. Adv. Parasitol. 40:279-316. Didier, E.S. 1998. State-of-the-Art Clinical Article Microsporidiosis. Clin. Infect. Dis. 27:1-7. Didier, P.J., E.S. Didier, and K.F. Snowden. 1998. Microsporidiosis Not just a disease of rabbits. Newsletter Amer. Comm. Lab. Anim. Dis. 19:3-7. Soave, R. and E.S. Didier. 1999. Cryptosporidium and Microsporidium. In Textbook of AIDS Medicine (2nd ed.). T.C. Merigan, J.G. Bartlett, and D. Bolognesi (eds.). Williams and Wilkins, Baltimore, MD. pp. 327-356. Didier, E.S. and G.T. Bessinger. 1999. Host-parasite relationships in microsporidiosis animal models and immunology. In:The Microsporidia and Microsporidiosis. M. Wittner (ed.). American Society for Microbiology, Washington, D.C. pp. 225-257. Didier, E.S. 1999. Immunology of Microsporidiosis. In Contributions to Microbiology. F. Petry (ed). S. Karger AG, Basel, Switzerland (in press). K.F. Snowden, E.S. Didier, J.M. Orenstein, and J.A. Shadduck. 1999. Animal models of human microsporidial infections. In Animal Models. Armed Forces Institute of Pathology, Washington, D.C. (in press).

Website: http://crisp.cit.nih.gov/crisp/Crisp_Query.Generate_Screen

- **Project Title: BIOELECTRICAL IMPEDANCE ANALYSIS HIV+ WOMEN WITH OR WITHOUT WASTING SYNDROME**

  Principal Investigator & Institution: Grunfeld, Carl; Professor of Medicine; University of California San Francisco 500 Parnassus Ave San Francisco, Ca 941222747

  Timing: Fiscal Year 2002; Project Start 01-DEC-2001; Project End 30-NOV-2002

  Summary: This abstract is not available.

  Website: http://crisp.cit.nih.gov/crisp/Crisp_Query.Generate_Screen

- **Project Title: BRAIN SIGNALING OF ESSENTIAL AMINO ACID DEFICIENCY**

  Principal Investigator & Institution: Gietzen, Dorothy W.; Professor; Vet Anatomy/Physiol/Cell Biol; University of California Davis Sponsored Programs, 118 Everson Hall Davis, Ca 956165200

  Timing: Fiscal Year 2003; Project Start 01-FEB-2003; Project End 30-NOV-2006

  Summary: (provided by applicant): Adequate amino acid (AA) nutrition is essential for the health and well being of humans and animals alike. Because AAs have no storage pool, the development of an indispensable AA (IAA) deficiency can occur rapidly, particularly if a mild state of protein deficiency already exists. IAA deficiencies have been shown to compromise growth and body function that depends on protein synthesis, such as wound healing. However, the growth reduction attributed to IAA imbalance is actually secondary to decreased food intake, an anorectic response to the IAA deficiency. Since AA supplements have become fashionable, and may be used particularly by "health food" faddists, dieters and athletes, IAA imbalance should be recognized as a potential health hazard. Moreover, individuals with cancer **cachexia,** disorders of AA metabolism, and other metabolic disorders may also suffer IAA disproportion, which could compromise their recovery. The long-term goal of the work in this laboratory is to determine how the brain recognizes IAA deficiency. Given the importance of AA nutrition, it is imperative that we gain a better understanding of the basic mechanisms by which IAA imbalance affects brain function. We are investigating these mechanisms with a well-described nutritional model using rats fed AA-imbalanced diets (IMB). Our recent work indicates that changes in behavior (rate of eating) in response to IMB occur within the first 12 min of feeding. Within this time period we have found increased glutamine and glutamate in the APC. Rapid changes in vitro include an activation of signal transduction pathways and mobilization of AA transporters. Based on our knowledge of this model, we propose the following specific aims: 1) to identify the initial metabolic signal(s) of IAA deficiency in the APC; 2) to identify the signal transduction pathways activated by the metabolic signals identified in Specific Aim 1; and 3) to identify the mechanisms of activation in the glutamatergic output cells of the APC that signal IAA deficiency. We hypothesize the following: The relative excess of AAs other than the limiting one increase AA metabolism and stimulate the glutamineglutamate cycle, leading to the activation of signaling pathways and the potentiation of APC neurons. When APC neurons are activated, their glutamatergic output first acts at AMPA receptors to signal AA deficiency to other parts of the brain for the anorectic responses.

Website: http://crisp.cit.nih.gov/crisp/Crisp_Query.Generate_Screen

- **Project Title: C/EBP BETA IN HEPATOCYTE GENE EXPRESSION & PROLIFERATION**

  Principal Investigator & Institution: Chojkier, Mario; Prof, Div of Gastroenterology; Veterans Medical Research Fdn/San Diego Foundation of San Diego San Diego, Ca 92161

  Timing: Fiscal Year 2002; Project Start 30-SEP-1998; Project End 31-AUG-2003

  Summary: This renewal proposal focuses on the signal transduction pathways that modulate hepatocyte gene expression and proliferation through site-specific phosphorylations of C/EBP-beta. Preliminary results show that TGF-alpha and phorbol esters/PKC-alpha mediate their effects on hepatocyte proliferation, at least in part, through the activation of ribosomal S6-kinase and phosphorylation of C/EBP-beta on its activation domain. In addition, **cachexia** and TNF-alpha inhibit albumin transcription, at least in part, throug an oxidative stress/NO cascade resulting in the activation of stress-activated protein (SAP)- kinase and phosphorylation of C/EBP-beta on its basic domain, which abolishes the binding of C/EBP-beta to the albumin enhancer/promoter DNA sequence. The specific aims are 1) assess the role of phosphorylation on hepatocyte proliferation, 2) examine the modulation of hepatocyte proliferatio in C/EBP-beta mice, 3) examine the regulation of the cell cycle by C/EBP-beta in hepatocytes, 4) assess the role of oxidative stress and NO on C/EBP-beta phosphorylation and inhibition of albumin transcription induced by **cachexia** an TNF-alpha, 5) examine the modulation of albumin expression in C/EBP-beta transgenic mice, and 6) examine the mechanisms that induce decreased albumin expression in human **cachexia.**

  Website: http://crisp.cit.nih.gov/crisp/Crisp_Query.Generate_Screen

- **Project Title: CALGB INSTITUTIONAL GRANT**

  Principal Investigator & Institution: Clamon, Gerald H.; Internal Medicine; University of Iowa Iowa City, Ia 52242

Timing: Fiscal Year 2003; Project Start 01-APR-1988; Project End 31-MAR-2009

Summary: (provided by applicant): The University of Iowa has been a member of CALGB since 1986. Accrual at the main member hospital is approximately 100 patients per year and approximately 20 more patients are accrued at two affiliates. Over the past 5 years, we have authored or co-chaired studies in non-small cell lung cancer, in chemoprevention of lung cancer, in experimental therapeutics for 506U78, and for omega-3 fatty acids in cancer **cachexia.** Administratively, Dr. Gerald Clamon has been vice chair of the Membership Committee and Dr. Raymond Hohl has been vice chair of the Institutional Performance Evaluation Committee (IPEC). In addition, Dr. Clamon is on the Respiratory Committee and is the liaison to the Cancer Control and Health Outcomes Committee, Dr. Hohl is on the Leukemia Committee and is the liaison to the Pharmacology and Experimental Therapeutics (PET) Committee, Dr. Brian Link is on the Lymphoma Committee, and Dr. Badrinath Konety is on the GU Committee. Dr. Nancy Rosenthal is reviewing slides for the Hematopathology Committee for a lymphoma trial, Dr. Shivanand Patel reviews cytogenetics for the Leukemia Committee, and Dr. Michael Vannier is serving on a new committee to evaluate new technologies in the imaging of tumors. New translational research at the University of Iowa has lead to the development of two new promising anti-cancer therapies. The HU 1D10 antibody developed in the laboratory of Dr. George Weiner at the University of Iowa has completed Phase I trials at the University of Iowa and demonstrated activity against lymphoma. The CpG oligodeoxynucleotide developed at the University of Iowa in the lab or Dr. Arthur Krieg is now completing Phase I trials at the University of Iowa. A pilot study of Pneumovax plus GM-CSF is being completed at the University of Iowa. This should lead to a phase III trial within CALGB and potentially improve success with vaccinations of the immune suppressed cancer patient.

Website: http://crisp.cit.nih.gov/crisp/Crisp_Query.Generate_Screen

- **Project Title: CHARACTERIZATION OF MYOSTATIN AND GDF-11**

  Principal Investigator & Institution: Lee, Se-Jin; Professor; Molecular Biology and Genetics; Johns Hopkins University 3400 N Charles St Baltimore, Md 21218

  Timing: Fiscal Year 2003; Project Start 08-DEC-1997; Project End 30-NOV-2007

  Summary: (provided by applicant): Myostatin (MSTN) and GDF-11 are secreted proteins that we originally identified in a screen for novel growth and differentiation factors related to transforming growth factor-Beta (TGF-B). The predicted sequences of MSTN and GDF-11 are greater than 90% identical in the mature, C-terminal portion of the proteins, and together, these molecules form their own subgroup within the larger TGF-B superfamily. We have been using a variety of in vitro and in vivo approaches, including gene targeting in mice, to attempt to identify the biological functions of MSTN and GDF-11. We have shown that mice lacking MSTN have dramatic and widespread increases in skeletal muscle mass, suggesting that MSTN normally functions as a negative regulator of muscle growth. We have also shown that mice lacking GDF-11 have extensive homeotic transformations of the axial skeleton, suggesting that GDF-11 normally acts as a global regulator of axial patterning. The overall aim of this proposal is to further investigate the biological functions of these molecules and the mechanisms by which their activities are regulated. The specific aims are: to investigate the functional redundancy of MSTN and GDF-11; to analyze the effect of postnatal loss of MSTN and GDF-11 on skeletal muscle mass; to further characterize the role of activin type II receptors in regulating MSTN and GDF-11 signaling; to identify other components of the MSTN and GDF-11 receptor complex; to further investigate the role of follistatin in regulating MSTN and GDF-11 activity; and to investigate the mechanism by which latent MSTN is activated. Taken together, these studies will provide important insights into the normal biological functions of these molecules and may suggest new strategies for modulating the activities of these molecules for human therapeutic applications in muscle wasting diseases, such as muscular dystrophy and **cachexia,** andmetabolic diseases, such as obesity and type II diabetes.

Website: http://crisp.cit.nih.gov/crisp/Crisp_Query.Generate_Screen

- **Project Title: CHEMICAL AND BIOLOGICAL STUDIES ON BIARYL PHENOLICS**

  Principal Investigator & Institution: Feldman, Ken S.; Professor; Chemistry; Pennsylvania State University-Univ Park 110 Technology Center University Park, Pa 16802

  Timing: Fiscal Year 2002; Project Start 01-JUL-1986; Project End 30-JUN-2006

  Summary: (provided by applicant): Continuing biological evaluation of potential anticancer and antisepsis chemotherapeutic analogues of members of the hydrolyzable tannin family of secondary plant metabolites is proposed. Characterization of the immunomodulatory properties of these species will proceed. Mechanism-of-action investigations at the molecular, cellular, and whole animal levels, coupled with structure/activity studies, are designed to reveal the basis for both up-regulation and down-regulation of cytokine (IL-lb and TNFa) secretion by certain tannins. A novel tumor targeting strategy for tannin delivery will be explored. Appreciation of the molecular-level details responsible for either triggering or suppressing cytokine release may serve as the basis for designing tannin-inspired chemotherapeutic agents for diseases as diverse as cancer and septic shock. Ongoing synthesis studies directed toward the potent marine anticancer principle diazonamide A will be brought to completion. In addition to providing a supply of this scarce material for further biological evaluation, successful execution of the plausibly biomimetic synthesis route will provide insight into the otherwise obscure biosynthesis of this complex peptide-based secondary metabolite. Finally, new studies on the synthesis of the architecturally complex 20S proteosome inhibitor TMC-95A and rationally designed analogues will be pursued. A possibly biomimetic (modified) tryptophan oxidative cyclization forms the centerpiece of the approach, and acquisition of the target and the aforementioned analogues will enable mechanism-of-action studies to move forward. Inhibition of the 20S proteosome can form the basis for chemotherapeutic intervention in a variety of disease states, including cancer, **cachexia,** and sepsis. The search for selective 20S proteosome inhibitors among the Ntn-type proteases will be advanced by these investigations.

  Website: http://crisp.cit.nih.gov/crisp/Crisp_Query.Generate_Screen

- **Project Title: CHRONIC RENAL INSUFFICIENCY IN NAPRTCS PATIENTS**

  Principal Investigator & Institution: Warady, Bradley; Children's Mercy Hosp (Kansas City, Mo) 2401 Gillham Rd Kansas City, Mo 64108

  Timing: Fiscal Year 2003; Project Start 30-SEP-2003; Project End 31-JUL-2008

  Summary: (provided by applicant): This application, a joint effort of 26 centers of the NAPRTCS, is entitled "Chronic Renal Insufficiency (CRI) in NAPRTCS Patients. We will enroll 300 children (1-16 years) with measured glomerular filtration rates (GFR) of 25-75 mL/min/1.73m2. Follow-up with annual GFR and 6 month physical examinations and determinations of hemoglobin, electrolytes, serum, albumin, serum calcium, serum phosphorus, parathyroid hormone and urinary indices will test the 1st hypothesis that this cohort will most accurately define the rate of and the risk factors for progression of

CRI, and that this progression will be correlated with proteinuria, albumin, blood pressure, nutritional status, growth and hyperparathyroidism. To test the 2nd hypothesis that cardiovascular disease develops in children with mild CRI and that its prevalence and severity increase in association with the progression of CRI, we will perform baseline and annual 24-hour ambulatory blood pressure monitoring, echocardiographic assessments to determine left-ventricular mass and LV function, and B-mode ultrasound of the carotid artery to determine the IMT and carotid artery compliance. To test the 3rd hypothesis that the neurocognitive outcome of children with CRI is influenced by the progression of renal insufficiency, a battery of validated neurocognitive tests will be conducted at study entry and at 6, 12 and 24 months to assess many cortical and subcortical areas of brain function. To test the 4th hypothesis that chronic inflammation contributes to **cachexia,** growth hormone resistance and growth retardation, we will examine the impact of circulating cytokine and neuropeptide concentrations on dietary intake, nutritional and growth parameters as well as growth hormone axis pertubations and responsiveness to growth hormone therapy. Finally, to test the 5th hypothesis that a correlation exist between bone histology, serum concentration of PTH and measured GFR, we will measure and characterize the biochemical and histologic features of renal osteodystrophy and determine the serum concentrations of PTH that are associated with normal rates of bone formation.

Website: http://crisp.cit.nih.gov/crisp/Crisp_Query.Generate_Screen

- **Project Title: COMBINED ANTI-ANGIOGENIC THERAPY AND SIRNA TARGETING OF CHOLINE KINASE**

  Principal Investigator & Institution: Bhujwalla, Zaver M.; Professor; Johns Hopkins University 3400 N Charles St Baltimore, Md 21218

  Timing: Fiscal Year 2003; Project Start 10-AUG-2003; Project End 31-JUL-2008

  Summary: Although the progression of cancer arrives at a common end point of organ failure, **cachexia** and death, common pathways are rare in cancer. Over the past decade one common pathway consistently revealed by MR spectroscopic studies is the elevation of phosphocholine and total choline in cancer cells and solid tumors. Data obtained by us demonstrate that phosphocholine in cancer cells is related to malignant transformation, endothelial cancer cell interaction, invasion and metatasis. Therefore the elevation of phosphocholine presents a unique target to exploit for therapy. In this proposal we intend to develop molecular biology strategies to target choline kinase in oxygenated as well as hypoxic cells using small interfering RNA (siRNA) to inhibit the transcription of choline kinase. We have chosen choline kinase as a target since it is the enzyme which converts choline to phosphocholine. Choline kinase inhibition will be induced in normoxic cells using a mifepristone inducible system or in hypoxic cells using the hypoxia response element to drive the formation of the siRNA. In vivo, the hypoxia inducible system will also be combined with anti-angiogenic treatment which will create hypoxia over a larger region of the tumor. The effects of choline kinase inhibition with or without anti-angiogenic therapy on invasion, metabolism and vascularization will be determined with combined MRI and MRSI. Optical imaging will be used to detect hypoxia, and histology to detect metastasis. Microarray analyses will be performed characterize molecular alterations. These studies will be performed with three human breast cancer cell lines and their transgenic counterparts, studied as cells and as solid tumors in vivo. Cells in hypoxic environments in solid tumors are the most resistant to radiation and chemotherapy, and are most likely to lead to recurrence of the disease. Our cancer invasion studies have shown that the presence of endothelial cells in the proximity of cancer cells under hypoxic conditions confers an advantage in invasion of the cancer cells. Approaches to enhance the action of anti-angiogenic therapy, by exploiting the hypoxia induced by anti-angiogenic therapy to further target a key pathway in cancer cells would minimize the risk of increased invasion and act synergistically with anti-angiogenic therapy in killing cancer cells.

Website: http://crisp.cit.nih.gov/crisp/Crisp_Query.Generate_Screen

- **Project Title: COMMUNITY BASED STUDY OF THE COURSE AND OUTCOMES OF ALZHEIMERS DISEASE**

  Principal Investigator & Institution: Stern, Yaakov; Professor; Columbia University Health Sciences Po Box 49 New York, Ny 10032

  Timing: Fiscal Year 2002; Project Start 15-JUL-2002; Project End 30-JUN-2003

  Summary: There have been very few community-based studies of progression of Alzheimer's disease (AD). None have used incident dementia patients and the later consequences of disease progression were rarely addressed. In the previous study period, we identified and initiated prospective follow-up of 601 AD patients, including 176 incident cases. We found that AD was associated with increased risk of mortality and hospitalization, and increased lifetime disability and paid service use. Male gender, more severe AD, **cachexia,** and extrapyramidal signs were each associated with increased risk of death. More rapid cognitive decline and mortality were associated with higher educational and occupational attainment. We also developed new measures of functional competence and quality of life, performance-based tests for functional change, and automated medical record retrieval for documenting in patient care. We propose to continue follow-up of the surviving patients and to initiate follow-up of an additional 150 incident and 200 prevalent cases in order to test specific hypotheses regarding determinants of disease course and outcomes. We will have the unprecedented opportunity to test all of our major hypotheses in a multi- ethnic cohort of incident dementia patients. We will determine the timing and occurrence of specific disease endpoints: change in CDR stage, use of paraprofessional care, increase in hours of ADL care, admission to nursing home, need for the equivalent of institutional care, and mortality. We will also characterize rapidity of disease course in AD by applying GEE and random effects models to prospectively obtained measures of cognitive function and ability to perform activities of daily living We will explore factors hypothesized to be associated with increased relative risk for the occurrence of the disease endpoints or with more rapid disease course; demographic features, particularly ethnicity, comorbid medical and sociocultural factors, behavioral manifestations, genetic information, as well as the rate of cognitive and functional decline and estrogen use information acquired prior to the incident dementia. We will compare hospitalization and mortality in demented patients to that observed in non-demented community patients. We will also identify what level of change in particular cognitive domains is associated with alteration in the functional task performance.

  Website: http://crisp.cit.nih.gov/crisp/Crisp_Query.Generate_Screen

- **Project Title: COMMUNITY CLINICAL ONCOLOGY PROGRAM**

  Principal Investigator & Institution: Loprinzi, Charles L.; Professor; Mayo Clinic Coll of Medicine, Rochester 200 1St St Sw Rochester, Mn 55905

  Timing: Fiscal Year 2002; Project Start 15-SEP-1983; Project End 31-MAY-2006

  Summary: (Applicant's Description) The Mayo Clinic, through the vehicle of the North Central Cancer Treatment Group (NCCTG), will serve as a primary research base for the following 15 CCOPs: Ann Arbor Regional CCOP, Carle Cancer Center CCOP, Cedar Rapids Oncology Project CCOP, Des Moines CCOP, Duluth CCOP, Merit Care Hospital CCOP, Geisinger CCOP, Metro Minnesota CCOP, Missouri Valley Cancer Consortium CCOP, Ochsner Clinic CCOP, Illinois Oncology Research Association CCOP, Scottsdale CCOP, Siouxland Community Cancer Consortium CCOP, Toledo CCOP, and the Wichita CCOP. We will also serve as a research base for cancer control protocol activity of non-CCOP participants and for the multiple CCOPs outside of our group who contribute to intergroup cancer treatment and cancer control protocols which we lead. We will cooperate with our affiliated CCOPs in planning their program and in conducting appropriate continuing education and workshops. We will provide training and active support for their data managers and oncology nurses. We will coordinate their multidisciplinary involvement in clinical cancer research protocols. This will include evolving and maintaining standard reporting procedures for surgery, pathology, and radiation therapy. We will hold regular meetings of the CCOPs for review of ongoing research, planning future research, and for related professional activities. We will continue the rigid quality control procedures which have proved so successful in the past, and upgrade these procedures as indicated. We will constantly monitor CCOP performance not only by timely review of patients, data sheets, pathology material, operative reports, and radiation therapy port films, but also by periodic randomly scheduled monitoring site visits. We will work with each CCOP participant to aid in their maturation as clinical investigators. We will assist them in developing new protocols for which they will share leadership, and we will work with them in preparing publications as well as presentations for national and regional meetings. We will make every effort to provide them with justifiable pride in their participation in the National Cancer Program. A high priority over this grant period will be the further expansion of our cancer control efforts with incorporation of associated basic laboratory support, leading to scientifically rigorous translational research efforts.

Website: http://crisp.cit.nih.gov/crisp/Crisp_Query.Generate_Screen

- **Project Title: COMPASSIONATE USE OF THALIDOMIDE IN ADULTS WITH HIV ASSOCIATED WASTING**

  Principal Investigator & Institution: Abrams, Donald; University of California San Francisco 500 Parnassus Ave San Francisco, Ca 941222747

  Timing: Fiscal Year 2002; Project Start 01-DEC-2001; Project End 30-NOV-2002

  Summary: This abstract is not available.

  Website: http://crisp.cit.nih.gov/crisp/Crisp_Query.Generate_Screen

- **Project Title: COMPLICATIONS OF HIV DISEASE AGENDA**

  Principal Investigator & Institution: Collier, Ann C.; Assistant Professor; University of Washington Grant & Contract Services Seattle, Wa 98105

  Timing: Fiscal Year 2003

  Summary: This abstract is not available.

  Website: http://crisp.cit.nih.gov/crisp/Crisp_Query.Generate_Screen

- **Project Title: COMPLICATIONS OF HIV DISEASE AGENDA**

  Principal Investigator & Institution: Delapanha, Robert; Howard University Washington, Dc 20059

  Timing: Fiscal Year 2002

Summary: SUBPROJECT ABSTRACT NOT AVAILABLE

Website: http://crisp.cit.nih.gov/crisp/Crisp_Query.Generate_Screen

- **Project Title: COMPLICATIONS OF HIV DISEASE AGENDA**

  Principal Investigator & Institution: Marigan, Thomas G.; Stanford University Stanford, Ca 94305

  Timing: Fiscal Year 2003

  Summary: SUBPROJECT NOT AVAILABLE

  Website: http://crisp.cit.nih.gov/crisp/Crisp_Query.Generate_Screen

- **Project Title: CYTOKINE AND HORMONE INTERACTIONS IN COMORBIDITY OF AIDS**

  Principal Investigator & Institution: Kelley, Keith W.; Professor; Animal Sciences; University of Illinois Urbana-Champaign Henry Administration Bldg Champaign, Il 61820

  Timing: Fiscal Year 2002; Project Start 01-SEP-2002; Project End 31-AUG-2006

  Summary: (provided by applicant): The anemia, neutropenia, loss of lean body mass and mortality of AIDS patients with wasting are associated with elevated levels of the proinflammatory cytokines TNFalpha and IL-1beta. AIDS patients with wasting are often given a 12- week therapy with very high doses of recombinant human growth hormone to increase plasma IGF-I, lean muscle mass and quality of life. However, the responsiveness of both hematopoietic and muscle cells to IGF-I has been documented to be defective in these patients. The central hypothesis of this application is that TNFalpha and IL-lbeta are responsible for inducing a state of IGF-I receptor resistance, which contributes to not only muscle wasting but also to the anemia and neutropenia of AIDS. IGF-I targets both hematopoietic myeloid progenitor cells and muscle myoblasts, and here we hypothesize that the molecular mechanism for IGF-I receptor resistance in wasting AIDS patients is caused by proinflammatory cytokines. Objective 1 will test the idea that IGF-I promotes promyeloid cell survival by blocking activation of the caspase family of serine proteases and whether this is inhibited by TNFa. Objective 2 focuses on the survival promoting activity of the tyrosine phosphorylated IGF-I receptor, including insulin-receptor substrate- 1 (IRS-1), IRS-2, PI 3-kinase and Akt. Objective 3 will determine if proinflammatory cytokines inhibit key IGF-I proliferative signals, including Shc, EFK1/2, AFX forkhead transcription factors and the cyclin-dependent kinase inhibitor 27. Finally, objective 4 will extend these results with myeloid progenitor cells to muscle myoblasts. Preliminary results indicate that low blood concentrations of TNFalpha and IL-1beta found in wasting AIDS patients inhibit the ability of IGF-I to promote both protein synthesis and differentiation into myotubes. This objective will also test the new idea that ceramide, a mediator of the actions of both TNFalpha and IL-1beta, induces resistance of the IGF-I receptor in muscle myoblasts. These studies are needed to understand how clinically-relevant concentrations of proinflammatory cytokines in wasting AIDS patients impair the functional ability of a major hormone receptor on both immune and muscle myoblast cells.

  Website: http://crisp.cit.nih.gov/crisp/Crisp_Query.Generate_Screen

- **Project Title: CYTOKINES AND NFKAPPABETA REGULATION OF CANCER CACHEXIA**

  Principal Investigator & Institution: Guttridge, Denis C.; Assistant Professor; Molecular Virology, Immunology & Medical Genetics; Ohio State University 1960 Kenny Road Columbus, Oh 43210

  Timing: Fiscal Year 2002; Project Start 20-MAR-2002; Project End 28-FEB-2007

  Summary: (provided by applicant): Elevated levels of the pro-inflammatory cytokine, tumor necrosis factor-alpha (TNF), is associated with certain cancers. TNF is thought to be a major contributor of cancer **cachexia,** a syndrome characterized by extreme weight loss, resulting from the wasting of skeletal muscle and adipose tissues. It is estimated that a majority of cancer patients exhibit **cachexia,** and strikingly, nearly one third of cancer mortalities result from **cachexia,** rather than tumor burden. Although the effects of TNF in cancer **cachexia** have long been studied, to date, very few if any cytokine-inducible molecular targets have been identified that mediate skeletal muscle and fat degeneration. NF-kappaB is a transcription factor which is potently activated by TNF. Previously, we identified that NF-kappaB functions as a negative regulator of skeletal muscle differentiation. Recent results reveal that TNF-induced activation of NF-kappaB leads to the repressed expression of MyoD, a skeletal muscle-specific transcription factor considered the "master switch" in the regulation of myogenic differentiation. It was also elucidated that TNF action requires additional signaling from the IFN- gamma pathway to elicit muscle wasting and that this degenerative process is completely prevented in the absence of NF-kappaB activity. Similar to skeletal muscle, very little is known at the molecular level about how TNF induces adipose tissue wasting. Preliminary data in this proposal demonstrate that TNF-induced fat loss correlates with a loss of C/EBP-alpha, a transcription factor whose expression is known to be critical for the maintenance of mature fat. Results also show that overexpression of NF-kappaB inhibits C/EBP-alpha expression, suggesting that analogous to skeletal muscle, cytokine-induced fat wasting may be mediated through the actions of NF-kappaB by targeting a key transcription factor. The main objective of this proposal is to better understand how cytokines, signaling through NF-kappaB, regulate tissue differentiation relevant in disease conditions such as cancer **cachexia.** This objective will be accomplished by performing the following three aims: AIM 1 will address how cytokines TNF + IFN-gamma and NF-kappaB lead to skeletal muscle decay; AIM 2 will investigate how TNF and NF-kappaB regulate the loss of adipocyte tissue; and AIM 3 will determine the requirement of TNF + IFN-gamma and NF-kappaB in skeletal muscle wasting in vivo. The completion of these AIMS will provide insight on the potential of NF-kappaB as a therapeutic target in cancer **cachexia.**

  Website: http://crisp.cit.nih.gov/crisp/Crisp_Query.Generate_Screen

- **Project Title: DEVELOPMENT OF A NATURAL CANNABINOID PRODUCT**

  Principal Investigator & Institution: Castor, Trevor P.; President & Chief Executive Officer; Aphios Corporation 3-E Gill St Woburn, Ma 01801

  Timing: Fiscal Year 2002; Project Start 01-JUN-2002; Project End 31-MAY-2003

  Summary: (provided by applicant): Marijuana (Cannabis sativa) and a number of cannabinoids including its primary psychoactive component, delta9-THC (delta9-tetrahydrocannabinol), show promise for treating pain and **cachexia** in cancer and AIDS patients. The overall goal of this research program is to develop a natural pharmaceutical grade delta9-THC product for medical use. While delta9-THC can be synthesized, the process is complex and expensive. It is our hypothesis that a natural delta9-THC product can be cost-effectively manufactured by utilizing supercritical fluids and near-critical fluids w/wo polar cosolvents such as alcohols (SuperFluids TM), and that such a process could also produce other bioactive cannabinoids and cannabinoid mixtures for future research and therapeutic use. In Phase I, we plan to establish "best" conditions for selective SuperFluids extraction and chromatographic purification (CXP) of delta9-THC from Cannabis sativa. The SuperFluids CXP process will be evaluated against conventional organic phase processes in terms of capital and operating costs as well as environmental impact. The results of our Phase I investigation will be used to perform engineering and economic analysis to determine the technical, economic and environmental feasibility of the proposed process. In Phase II, we will scale-up and pilot the process for producing cannabinoids for commercialization by Molecular Delivery Corporation, Pleasanton, CA.

Website: http://crisp.cit.nih.gov/crisp/Crisp_Query.Generate_Screen

- **Project Title: EXERCISE INDUCED GROWTH OF SKELETAL MUSCLE**

  Principal Investigator & Institution: Booth, Frank W.; Professor; Veterinary Biomedical Sciences; University of Missouri Columbia 310 Jesse Hall Columbia, Mo 65211

  Timing: Fiscal Year 2002; Project Start 01-AUG-1979; Project End 30-APR-2004

  Summary: (Adapted from the applicant's abstract):Promoting skeletal muscle growth is extremely important for medical conditions in which muscle wasting contributes to low quality of life, high health care costs, and institutionalization (i.e. aging, **cachexia,** congestive heart failure, etc.). It is well known that skeletal muscle hypertrophies in response to increased loading; however the mechanisms underlying this phenomenon remain poorly understood. In this respect, there is accumulating evidence that hormonal signaling and mechanical signaling (via focal adhesion complex proteins) may act synergistically and share common pathway intermediates such as focal adhesion kinase (FAK), serum response factor and other upstream/downstream elements. To examine this possibility, the current proposal consists of a strategy to tease out the individual and combined effects of angiotensin II signaling, insulin-like growth factor-I (IGF-1) signaling and integrin (mechanical) signaling in skeletal muscle hypertrophy. In the first specific aim, the PI proposes to confirm and extend upon two pilot experiments in which, using an overload model (via synergistic gastrocnemius ablation), compensatory hypertrophy of the rat soleus muscles is almost completely inhibited by the use of an ACE inhibitor. Although angiotensin II is a known stimulus to cardiac and smooth muscle growth, these findings in skeletal muscle are novel. The second specific aim consists of multiple experiments designed to a) in living rats, test the effect of angiotensin II alone, IGF-1 alone, and mechanical loading alone (rat resistance exercise model) on the acute (1 hr post stimulus) response of multiple downstream signaling elements common to these 3 stimuli in skeletal muscle; b) in living rats, test the effect of skeletal muscle loading on these downstream elements while either blocking endogenous angiotensin II input (receptor blockade or ACE inhibition), blocking endogenous IGF-1 input (receptor blockade), or blocking mechanical signaling (disrupting the integrin/extracellular matrix interface with RGD peptide); and, c) in cultured rat skeletal myotubes, test the effect of exogenous angiotensin II alone, exogenous IGF-1 alone, and stretch alone on these downstream elements. Finally, the third specific aim utilizes microarray technology to examine the overlap between these growth factor and mechanical stimuli at the level of mRNA expression in skeletal muscle of living rats. Elucidation of the mechanisms signaling skeletal muscle growth may lead to drugs, gene therapy, or other countermeasures against skeletal muscle wasting in individuals for whom exercise is perhaps impossible.

Website: http://crisp.cit.nih.gov/crisp/Crisp_Query.Generate_Screen

- **Project Title: EXERCISE INTERVENTIONS IN HIV INFECTED ADULTS**

  Principal Investigator & Institution: Roubenoff, Ronenn; Associate Professor of Medicine and Nutr; Tufts University Boston Boston, Ma 02111

  Timing: Fiscal Year 2002

  Summary: This project will examine the effect of exercise training on functional status in patients with HIV wasting; and the effect of exercise on abdominal visceral fat and insulin resistance in patients with HIV-associated fat redistribution. In the past several years, we have shown that 1) one bout of hard exercise does not raise HIV RNA levels; 2) progressive resistance exercise (RE) leads to increase in lean mass, comparable to that seen with growth hormone or androgen therapy; 3) RE leads to fat loss in normal-weight subjects, but to fat (and total mass) gain in wasted subjects; 4) in patients with fat redistribution, aerobic plus resistance exercise (ARE) leads to significant decline in trunk fat mass without loss of lean body mass or peripheral fat mass. In addition, we have preliminary evidence that 5) RE improves functional status via increases in strength and lean mass; 6) the protein metabolic response to one bout of hard exercise differs substantially between wasted and non-wasted patients; and 7) that this response can be used to predict who will benefit from RE with a gain in lean mass. Thus exercise potentially offers singular advantages in treatment and prevention of both wasting and abdominal obesity in HIV infection. The long-range goal of this research is to develop practical ways of using exercise to prevent and treat body composition abnormalities caused by HIV infection. We propose to recruit 100 patients with HIV infection with either wasting or fat redistribution, and enroll them in a long-term, randomized, outpatient study of exercise and diet. The major outcomes for the wasting group will be increased in lean mass and functional status, and whether the protein metabolic response to one bout of acute exercise predicts the response to RE. For the fat redistribution group, the expected outcomes are a decrease in abdominal visceral ft, improved insulin resistance, increased muscle glucose transporter-4 (GLUT-4) levels, and improved lipoprotein status.

  Website: http://crisp.cit.nih.gov/crisp/Crisp_Query.Generate_Screen

- **Project Title: EXTRACELLULAR MATERIALS AND EMBRYONIC ORGAN FORMATION**

  Principal Investigator & Institution: Bernfield, Merton R.; Clements Smith Professor of Pediatrics; Children's Hospital (Boston) Boston, Ma 021155737

  Timing: Fiscal Year 2002; Project Start 01-MAR-2000; Project End 30-APR-2002

  Summary: (adapted from investigator's abstract): Syndecans, cell surface heparan sulfate proteoglycans, (HSPG) bind and modulate the activity of a large number of extra-cellular effectors. The ectodomains of the syndecans can be shed, generating soluble HSPGs that can inhibit these cell surface interactions. Several transgenic mouse lines that express high levels of cell surface syndecan- 1 under the control of a CMV promoter/enhancer were generated to evaluate its functions in vivo. Syndecan- 1 was expressed in multiple somatic tissues and in the hypothalamic areas that regulate body weight. The transgenic mice mimic (i) obese mice with abnormalities in melanocortin-4 receptor function and (ii) humans with the Bardet-Biedl syndrome, a genetic malformation and obesity syndrome of unknown etiology. Transgenic expression of syndecan- 1 appears to have has uncovered a physiological control of feeding behavior. These studies define new functions for syndecans and have important implications for understanding eating disorders, both obesity and **cachexia.** Obesity is a significant public health hazard; about half of U.S. women and men are now considered overweight and the IOM indicates that this costs more than $70 billion annually in the U.S. Thus, syndecan induction and syndecan interactions are potentially important new targets for pharmacological control of body weight. Specifically, the investigators aim to explore the remarkable phenotypes produced by syndecan- 1 overexpression: (i) establish the role of syndecans in melanocortin receptor function by characterizing the interaction of syndecans with agouti/AGRP peptides and analyzing how this interaction modulates melanocortin receptor signaling both in vitro and in vivo. (ii) evaluate whether hypothalamic expression of syndecan-3 is a physiological regulator of feeding behavior by characterizing the induced expression of hypothalamic syndecan-3. analyzing feeding behavior in syndecan-3 null mice and identifying potential regulators of hypothalamic synce~an-3 expression. (iii) analyze the obesity and morphogenetic abnormalities of the syndecan- 1 overexpressing mouse by evaluating the mouse as a genetic model of the Bardet-Biedl syndrome and by identifying the genes responsible for morphogenetic abnormalities and for reducing the obesity.

Website: http://crisp.cit.nih.gov/crisp/Crisp_Query.Generate_Screen

- **Project Title: FAT DISTRIBUTION AND INSULIN RESISTANCE IN HIV**

  Principal Investigator & Institution: Kotler, Donald P.; Professor of Medicine; St. Luke's-Roosevelt Inst for Hlth Scis Health Sciences New York, Ny 100191102

  Timing: Fiscal Year 2002

  Summary: Myostatin, uncoupling proteins, and ACE polymorphisms are recently discovered regulators of skeletal muscle growth, metabolism, and function. Skeletal muscle, the largest body compartment in normal weight humans, is increasingly a research focus of molecular genetic, and clinical investigations. Despite this intense research interest, methods of non-invasively characterizing regional and total body skeletal muscle distribution, mass, and composition remain remarkably limited. The first phase of this study in Program Project II developed and refined skeletal muscle evaluation methods and models in a cross-sectional cohort of normal and overweight ethnically-mixed adults. In progressing towards this aim in adults we observed and reported, using reference body composition methods, that; older adults have less relative skeletal muscle mass than young subjects; that skeletal muscle mass than young subjects; that skeletal muscle mass and distribution are functions of gender, age, and body mass; and that at all adult ages, African Americans have a larger skeletal muscle and related bone compartment than Caucasians, even after controlling for other known skeletal muscle determinants. With these biological observations as a basis, we validated, improved older, or developed new skeletal muscle mass measurement methods including those based on magnetic resonance imaging, or developed new skeletal muscle mass measurement methods including those based on magnetic resonance imaging, dual-energy x-ray absorptiometry, 40K counting, bioimpedance analysis, anthropometry, and urinary metabolite markers. These efforts led to important collaborations with members of the other projects, development of new laboratory resources in the core units, and outreach to engineers with modeling experience in the new Columbia Department of Biomedical Engineering. Important gaps, however, remain: our method and models are applicable only in adults; models were developed in normal and overweight adults and not at body mass extremes; and our methods were validated only in cross-sectional samples and not in longitudinal cohorts with skeletal muscle changes secondary to growth in children or interventions. The clinical and research importance of all 3 of these areas led us to advance 6 new hypotheses and related aims divided into 3 separate human and animal studies.: Study 1 proposes to advance method development in 240 African American and Caucasian males & females in Tanner Stages 1-5; 48 will be followed up at 2-3 years with growth; Study 2 proposes to cross-validate models in adult patients with underweight (anorexia nervosa) and obesity, in Projects 2 and 3, before and during treatments designed to produce weight change; Study 3 is designed to non-invasively evaluate aspects of muscle composition across the human lifespan in subjects from all four projects; and to establish, for the first time, relevant electrical properties of isolated rodent skeletal muscle before and following specific hypothesis-based interventions. In addition, to interact projects, this study will also provide important new information on adiposity and energy expenditure-related issues in children. The composite developed methods and the biological issues that they touch upon would provide a foundation for human skeletal muscle studies anticipated in the near future, particularly in children.

Website: http://crisp.cit.nih.gov/crisp/Crisp_Query.Generate_Screen

- **Project Title: FISH OIL MODULATION OF TUMOR INFLAMMATION**

  Principal Investigator & Institution: Espat, Nocif J.; Surgery; University of Illinois at Chicago 1737 West Polk Street Chicago, Il 60612

  Timing: Fiscal Year 2002; Project Start 01-SEP-2002; Project End 31-AUG-2007

  Summary: (provided by applicant): The primary purpose of this mentored award is to prepare the applicant for a career as an independent physician scientist. The applicant proposes to acquire additional skills in cell biology and molecular analysis in the context of a project that is directly relevant to his clinical specialty. The-long term goals are: 1) to investigate the mechanism(s) and define the relationship between tumor related inflammation and cancer associated **cachexia;** and 2) to develop safe and effective anti-inflammatory treatment strategies for patients with progressive malignancy using (nutritional) eicosapentaenoic acid, (EPA)) and/or (pharmacologic) selective cyclo-oxygenase-II (COX-II) inhibitor agents. Anorexia, weight loss and the catabolism of lean body mass define the clinical syndrome of cancer-associated **cachexia.** Preventing or delaying **cachexia** is a clinically significant goal, since improved outcome and survival for cancer patients has been consistently demonstrated to parallel the preservation of lean body mass. 1-4 Clinical and experimental evidence from our lab and others supports the use of EPA as an anti-inflammatory therapy. EPA is a w-3 fatty acid that may attenuate the production of pro-inflammatory cytokines, growth factors and inflammatory mediators, in response to inflammatory stimuli, however the mechanism(s) remain to be defined. Hypothesis: EPA alone or in combination with COX-II inhibitors attenuate the tumor-related inflammation of progressive malignancy. To test this hypothesis we will use the in vitro RAW 264-7 cell culture model and the well-established rodent model of progressive malignancy resulting in cancer-cachexia, the methyl-cholanthrene (MCA) fibrosarcoma, with the following specific aims. AIM1: To evaluate in vitro EPA and/or COX-II inhibition of macrophage TNF-alpha, IL-1beta, prostaglandin E2, COX-II enzyme production, NF-kB activity and apoptosis. AIM 2: To evaluate in vivo EPA and/or COX-II inhibition therapies of tumor-related TNF-alpha, IL-1beta, prostaglandin E2, COX-II enzyme production, NF-kB activity, apoptosis and regulation of the ubiquitin proteasome proteolytic pathway in response to progressive non-metastasizing malignancy.

  Website: http://crisp.cit.nih.gov/crisp/Crisp_Query.Generate_Screen

- **Project Title: FOLATE PATHWAY POLYMORPHISMS AND PANCREATIC CANCER RISK**

  Principal Investigator & Institution: Goggins, Michael G.; Associate Professor; Pathology; Johns Hopkins University 3400 N Charles St Baltimore, Md 21218

  Timing: Fiscal Year 2002; Project Start 22-AUG-2001; Project End 30-JUN-2003

  Summary: Pancreatic cancer is the fifth leading cause of cancer death in the USA. Currently, there is no effective screening test for asymptomatic individuals and the vast majority of patients with pancreatic cancer present with advanced incurable disease. To reduce the burden of pancreatic cancer, we need to detect early pancreatic cancers and define those at risk of developing the disease. This is particularly true of individuals with a family history of pancreatic cancer, with germline mutations of BRCA2, with germline mutations in p16, or with familial pancreatitis who have lifetime risks of developing pancreatic cancer ranging from 5-40%. Identifying modifiable risk factors may help reduce the burden of this deadly disease. Low folate status has been shown to increase the risk of several cancers and genetic polymorphisms in the folate pathway alter this risk. Since pancreatic cancer leads to **cachexia,** weight loss and maldigestion, identifying nutrient risk factors for pancreatic cancer utilizing a case-control design has limitations. Studies of genetic polymorphisms that impair folate metabolism and mirror environmental exposures can predict the significance of folate status on pancreatic cancer risk. Several studies have demonstrated that common and functionally significant polymorphisms in the methylene tetrahydrofolate reductase gene (MTHFR) and methionine synthase are associated with a reduced risk of several cancers. MTHFR impairment preferentially maintains folates as 5, 10 methylene THF, thereby maintaining optimal thymidine production, at the expense of less methylTHF, needed for DNA methylation. If DNA hypomethylation is an important predisposing factor to cancer formation, polymorphisms in the folate pathway that impair the formation of SAM such as methionine synthase (MS) should increase cancer risk. We hypothesize that defective MTHFR and MS function arising from genetic polymorphisms will protect against pancreatic cancer. If true, it would suggest that thymidine incorporation is more important for cancer protection than reduced methyl group availability for DNA methylation. Carriers of polymorphisms in MTHFR and MS may also be more likely to harbor DNA hypomethylation in their pancreatic cancers of individuals. We will determine i) the prevalence of polymorphisms in the folate pathway (the 677C>T, 1298A>C MTHFR and the 2756A>G MS polymorphisms) in 350 pancreatic cancer cases and in 350 non-cancer controls and ii) determine if DNA hypomethylation in pancreatic cancer xenograft DNA is related its' MTHFR and MS status.

  Website: http://crisp.cit.nih.gov/crisp/Crisp_Query.Generate_Screen

- **Project Title: G PROTEIN-EFFECTOR INTERACTIONS IN GUSTATION**

  Principal Investigator & Institution: Margolskee, Robert F.; Professor; Physiology and Biophysics; Mount Sinai School of Medicine of Nyu of New York University New York, Ny 10029

  Timing: Fiscal Year 2002; Project Start 01-AUG-1996; Project End 31-JUL-2007

  Summary: (provided by applicant): The long-term objective of our research program is to understand how the vertebrate gustatory system transduces signals and encodes information. Of particular importance are taste cell guanine nucleotide binding regulatory proteins (G proteins) and the seven transmembrane helix receptors that couple to them. G proteins regulate effector enzymes such as phosphodiesterase (PDE) and phospholipase C (PLC) to effect taste cell changes in intracellular second messengers. We have used molecular cloning to identify a number of the key components of taste transduction pathways, including Alpha-gustducin, a taste specific G protein Alpha -subunit closely related to the Alpha-transducins. The scope of this Competing Continuation encompasses the roles in taste transduction and coding of heterotrimeric gustducin?s component subunits and the downstream effector enzymes to which they couple. To elucidate the specific roles in taste transduction and coding of Alpha-gustducin, BetaGamma-gustducin, Ggamma13, taste-expressed PDEs and PLCBeta2 we will use a multidisciplinary approach applying biochemical, transgenic, behavioral, and electrophysiological techniques. The Experimental Goals of the proposal are the following. 1. To determine which PDEs present in taste tissue can be activated by alpha-gustducin. 2. To determine if these PDEs are co-expressed with alpha-gustducin in taste cells. 3. To determine if these PDEs can be activated by any other G protein alpha-subunits co-expressed with them in taste cells. 4. To generate alpha-gustducin mutants selectively deficient in the ability to activate the taste PDEs. 5. To generate transgenic mice expressing such an alpha-gustducin mutant. 6. To biochemically characterize taste transduction responses of the alpha-gustducin mutant mice. 7. To behaviorally characterize the alpha-gustducin mutant mice. 8. To electrophysiologically characterize the alpha-gustducin mutant mice. 9. To generate transgenic mice lacking signals mediated by gustducin?s beta, gamma-subunits. 10. To biochemically characterize taste transduction responses of the beta gamma-gustducin deficient mice. 11. To behaviorally characterize the beta, gamma-gustducin deficient mice. 12. To electrophysiologically characterize the beta, gamma-gustducin deficient mice. The results of these studies will provide significant new insights into the molecular mechanisms underlying taste transduction and coding. Gustatory and metabolic disorders such as malgeusia, dysgeusia and **cachexia** frequently occur in conjunction with several types of cancer. The knowledge gained from this proposal should further our understanding of the molecular bases of the taste disorders and may lead to effective intervention.

Website: http://crisp.cit.nih.gov/crisp/Crisp_Query.Generate_Screen

- **Project Title: HYPOTHALAMIC MECHANISMS IN CACHEXIA**

  Principal Investigator & Institution: Marks, Daniel L.; Pediatrics; Oregon Health & Science University Portland, or 972393098

  Timing: Fiscal Year 2004; Project Start 01-JUN-2004; Project End 31-MAY-2009

  Summary: To achieve normal growth, development, and quality of life, individuals must maintain adequate intake of nutrition and be free from prolonged metabolic derangement. Unfortunately, people affected with either acute or chronic diseases often show disorders of nutrient balance. In some cases, a devastating state of malnutrition known as **cachexia** arises, brought about by a synergistic combination of a dramatic decrease in appetite and an increase in metabolism of fat and lean body mass. This combination is found in a number of disorders including cancer, cystic fibrosis, AIDS, rheumatoid arthritis, and renal failure, and is an important determinant of morbidity and mortality in these conditions. Experimental models have demonstrated the importance of cytokines in mediating illness-induced anorexia and **cachexia** but the neuronal systems involved in transducing this signal have not been fully defined. Work in this lab and in others has demonstrated that hypothalamic melanocortin receptors play a critical role in regulating feeding behavior, linear growth, metabolic rate, and insulin sensitivity. Stimulation of the hypothalamic melanocortin-4 receptor (MC4-R) produces relative anorexia, while prolonged antagonism of this receptor stimulates feeding and results in excessive weight gain and growth. More recently, we have been able to demonstrate that in both acute and chronic disease models, blockade of the MC4-R results in a dramatic attenuation of **cachexia.** We have also demonstrated that blockade of the melanocortin-3 receptor (MC3-R) leads to enhanced disease-associated **cachexia** whereas stimulation of the MC3-R leads to increased food intake. Current research goals fall into two general areas as described in this grant. First, we will examine the contribution and unique function the MC3-R in acute and chronic **cachexia.** Second, the mechanisms by which circulating cytokines and tumor-derived factors activate the hypothalamic melanocortin system will be defined. Additionally, the process of habituation to cytokine-mediated anorexia will be investigated in the context of central melanocortin function. Ultimately, this work may lead to investigation of drug therapy for this widespread medical problem.

Website: http://crisp.cit.nih.gov/crisp/Crisp_Query.Generate_Screen

- **Project Title: INTERLEUKIN-6 EXPRESSION AND FUNCTION IN ADIPOSE CELLS**

  Principal Investigator & Institution: Harp, Joyce B.; Associate Professor; Nutrition; University of North Carolina Chapel Hill Aob 104 Airport Drive Cb#1350 Chapel Hill, Nc 27599

  Timing: Fiscal Year 2002; Project Start 01-APR-2002; Project End 31-MAR-2007

  Summary: Elevated interleukin-6 (IL-6) is associated with fat wasting in systemic infection and cancer **cachexia.** However, important new data indicates that circulating IL-6 is also elevated in human obesity, and adipose tissue is the principal source of this elevation. Because obesity is among the most prevalent public health challenges in the United States, it is important to understand IL-6 expression and function in adipose tissue, and to determine whether dysregulated expression of adipose tissue IL-6 is involved in the development of obesity and obesity-related co-morbidities. IL-6 traditionally signals through STAT3 activation, but in differentiating preadipocytes, IL-6 inhibits and STAT3 appears to be necessary for adipocyte formation. In this proposal we propose the following Specific Aims. Aim 1: To determine mechanisms involved in IL-6-induced inhibition of adipogenesis. We hypothesize that greater than or equal to 10 ng/ml IL-6 inhibits the preadipocyte to adipocyte conversion by altering normal cell cycle progression and subsequent adipogenic transcription factor expression. We will determine in 3T3-L1 preadipocytes the effect of IL-6 on cell cycle progression and differentiation. Using chimeric GM-CSF- gp130 receptor transfections, the signaling mechanisms involved to transduce IL-6 effects will be explored. To explore the physiological relevance of IL-6 in adipose tissue, we will determine whether IL-6 knockout mice have altered adipose tissue growth, glucose, and lipid metabolism on normal and high fat diets. Aim 2: To characterize adipose tissue IL-6 expression in animal models of obesity. We find IL-6 mRNA is expressed in adipose tissue of lean mice, but it has been reported that obese db/db mice do not express IL-6 mRNA in adipose tissue. Since glucocorticoids repress IL-6 expression, we hypothesize that IL-6 expression is depressed in adipose tissue of ob/ob and db/db mice by high systemic corticosterone levels that are characteristic of these models of obesity. We also predict that IL-6 expression is elevated in adipose tissue of diet-induced obese (DIO) mice, similarly to obese humans. DIO mice retain normal corticosterone levels with the development of obesity. We will characterize IL- 6 expression in adipose tissue of lean control, DIO, ob/ob, and db/db all on a C57BL/6J background at baseline and in response to glucocorticoid agonists and antagonists, and thiazolidinediones. Aim 3: To identify the differentiation-induced STAT3 activating ligand. Our new pilot data indicate that IL-6 is not the autocrine factor responsible for MDI-induced STAT3 activation, but that the heparin binding ligand midkine (MK) is. In this Aim, we will confirm our preliminary studies, and determine whether midkine is the sole STAT3 activating ligand released upon MDI stimulation of 3T3-LI cells. Aim 4: To determine the role of STAT3 activation in adipogenesis. We hypothesize that activation of STAT3 is necessary for adipogenesis. We will block MDI-induced STAT3 activation by overexpression of PIAS3. Alternately, we will mimic STAT3 activation by overexpression of a constitutively active STAT3 to determine whether STAT3 activation alone is necessary and sufficient to induce adipogenesis. The role of STAT3 in fat pad formation will be investigated by implantation into the subcutaneous space of nude mice human preadipocytes that express vector, PIAS3, or constitutively active STAT3.

Website: http://crisp.cit.nih.gov/crisp/Crisp_Query.Generate_Screen

- **Project Title: INTESTINAL IMMUNE DYSFUNCTION AND WASTING**

  Principal Investigator & Institution: Lackner, Andrew A.; Professor & Director; Harvard University (Medical School) Medical School Campus Boston, Ma 02115

  Timing: Fiscal Year 2002

  Summary: There is no text on file for this abstract.

  Website: http://crisp.cit.nih.gov/crisp/Crisp_Query.Generate_Screen

- **Project Title: MECHANISM OF TCDD-INDUCED WASTING SYNDROME**

  Principal Investigator & Institution: Matsumura, Fumio; Professor; None; University of California Davis Sponsored Programs, 118 Everson Hall Davis, Ca 956165200

  Timing: Fiscal Year 2002; Project Start 09-AUG-1990; Project End 31-JUL-2006

  Summary: This abstract is not available.

  Website: http://crisp.cit.nih.gov/crisp/Crisp_Query.Generate_Screen

- **Project Title: MECHANISMS AND THERAPEUTICS IN CANCER ANOREXIA/CACHEXIA**

  Principal Investigator & Institution: Jatoi, Aminah; Assistant Professor; Mayo Clinic Coll of Medicine, Rochester 200 1St St Sw Rochester, Mn 55905

  Timing: Fiscal Year 2002; Project Start 20-SEP-2002; Project End 31-JUL-2005

  Summary: (provided by applicant): The anorexia/cachexia syndrome occurs in greater than 50 percent of patients with advanced cancer. The investigators propose a 2-pronged approach to dissect the pathophysiology of this debilitating syndrome: palliation of anorexia and abrogation of lean tissue wasting. First, they hypothesize that inhaled neuropeptide y (NPY) palliates anorexia, presumably by means of NPY-G protein receptor interactions. Since their preliminary data suggest circulating concentrations of this potent orexigenic hormone are depressed in anorexic cancer patients, they propose to launch a clinical trial in NPY. Second, they hypothesize that the TNFalpha inhibitor, etanercept, suppresses the ubiquitin-proteasome system -- a TNFalpha-driven pathway of muscle wasting -- and thereby allows cancer patients to regain lean tissue. The investigators propose to test whether etanercept leads to decreased muscle ubiquitin conjugates and preservation of lean tissue in advanced cancer patients. The specific aims of this proposal emphasize this 2-pronged approach to the cancer anorexia/cachexia syndrome at the levels of intake and lean tissue wasting and include: 1) To determine a non-toxic, biologically active dose of intranasal NPY. Such knowledge would lay the groundwork for larger clinical trials with this hormone in anorexia in cancer. 2) To explore whether NPY1 and Y5 receptor polymorphisms are associated with aneroxia in patients with advanced cancer independent of serum NPY. 3) To explore whether the TNFalpha inhibitor, etanercept, blocks the development of muscle ubiquitin-protein conjugates, preserves lean tissue and improves appetite. Such a trial would provide the scientific underpinnings for the investigation of cytokine blockade in the treatment of the cancer anorexia/cachexia syndrome. The principal investigator, Dr. Aminah Jatoi, has unique dual training in medical oncology and nutrition. This K23 grant application will serve as a springboard to allow her to delve into the pathophysiology of this syndrome and to develop into an independent clinical investigator.

Website: http://crisp.cit.nih.gov/crisp/Crisp_Query.Generate_Screen

- **Project Title: MECHANISMS OF ACTION OF HAF--KAPOSI'S SARCOMA**

  Principal Investigator & Institution: Gallo, Robert C.; Professor and Director; University of Md Biotechnology Institute Baltimore, Md 212023101

  Timing: Fiscal Year 2002

  Summary: In the course of studies on the pathogenesis of Kaposi's Sarcoma (KS), we observed an unusual phenomena: regression of malignant [sarcoma] tumors derived from xeno-transplanted neoplastic human KS cells [KS Y-1 and KS SLK] and immunodeficient mice during early pregnancy. This led us to experiments designed to determine the identity and mechanism(s) of action of the active factor(s) subsequent found in both urine and sera of mice and women in early pregnancy. These factor(s) have the following effects: (1) kill KS tumor cells in vitro and in mice with the transplanted tumors by inducing programmed cell death; (2) inhibit angiogenesis in three different test systems; (3) promote growth of bone marrow hematopoietic precursors; (4) are anti-wasting; (5) inhibit HIV-1 expression in vitro, in HIV-1 transgenic mice, and inhibit SIV infection of monkeys; and (6) are not toxic within the concentration range used in these experiments. This factor(s), tentatively called hCG-associated factor [HAF], is present in some clinical grade crude commercial preparations of hCG and some commercial preparations of hCG and some commercial preparations of the beta chain of hCG [betahCG], is protein in nature, can be separated from hCG and betahCG [and to date the partially purified material retains all biological activities], can be mimicked by certain synthetic peptides of betahCG we call Satellins, and utilizing the crude active hCG preparations have been demonstrably active in clinical trials. Our suspicion is that HAF may be an internal fragment of betahCG resulting from a specific proteolysis and that this fragment is a variable containment of some commercial preparations of hCG and betahCG. Work in this proposal will: (1) confirm these observations, many of which are preliminary; (2) define some of the general mechanisms involved for some of these diverse biological effects, utilizing partially purified [hCG-free] poly or oligo peptide fractions and the Satellins; (3) explore the possibility that several of these effects [anti-KS, anti-angiogenic, anti-HIV activities, and even the pro-hematopoietic effect] may be due to a common mechanism, HAF-induction of programmed cell death; (4) carry out some of the bioassays for the chemical purification steps [in Project 2]; and, (5) characterize the biological effects of purified HAF.

  Website: http://crisp.cit.nih.gov/crisp/Crisp_Query.Generate_Screen

- **Project Title: MECHANISMS OF TNF/CYTOKINE ACTIONS**

  Principal Investigator & Institution: Vilcek, Jan T.; Professor; Microbiology; New York University School of Medicine 550 1St Ave New York, Ny 10016

  Timing: Fiscal Year 2002; Project Start 15-APR-1998; Project End 31-JAN-2004

Summary: Tumor necrosis factor (TNF) plays important roles in host resistance to cancer and infections, but this cytokine also acts as a key mediator of pathologies in autoimmunity, septic shock and **cachexia.** The long-term goal of our studies is to explain the molecular mechanisms whereby TNF produces its important biological actions. Elucidation of intracellular signaling pathways is essential for understanding how TNF and other related cytokines produce the multitude of their actions as well as for the design of methods that would inhibit their undesirable effects in the intact organism. In this application we propose to determine the roles played by members of the large family of mitogen activated protein (MAP) kinases in TNF actions. The hypothesis to be examined is that the ERK, JNK/SAPK and p38 MAP kinases are important mediators of TNF actions and that each of these MAP kinase subfamilies plays specific roles in the different cellular functions activated by TNF. The first specific aim is to determine the roles of the major MAP kinase subfamilies in the activation of gene expression by TNF. Toward this end we shall analyze the involvement of MAP kinases in the TNF-induced activation of the IL-6 and IL-8 genes in which the roles of specific transcription factors (especially NF-kappaB and NF-IL6) have been extensively documented. We shall also determine the roles of MAP kinases on the activation of genes responsive to the AP-1 and IRF-1 transcription factors. The second specific aim is to determine the mechanism whereby the p38 kinase mediates inhibition of TNF-induced NF-kappaB activation. We shall determine whether p38 activation alone is sufficient to inhibit TNF- induced I-kappaBalpha phosphorylation and degradation, and which of the intracellular signaling proteins known to mediate NF-kappaB activation by the p55 TNF receptor is the target of the inhibitory action mediated by p38. These studies will help to understand signaling pathways activated by TNF and will contribute to the design of methods for the inhibition of undesirable side effects of TNF in pathological conditions.

Website: http://crisp.cit.nih.gov/crisp/Crisp_Query.Generate_Screen

- **Project Title: METABOLIC PATHWAYS, MONOKINES, AND WASTING IN HIV INFECTION**

  Principal Investigator & Institution: Hellerstein, Marc K.; University of California San Francisco 500 Parnassus Ave San Francisco, Ca 941222747

  Timing: Fiscal Year 2002

  Summary: This abstract is not available.

  Website: http://crisp.cit.nih.gov/crisp/Crisp_Query.Generate_Screen

- **Project Title: METABOLIC PROCESSES BEHIND CANCER CACHEXIA**

  Principal Investigator & Institution: Tayek, John A.; Associate Professor; Harbor-Ucla Research & Educ Inst 1124 W Carson St Torrance, Ca 905022052

  Timing: Fiscal Year 2003

  Summary: This abstract is not available.

  Website: http://crisp.cit.nih.gov/crisp/Crisp_Query.Generate_Screen

- **Project Title: METABOLIC REGULATION IN THE ACUTE PHASE**

  Principal Investigator & Institution: Ron, David; Professor; Cell Biology; New York University School of Medicine 550 1St Ave New York, Ny 10016

  Timing: Fiscal Year 2002; Project Start 01-FEB-1993; Project End 30-JUN-2003

  Summary: Nutritional deprivation of cells plays an important role in human diseases ranging from stroke and ischemic heart disease to the **cachexia** of cancer and chronic infection. In addition to their ability to react to lack of specific nutrients, cells have evolved more general stress-response pathways that are activated by many forms of cellular malnutrition and other metabolic perturbations. The gene encoding the transcription factor CHOP/GADD153 is induced by a pathway that is activated when cells are deprived of oxygen, energy sources or essential amino-acids. Chop gene knock-out in mice and other experiments indicate that this pathway regulates adaptation to malnutrition in terms of changes in cell growth, differentiation and programmed cell death. Therefore, there is reason to believe that manipulating this response may impact on a broad range of medical conditions associated with cellular malnutrition. The goal of this study is to identify components of the signaling pathways that regulate Chop expression in starved cells and, utilizing genetic tools, to define their role in effecting cellular adaptation to this stressful state. Previous experiments implicate a stress-signal emanating from the endoplasmic reticulum (ER) in Chop induction in response to nutritional and metabolic stress. We have cloned two novel murine genes that are candidates for playing a role in regulating responses to ER stress in mammalian cells. The first, Ire1, encodes a murine homologue of the yeast protein Ire1p, implicated in activating gene expression in response to ER stress in that organism. The second, Perk, plays a role in attenuating translation in response to the accumulation of unfolded proteins in the ER and as such would be expected to play a role in reducing stress in that compartment. We will examine the hypothesis that Ire1 positively regulates Chop expression whereas Perk, by attenuating ER stress, negatively regulates it. We will examine the consequences of interfering with signaling by these two proteins in the context of mouse models of human diseases associated with ER stress. These will include a stroke model, models for renal acute tubular necrosis and mouse models for Pelizaeus-Merzbacher Leukodystrophy. A screen for other genes regulating Chop's response to malnutrition will also be carried out and these new components of the pathway will be examined functionally in cellular assays. If successful, these studies will shed light on basic biological principles that regulate the function of the secretory pathway in mammalian cells and on a poorly understood but broadly-utilized stress-response that is activated in many disease states. The anchoring of these studies in animal-based disease models will hopefully provide clues as to the likely outcome of interfering with the function of specific components of the pathway. This information will be invaluable for rational selection of targets for therapeutic interventions that rely on manipulating the cellular response to ER stress.

Website: http://crisp.cit.nih.gov/crisp/Crisp_Query.Generate_Screen

- **Project Title: MOLECULAR BASIS FOR MUSCLE PROTEIN LOSS IN CACHEXIA**

  Principal Investigator & Institution: Lecker, Stewart H.; Assistant Professor of Medicine; Cell Biology; Harvard University (Medical School) Medical School Campus Boston, Ma 02115

  Timing: Fiscal Year 2002; Project Start 01-AUG-1999; Project End 31-JUL-2004

  Summary: Muscle wasting, which occurs mainly by an activation of the ubiquitin-proteasome degradative pathway, is a prominent, debilitating feature of many disease states, including diabetes mellitus and renal failure. Recently, using a newly established cell-free system, we have been able to demonstrate that rates of ubiquitin (Ub) conjugation increase in atrophying muscles from septic; tumor-bearing, diabetic and uremic rats, and that a subset of Ub conjugating enzymes, the N-end rule pathway, is responsible for most of the enhanced Ub conjunction in these atrophying muscles. This is an interesting, unexpected discovery because the N-end rule pathway has been viewed as a minor ubiquitination system that was only involved in the elimination of certain abnormal polypeptides. These results raise the possibility that in **cachexia,** muscle proteins may be modified to become substrates for this pathway. We propose to use our newly developed cell-free system to further characterize this process. We will measure the abundance and activity of the N-end rule pathway enzymes (E1, E2/14K, and E3alpha) to identify the ones which are responsible for the enhanced proteolysis, and identify the substrates in muscle for these enzymes. In collaborative studies, we will genetically produce animals in which these enzymes are deleted to directly show their requirement in muscle atrophy. Finally, since most of the loss of muscle protein during muscle atrophy is from myofibrillar components, we will begin to study how the myofibril may serve as a source of substrates of the Ub-proteasome pathway by developing an assay for myofibril disassembly. Defining the components of the Ub-proteasome pathway and myofibril disassembly which are modulated in diabetes and renal failure should not only help to illuminate the regulation of muscle protein turnover, but also may allow the development of inhibitors that could combat the morbidity of these catabolic diseases. These studies will be performed in the laboratory of Dr. Alfred Goldberg, a leader in the fields of muscle proteolysis and the Ub-proteasome pathway. The applicant is a graduate of the M.D./Ph.D. program at UCLA, completing a Nephrology fellowship at the Beth Israel Deaconess Medical Center and Harvard Medical School. His long-term goal is to develop a research program centered on problems of protein folding and degradation relevant to kidney disease. This proposal offers the unique opportunity for the applicant to obtain further cell biology training, gaining experience in animal physiology, DNA technology, and biochemistry, while studying clinically relevant problems in renal disease.

Website: http://crisp.cit.nih.gov/crisp/Crisp_Query.Generate_Screen

- **Project Title: MOLECULAR PATHOGENESIS OF MNGIE**

  Principal Investigator & Institution: Hirano, Michio; Assistant Professor; Columbia University Health Sciences Po Box 49 New York, Ny 10032

  Timing: Fiscal Year 2003; Project Start 01-DEC-2002; Project End 30-NOV-2007

  Summary: Mitochondria are the main sources of energy in the cell. They are unique mammalian organelles because they contain their own DNA (mtDNA), whose genes encode components of the respiratory chain/oxidative phosphorylation system. They are essential for the normal functioning of all cells in the body, and are absolutely critical for the function of those tissues that are highly dependent on aerobic metabolism, including heart, skeletal muscle, and brain. Since 1988, single large-scale mtDNA rearrangements, more than 100 mtDNA point mutations, as well as mendelian-inherited multiple mtDNA deletions have been associated with human diseases. Mitochondrial neuro-gastrointestinal encephalomyopathy (MNGIE) is an autosomal recessive disorder associated with multiple deletions and depletion of mtDNA in skeletal muscle. The major clinical features are: ptosis, external ophthalmoparesis, gastrointestinal dysmotility, **cachexia,** peripheral neuropathy, and leukodystrophy. We mapped the disease to chromosome 22q13.32-qter and subsequently identified loss-of-function mutations in the thymidine phosphorylase (TP) gene as the cause of the disorder. With the support of a NIH grant, we have continued our investigation of MNGIE. Clinicians from around the world have sent us blood samples to test for defects in thymidine phosphorylase. To date, we have identified 51 MNGIE patients. All patients tested have shown very low or no detectable activity of thymidine phosphorylase in huffy coat samples. In addition, we have identified dramatic increases of thymidine levels in plasma from patients. These findings led us to hypothesize that elevated intracellular levels of thymidine cause alterations of mitochondrial nucleotide pools that, in turn, induce point mutations, multiple deletions, and depletion of mtDNA. To test our hypothesis, we propose to study this disorder in vivo using human autopsy samples and in vitro using fibroblasts from patients. In addition, we have produced thymidine phosphorylase knock-out mice as a model for MNGIE. Our proposed studies of the pathogenesis of MNGIE are likely to enhance our understanding of nucleotide metabolism and will likely lead to more rational therapies for this uncommon, but devastating illness.

Website: http://crisp.cit.nih.gov/crisp/Crisp_Query.Generate_Screen

- **Project Title: MOLECULAR TYPING OF TASTE CELLS USING MICROARRAYS**

  Principal Investigator & Institution: Huang, Liquan; Physiology and Biophysics; Mount Sinai School of Medicine of Nyu of New York University New York, Ny 10029

  Timing: Fiscal Year 2002; Project Start 01-APR-2002; Project End 31-AUG-2002

  Summary: (provided by applicant): The long-term objective is to understand the molecular mechanisms that different types of morphologically and physiologically heterogeneous taste cells utilize in receiving, processing and transmitting gustatory signals. Using a set of known genes we have successfully applied single cell RT-PCR amplification and filter hybridization methods to determine limited gene expression patterns for some taste cells, and to identify several taste cell type selective signaling elements thought to play a critical role in bitter sensation. In this application, we will use single cell RT-PCR products to probe DNA arrays to establish global gene expression profiles for many taste cells, to determine and predict taste cell types/subtypes based on their expression profiles, to identify additional taste type or subtype- selective genes or clusters of genes that define this type or subtype's physiological functions in taste perception. The specific goals of this application are: 1. To generate DNA probes from taste buds, filiform papillae and 100 individual taste cells using both an aRNA amplification method and a modified single cell RT-PCR procedure; 2. To screen genome-wide DNA arrays with both taste bud and filiform probes, to identify and re-array genes that are enriched in taste buds over filiform papillae to prepare taste DNA arrays (taste chips); 3. To screen the taste chips in pair wise fashion with a taste bud probe paired with one of the 100 single taste cell probes to be generated, and to establish the gene expression profiles of the individual taste cells by identifying the expressed genes on the taste chips in each single cell probe, to determine and discover taste cell types or subtypes using unsupervised partitional clustering method, and to identify additional gene classifiers with the neighborhood analysis method. The results of these studies will contribute to the development of new technologies in pursuing post-genomic biomedical research, provide genetic bases for taste cell classification and yield significant novel insights into the molecular mechanisms underlying taste transduction. The knowledge gained from this application should further our understanding of genetic differences in taste sensitivity, and the gustatory and metabolic disorders such as malgeusia, dysgeusia and **cachexia.**

  Website: http://crisp.cit.nih.gov/crisp/Crisp_Query.Generate_Screen

- **Project Title: MOUSE MODELS TO STUDY GONADAL TUMOR DEVELOPMENT**

  Principal Investigator & Institution: Matzuk, Martin; Professor; Pathology; Baylor College of Medicine 1 Baylor Plaza Houston, Tx 77030

  Timing: Fiscal Year 2002; Project Start 01-AUG-1993; Project End 31-MAR-2006

  Summary: Cancer is a major cause of morbidity and mortality in our society. Like other malignancies, ovarian and testicular cancers arise through multiple genetic alterations.

Using a knockout mouse model, we discovered that the inhibins, alpha:beta heterodimeric members of the transforming growth factor beta superfamily, are tumor suppressors with specificity for the gonads and adrenal cortex. In mice lacking alpha inhibin, neither inhibin A (alpha:betaA) nor inhibin B (alpha:betaB) is produced, and granulosa/Sertoli cell tumors of the ovaries and testis develop as early as 4 weeks of age with 100% penetrance. The ovarian tumors are often mixed tumors consisting of both granulosa cell and Sertoli cell components. Castration of male and female inhibin a knockout mice leads to a high incidence of sex steroidogenic adrenal cortical tumors (66 of 67 mice). Mice with gonadal or adrenal tumors are rapidly affected by a cancer wasting syndrome which mimics the **cachexia** syndromes associated with human cancer cases. Using a genetic approach to generate double mutant mice lacking both alpha inhibin and activin receptor type IIA (ActRIIA), we showed that tumor-produced activin directly signals through ActRIIA in the liver and stomach to cause this wasting syndrome. Using similar genetic approaches, we have shown the following: (1) Overexpression of the activin antagonist follistatin alleviates some of the cachexia-like symptoms caused by the circulating activins and slows the tumor development; (2) Absence of gonadotropins FSH and LH, prevents tumor development; (3) Lack of only FSH slows tumor development in both sexes, but mortality rates are sexually dimorphic (0% survival of females, 70% survival of males) demonstrating that FSH functions differentially in ovarian and testicular tumorigenesis; and (4) Absence of the cyclin-dependent kinase (Cdk) inhibitor p27(Kip1) speeds the process of gonadal tumorigenesis. The studies in this competitive renewal proposal will continue to define the inhibin signaling process and the mechanism of inhibin action in gonadal and adrenal function in vivo.

Website: http://crisp.cit.nih.gov/crisp/Crisp_Query.Generate_Screen

- **Project Title: MUSCLE AMINO ACID METABOLISM IN AIDS CACHEXIA**

  Principal Investigator & Institution: Yarasheski, Ke; Washington University Lindell and Skinker Blvd St. Louis, Mo 63130

  Timing: Fiscal Year 2002

  Summary: Muscle protein wasting occurs in HIV-infected individuals and is often the initial indication of AIDS. The alterations in muscle protein metabolism that explain AIDS-wasting are unknown. Seven subjects with AIDS-wasting (CD410% weight loss, 10 HIV-infected men and 1 woman (CD4>200/mm3, HIV mRNA= 3.3x103 copies/ml) without wasting or OI (asymptomatic), and 6 HIV-negative lean men (control) were studied. Constant intravenous infusions of 1-[13C]-leucine and 2-[15N]-glutamine were used to assess plasma leucine and glutamine rate of appearance (Ra), whole-body leucine oxidation rate, and 13C-leucine incorporation rate into whole-body and mixed muscle protein. Fasting whole-body proteolysis and synthesis rates were increased (P<0.05) above control in the asymptomatic HIV-infected subjects, and further increased (P<0.05) in AIDS-wasting. Fasting mixed muscle protein synthesis rate was increased in the asymptomatic subjects (P<0.05), but similar in AIDS-wasting and control subjects. Plasma glutamine Ra was increased (P<0.001) in AIDS-wasting subjects, but similar in control and asymptomatic subjects. These findings suggest that AIDS-wasting results from; (a) a preferential reduction in muscle protein, (b) a failure to sustain an elevated rate of mixed muscle protein synthesis while whole-body protein turnover is increased, and (c) a significant increase in glutamine release into the circulation, probably from muscle proteolysis. The reason for the increased glutamine Ra in AIDS-wasting is unknown, but several interesting possibilities exist.

  Website: http://crisp.cit.nih.gov/crisp/Crisp_Query.Generate_Screen

- **Project Title: MUSCLE AMINO ACID METABOLISM IN AIDS CACHEXIA**

  Principal Investigator & Institution: Yarasheski, Kevin E.; Associate Professor; Internal Medicine; Washington University Lindell and Skinker Blvd St. Louis, Mo 63130

  Timing: Fiscal Year 2002; Project Start 15-MAY-1998; Project End 30-APR-2005

  Summary: (adapted from the Abstract): The Principal Investigator proposes to test five objectives based on his preliminary observations. He and his associates have published that increased muscle proteolysis and failure to sustain muscle protein synthesis exists in AIDS-cachexia. The first aim of this project, therefore, is to determine if the increased mediators of muscle proteolysis in this population is due to contractile muscle protein breakdown by way of the ubiquitin-proteasome pathway or whether increased proteolysis is due to the overproduction of cytotoxic nitric oxide/NO reactive intermediates in skeletal muscle. These researchers have demonstrated that not only is the rate of appearance (Ra) of glutamine (70% derived from muscle) in the circulation increased but serum glutamine concentrations are low in patients with HIV-associated wasting. The Investigator hypothesizes that the overproduction of glutamine serves to provide nitrogen to other important biochemical processes. Hence, he plans to determine (1) if glutamine is used at a more rapid rate by for CD4 and CD8 lymphocytes (approximately 10~9 cells are produced each day to combat HIV); (2) if excess glutamine nitrogen is transported to the liver for urea synthesis; and (3) if excess glutamine is used by the liver for antioxidant activity (i.e., glutathione synthesis). Finally, the researchers have preliminary data suggesting that serum levels of HIV RNA are associated with greater rates of muscle proteolysis. The Investigator hypothesizes that reducing HIV viral burden will reduce muscle wasting. In this phase of the project, he proposes to assess whether a reduction of HIV with highly active antiviral drugs will be associated with significant reductions in muscle proteolysis, reduced plasma glutamine Ra, increased muscle protein synthetic rate and increased muscle mass in patients with wasting.

  Website: http://crisp.cit.nih.gov/crisp/Crisp_Query.Generate_Screen

- **Project Title: MUSCLE PROTEIN SYNTHESIS AND GH/IGF AXIS IN AIDS**

  Principal Investigator & Institution: Gelato, Marie C.; Professor of Medicine; State University New York Stony Brook Stony Brook, Ny 11794

  Timing: Fiscal Year 2003

  Summary: This abstract is not available.

  Website: http://crisp.cit.nih.gov/crisp/Crisp_Query.Generate_Screen

- **Project Title: MUSCLE PROTEIN TURNOVER AND AMINO ACID UPTAKE IN SEPSIS**

  Principal Investigator & Institution: Hasselgren, Per-Olof J.; Beth Israel Deaconess Medical Center St 1005 Boston, Ma 02215

  Timing: Fiscal Year 2002; Project Start 01-JAN-1987; Project End 31-JUL-2004

  Summary: Previous studies suggest that sepsis-induced muscle catabolism reflects ubiquitin-proteasome-dependent degradation of myofibrillar proteins regulated by glucocorticoids. Because intact myofibrils are not degraded by the proteasome, it is possible that actin and myosin are dissociated from the myofibrils before they are ubiquitinated and degraded by the proteasome. We will test the hypotheses: 1) sepsis results in glucocorticoid-mediated calcium/calpain-dependent Z-band disintegration and release of myofilaments in skeletal muscle; 2) sepsis results in increased N-end rule pathway-dependent ubiquitination and breakdown of muscle proteins and upregulated expression and activity of the ubiquitin- conjugating enzyme E2/14k and ubiquitin ligase E3alpha; 3) sepsis- induced muscle **cachexia** can be inhibited by proteasome blocker in vivo; 4) muscle **cachexia** in patients with sepsis is associated with increased expression and activity of calpains, release of myofilaments and upregulated protein breakdown in the N-end rule pathway. A septic model in rats consisting of cecal ligation and puncture is used in the majority of experiments. Total and myofibrillar protein breadkdown rates are measured in incubated muscles by determining net release of tyrosine and 3-methylhistidine respectively. Integrity of sarcomeric Z-bands is studied by electron microscopy. Gene and protein expression of calpain and calpastatin are determined by Northern and Western blot analysis, respectively. The role of calcium/calpain-dependent proteolysis is assessed by the effect of dantrolene and diltiazem on sepsis-induced morphologic and metabolic changes. The role of glucocorticoids in sepsis- induced changes in muscle calcium levels and release of myofilaments is determined by the glucocorticoid receptor antagonist RU38486. To test the role of the N-end rule pathway, expression and activity of E2/14k and E3alpha are determined and specific E3albha inhibitors are used in a cell- free system. Similar determinations are performed in muscle from patients with sepsis. The proposal is novel because it suggests that muscle **cachexia** during sepsis is caused by two distinct mechanisms, i.e., calcium/calpain-dependent release of myofilaments from the sarcomere followed by ubiquitination of myofilaments in the N-end rule pathway and subsequent degradation of ubiquitinated filaments by the 26S proteasome. The hypothesis implies two levels at which sepsis-induced muscle **cachexia** may be prevented/treated, i.e., inhibition of myofilament release by treatment with a calcium antagonist and inhibition of ubiquitin/proteasome-dependent degradation of the released myofilaments by a proteasome blocker.

Website: http://crisp.cit.nih.gov/crisp/Crisp_Query.Generate_Screen

- **Project Title: MYOGENIC GROWTH AND DIFFERENTIATION**

  Principal Investigator & Institution: Olwin, Bradley B.; Professor; Molecular, Cellular & Dev Biol; University of Colorado at Boulder Boulder, Co 80309

  Timing: Fiscal Year 2002; Project Start 15-JUL-1999; Project End 30-JUN-2004

  Summary: Aging, severe injury and skeletal muscle diseases all result in the loss of skeletal muscle tissue. Although skeletal muscle has a large regenerative capacity, a permanent loss of skeletal muscle tissue can occur in each of these clinical occurrences. The molecular mechanisms that regulate skeletal muscle regeneration are largely unknown. Implicated in skeletal muscle growth and regeneration are extracellular factors that include the insulin-like growth factors (IGFs), the fibroblast growth factor (FGFs), the transforming growth factor family (TGFs and GDFs), and hepatocyte growth factor (HGF). The loss of skeletal muscle function occurring in humans with muscular dystrophy and aging has been attributed to a loss of muscle regenerative capacity, but little is known concerning the mechanisms involved in this process. Myoblast transfer therapy to alleviate these symptoms is largely unsuccessful in animals and humans due to the death of greater than or equal to 95 percent of myoblasts following injection and the poor proliferative potential of the remaining cells. As an alternative, gene therapy with adenoviruses may be difficult due to the large mass of muscle tissue. It is likely that a combination of these procedures will be required to eventually cure muscle diseases and recover muscle tissue in patients exhibiting severe **cachexia.** In order to make myoblast transfer therapy successful, it will be necessary to manipulate the decision of a committed myoblast to proliferate, remain quiescent and undifferentiated, or to terminally differentiate and undergo cell fusion. A primary goal of the proposed research is to understand the relationships that regulate proliferation and differentiation in myogenic cells. The specific aims are to: 1. characterize the molecular mechanisms that are utilized by intracellular FGF-2 to promote myoblast proliferation; 2. analyze potential MAPK phosphatase 1 (MKP1) substrates and determine their involvement in FGF-mediated repression of skeletal muscle differentiation; 3. identify unknown MKP1 substrates that may act to mediate repression of differentiation by FGFs; 4. characterize MKP1 substrates identified in aim 3 and determine their involvement in repression of skeletal muscle differentiation. These goals will be accomplished by a combination of approaches that include the use of novel FGF-2 fusion proteins that partition into the cytoplasm via a receptor-independent mechanism, expression of mutant signal transducers, identification of unknown substrates by nanospray mass spectrometry, and determination that the identified MKP1 substrates are clinical regulators of skeletal muscle differentiation.

Website: http://crisp.cit.nih.gov/crisp/Crisp_Query.Generate_Screen

- **Project Title: NANDROLONE IN HIV ASSOCIATED WEIGHT LOSS**

  Principal Investigator & Institution: Mulligan, Kathleen; Associate Professor; University of California San Francisco 500 Parnassus Ave San Francisco, Ca 941222747

  Timing: Fiscal Year 2002; Project Start 01-DEC-2001; Project End 30-NOV-2002

  Summary: This abstract is not available.

  Website: http://crisp.cit.nih.gov/crisp/Crisp_Query.Generate_Screen

- **Project Title: NATURAL CONTROL OF M AVIUM IN SAIDS**

  Principal Investigator & Institution: Didier, Peter J.; Tulane University of Louisiana New Orleans, La New Orleans, La 70112

  Timing: Fiscal Year 2002

  Summary: The objectives of this pilot project are to establish the source of Mycobacterium avium infection in SIV-infected monkeys, characterize immune correlates of disease, and determine the feasibility of vaccination to prevent opportunistic infection of SAIDS animals with M. avium. The incidence of M. avium infection (MAI) in the SAIDS colony has increased from undetectable levels in 1988 to 18-25% in recent years. This opportunistic infection produces diarrhea, **cachexia,** and sometimes pneumonia in severely immunocompromized monkeys with remarkable similarity to MAI in children with AIDS. We detect M. avium by culture and PCR and characterize isolates from the environment (soil and water) and monkeys by molecular fingerprint analysis. To date, isolates from the environment rarely infect deep tissues of monkeys. In vitro testing of monkey macrophages demonstrates that cells co-infected with SIV and a common strain of pathogenic M. avium found in our monkey colony produces higher than expecte d levels of virus. Protein components of our pathogenic strain are being characterized. We have demonstrated that animals infected with SIV and severely immunodeficient can be infected with our pathogenic strain (MavK128) while inoculation with a human strain of M. avium (Serovar 4) fails to infect immunodeficient monkeys. In a pilot study vaccination of four animals with sonicated M. avium prior to SIV-infection failed to protect them from challenge with MavK128 but lesions contained more lymphocytes than expected. Future studies could look for promising formulations of M. avium and adjuvant that might provide protection against opportunistic infection. FUNDING Venture Research PUBLICATIONS Greenberg SS, Xie JM, Kolls J, Mason C, Didier P. Rapid induction of mRNA for nitric oxide synthase II in rat alveolar macrophages by intratracheal administration of Mycobacterium tuberculosis and Mycobacterium avium. Proc Soc Exp Bio Med, 209:46-53, 1995. Didier P, Ramesh G, Newman G, Maslow J. Detection of M. avium by PCR in rhesus monkeys. [Abstract #2486]. FASEB J, 10(6):A1431, 1996. Brar I, Didier P, Murphey-Corb M, Newman GW, Maslow JN. Prevalence of Mycobacterium avium complex (MAC) infection in SIV infected monkeys. [Abstract]. Infectious Diseases Society Meeting, September 1996, New Orleans, LA. Brar I, Didier P, Murphey-Corb M, Maslow JN. Epidemiology of Mycobacterium avium complex (MAC) infection in simian immunodeficiency virus (SIV) infected rhesus monkeys. [Abstract #655], p185, 4th Conference on Retroviruses and Opportunistic Infections, Washington, DC, January 22-26, 1997.

Website: http://crisp.cit.nih.gov/crisp/Crisp_Query.Generate_Screen

- **Project Title: NEURAL HIERARCHY IN THE MODULATION OF INGESTIVE BEHAVIOR**

Principal Investigator & Institution: Grill, Harvey J.; Professor; Psychology; University of Pennsylvania 3451 Walnut Street Philadelphia, Pa 19104

Timing: Fiscal Year 2002; Project Start 01-JUL-1983; Project End 29-FEB-2004

Summary: Understanding the role of the nervous system in feeding control is an important goal for basic and clinical science. In humans, the excessive feeding associated with some obesities increases the probability of diabetes, hypertension, and heart disease. Other feeding-related problems (failure to thrive, early satiety, dyspepsia, gastroesophageal reflux, dysphagia, **cachexia,** anorexia, bulimia) account for a significant portion of health-care expenditures in the U.S. Clearly, basic research into the location and operating characteristics of the neural substrates that control feeding behavior is essential for: an understanding of the basic physiology of intake control, an appreciation of the CNS underpinnings of various feeding pathologies, and the development of effective pharmacological treatments. We believe, as did Sherrington that the most fruitful approach to analyzing a complex distributed neural control system, such as that controlling feeding behavior, begins at the anatomical level(s) of the relevant sensory inputs and motor outputs. It is a given that many of the relevant sensory inputs (taste, visceral) enter, and all of the consummatory motor outputs (somatic and autonomic) emerge, at the level of the caudal brainstem (CBS). To address the issue of integration, we developed a chronic decerebrate rat (CD) model and have provided data that call attention to a CBS contribution to intake control. When the CD and intact rat respond similarly to selective treatments we can infer that the CBS--neurally disconnected from the hypothalamus long held to be the seat of intake control--is sufficient for all elements of the integrated response. In addition, with 4th icv infusion of orexigenic agents we will explore the relevance of CBS receptor systems to the integrated behavioral response of the neurologically intact rat. Finally, we approach a more anatomically resolved analysis of the intake-relevance of specific CBS structures through intraparenchymal infusion, cFos immunohistochemical, and NPY mRNA expression studies. The proposed experiments address the following specific aims evaluate: (1) the sufficiency of the CBS for response to signals that underlie short-term intake control; (2) the role of CBS structures in long-term intake control and (3) the relevance of CBS receptors to the feeding response evoked by selected orexigenic agents.

Website: http://crisp.cit.nih.gov/crisp/Crisp_Query.Generate_Screen

- **Project Title: NOVEL INHALATION DEVICE FOR DELIVERING VAPOR-STATE DRUGS**

  Principal Investigator & Institution: Rabinowitz, Joshua D.; Alexza Molecular Delivery Corporation 1001 E Meadow Cir Palo Alto, Ca 94303

  Timing: Fiscal Year 2003; Project Start 01-NOV-2001; Project End 31-MAR-2005

  Summary: (provided by applicant): Poor appetite is one of the subjective symptoms that cancer patients find most frustrating, and resulting **cachexia** is a common cause of death from cancer. In addition, nausea is a frequent side effect of cancer treatment. Oral delivery of the cannabinoid agonist dronabinol is approved by the FDA as both an anti-emetic agent and an appetite-enhancer. Its clinical utility, however, is limited by extensive first pass metabolism and resulting inconsistent oral bioavailability. In Phase I of this grant application, we have demonstrated the ability to form high purity, small particle size aerosols of dronabinol for reliable systemic delivery through inhalation. These aerosols can be produced by simple, breath-actuated devices. In Phase II of the grant, we now propose to prove the consistency of systemic absorption of these aerosols when inhaled by dogs. In addition, we plan to conduct the animal toxicology experiments and produce the clinical trial materials required to initiate human studies of inhaled dronabinol. Accomplishment of these goals of Phase II will lead directly to human clinical testing of a cost effective, commercially viable dronabinol inhalation delivery system. Beyond providing for improved dronabinol delivery, this drug product addresses a major unmet need in the cancer area: an appetite-enhancing and nausea-decreasing medication that works rapidly and does not require painful injection or for patients with gastrointestinal distress to consume oral medication.

  Website: http://crisp.cit.nih.gov/crisp/Crisp_Query.Generate_Screen

- **Project Title: NOVEL INHALATION SYSTEM FOR DELIVERING VAPOR-STATE DRUGS**

  Principal Investigator & Institution: Mufson, Daniel; Alexza Molecular Delivery Corporation 1001 E Meadow Cir Palo Alto, Ca 94303

  Timing: Fiscal Year 2002; Project Start 27-AUG-2002; Project End 31-OCT-2002

  Summary: Delta-9-tetrahydrocannibinol (THC) is approved for AIDS-related anorexia, chemotherapy-related nausea and vomiting, and clinical evidence supports efficacy of THC in pain, even suggesting an opioid sparing strategy with equivalent analgesia. Current THC formulations have significant disadvantages, including imprecise dosing, variable absorption, poor bioavailability, slow onset of action, and toxic components and legal issues if smoked. Medical experts agree that a rapid-onset, reliable and safe delivery system for THC represents an unmet patient need. MDC proposes its hand-held inhaler to meet this need. The inhaler is the first to deliver vapor-state drug without excipients. The inhaled, reproducible dose will be absorbed from the lung rapidly with high bioavailability, providing effective blood levels, and rapid-onset of action. Utilizing an in vitro test apparatus, MDC demonstrate feasibility by generating ultrafine particles of optimal size and distribution, without degradation, for vapor-state inhalation delivery. In Phase I we propose developing a benchtop prototype device and conducting in-vitro verification. Phase I AIMS include: 1) designing, constructing and testing a benchtop prototype producing acceptable, ultrafine particle sizes and PSD, 2) producing doses reproducibly without degradation, and 3) analyzing economical scale-down for hand-help operation. The ultimate goal is clinical evaluation of efficacy and safety leading to an NDA and regulatory approval. PROPOSED COMMERCIAL APPLICATION: The commercial market potential for the MDC Inhalation Delivery of

THC alone includes, among others, millions of cancer patients and thousands of AIDS patients who would benefit from improved management of pain, **cachexia,** nausea, and other symptoms using inhaled analgesia medications (as prescribed by their doctors) in the United States and other countries.

Website: http://crisp.cit.nih.gov/crisp/Crisp_Query.Generate_Screen

- **Project Title: NUTRITIONAL ASSESSMENT AND INTERVENTIONS FOR HIV INFECTED INFANTS AND CHILDREN**

  Principal Investigator & Institution: Miller, Tracie L.; University of Rochester Orpa - Rc Box 270140 Rochester, Ny 14627

  Timing: Fiscal Year 2002

  Summary: This abstract is not available.

  Website: http://crisp.cit.nih.gov/crisp/Crisp_Query.Generate_Screen

- **Project Title: NUTRITIONAL INTERVENTION FOR CANCER CACHEXIA**

  Principal Investigator & Institution: Fuller, John C.; Metabolic Technologies, Inc. 2625 N Loop Dr, Ste 2150 Ames, Ia 50010

  Timing: Fiscal Year 2002; Project Start 01-AUG-1999; Project End 28-FEB-2004

  Summary: (Scanned from the applicants description) The American Cancer Society estimates 564,800 Americans will die of cancer this year. Evidence suggests that up to one-third of those deaths are related to malnutrition and **cachexia** for which there are currently no effective nutritional interventions. Weight loss is a predictor of survival in patients receiving cancer therapy and supplemental nutrition is often indicated in patients undergoing surgery, chemotherapy, or radiation therapy. Phase I research has clearly shown that daily supplementation with HMB/Arg/Gln was effective in preventing and reversing the weight and muscle mass losses in stage IV cancer patients who were undergoing various regimens of chemotherapy. In this Phase II multicenter trial, it is proposed to include a more homogenous group of cancer patients, with diagnoses limited to lung and proximal GI-tract cancers which are notoriously known to result in significant wasting. The proposal will determine if early therapeutic interventions with HMB/Arg/Gln will result in (a) decreasing weight loss, (b) reversing muscle wasting, (c) decreasing protein turnover, (d) decreasing toxicity to chemotherapeutic agents and better adherence to chemotherapeutic regimens, and (e) improving overall feeling of well being. If as expected Phase II results confirm the effectiveness of the nutrient mixture in cancer patients, a product would be marketed for this purpose. PROPOSED COMMERCIAL APPLICATION: Since over 1.2 million cases of cancer are expected to be diagnosed this year alone (American Cancer Society), the market potential for the proposed nutritional product is very large. It is expected that Phase II will continue to support the positive findings of Phase I and that a product containing the nutrient combination in a ready-to-drink formulation would be marketed upon this confirmation. A balanced nutritional product containing high quality protein and other nutrients would likely be developed. It is envisioned that these products will be highly effective over-the-counter and/or prescription nutritional supplements for cancer patients with **cachexia** to improve quality of life of cancer patients.

  Website: http://crisp.cit.nih.gov/crisp/Crisp_Query.Generate_Screen

- **Project Title: OPPORTUNISTIC INFECTIONS IN INTESTINAL DYSFUNCTION & WASTING**

  Principal Investigator & Institution: Tzipori, Saul W.; Harvard University (Medical School) Medical School Campus Boston, Ma 02115

  Timing: Fiscal Year 2002; Project Start 01-MAR-2002; Project End 28-FEB-2003

  Summary: There is no text on file for this abstract.

  Website: http://crisp.cit.nih.gov/crisp/Crisp_Query.Generate_Screen

- **Project Title: PAMIDRONATE TRIAL IN AIDS WASTING SYNDROME PATIENTS**

  Principal Investigator & Institution: Postlethwaite, Arnold E.; Professor; University of Tennessee Health Sci Ctr Memphis, Tn 38163

  Timing: Fiscal Year 2003

  Summary: This abstract is not available.

  Website: http://crisp.cit.nih.gov/crisp/Crisp_Query.Generate_Screen

- **Project Title: PGC-1 AND NUCLEAR RECEPTORS IN ADAPTIVE THERMOGENESIS**

  Principal Investigator & Institution: Spiegelman, Bruce M.; Professor; Dana-Farber Cancer Institute 44 Binney St Boston, Ma 02115

  Timing: Fiscal Year 2002; Project Start 10-SEP-1998; Project End 31-JUL-2006

  Summary: (provided by applicant): During the past several years, we have shown that the coactivator PGC-1 can activate and coordinate several key aspects of energy and glucose metabolism. It does this by binding to and coactivating a large number of nuclear receptors such as PPARgamma, HNF-4alpha, GR and other tissue-selective transcription factors such as MEF2C and NRF-1. Our emphasis in the next 5 years will be to determine in detail the physiological role of PGC-1 and key mechanisms that are used to activate its transcriptional properties. Our first Aim will be to determine with "state of the art" precision how PGC-1 alters respiration, mitochondrial uncoupling and the control of reactive oxygen species (ROS). Our second Aim will utilize "knock-out" mice (general and tissue-specific) for PGC-1 to determine the precise role of this protein in several processes where a function has been suggested - mitochondrial biogenesis, thermogenesis and glucose homeostasis. Physiological studies will utilize clamp technique to determine functions of specific tissues. Aim 3 investigates the molecular mechanisms whereby p38 MAP kinase can regulate both the degradation of PGC-1 and its transcriptional activity. In particular we will investigate whether and how p38 can modulate the ability of the APC ubiquitin ligase to interact with PGC-1. In a related Aim (4), we will use knock-out mice to investigate the rote of PGC-1 in the **cachexia** and hypermetabolism brought about in physiological states associated with elevated cytokines and p38 activation: infection and cancer. The last Aim (5) will begin studies of the biological role of a new, close homolog of PGC-1 we have termed PGC-1-beta. We will investigate the activities of this protein, which is expressed at very high levels in BAT and heart, on mitochondrial biogenesis, respiration and the determination of brown adiopytes. Disorders of energy balance and glucose homeostasis are key componenets of obesity and Type 2 diabetes, the most common metabolic disorders in the industrial world. These studies should elucidate key regulatory steps that may lead to new targeted therapies.

  Website: http://crisp.cit.nih.gov/crisp/Crisp_Query.Generate_Screen

- **Project Title: PHYSIOLOGY OF RESPIRATORY MUSCLE CELLS**

  Principal Investigator & Institution: Reid, Michael B.; Professor & Chair; Medicine; Baylor College of Medicine 1 Baylor Plaza Houston, Tx 77030

  Timing: Fiscal Year 2002; Project Start 10-APR-1998; Project End 30-NOV-2005

  Summary: (provided by applicant): Tumor necrosis factor-alpha (TNF-alpha) is suggested to promote atrophy and weakness of respiratory and limb skeletal muscles in diseases that range from chronic obstructive pulmonary disease to cancer, from congestive heart failure to AIDS. Despite its putative pathophysiological significance, surprisingly little is known about the mechanisms of TNF-alpha action in skeletal muscle. The long-term goal of this project is to determine the redox mechanisms by which TNF-alpha compromises muscle performance. Thus far, we have established that clinically-relevant levels of TNF-alpha act directly on skeletal muscle cells to stimulate loss of muscle protein without inducing apoptotic or necrotic cell death. Early signaling events in this catabolic response include activation of nuclear factor-kB (NFkB). Over several days, TNF-alpha/NFkB signaling accelerates degradation of muscle protein, causing a net protein loss. The current project extends our work on this pathway to address the underlying signaling events in greater depth and to evaluate the mechanism of accelerated protein degradation. We have three Specific Aims: 1.) To define receptor-mediated signaling events by which TNF-alpha activates NFkB in skeletal muscle. 2.) To evaluate regulation of ubiquitin conjugating activity by TNF-alpha. 3.) To evaluate the ubiquitin conjugating enzyme UbcH2 as an essential element of TNF-alpha/NFkB-regulated catabolism. These aims will be addressed using an integrative approach that incorporates muscle preparations ranging from cultured myotubes to TNF-alpha treated animals. Cause/effect relationships will be evaluated using a panel of pharmacologic, immunologic, and genetic interventions. Results of the proposed studies will help establish molecular mechanisms whereby TNFalpha stimulates catabolism of respiratory and limb skeletal muscle.

  Website: http://crisp.cit.nih.gov/crisp/Crisp_Query.Generate_Screen

- **Project Title: PHYTOMELATONIN AND CANCER PREVENTION**

  Principal Investigator & Institution: Blask, David E.; Mary Imogene Bassett Hospital Cooperstown, Ny 13326

  Timing: Fiscal Year 2002; Project Start 15-SEP-1997; Project End 30-APR-2005

  Summary: (provided by applicant): The long-term goal of this research project is to better understand the role of melatonin derived from the pineal gland, in conjunction with phytomelatonin ingested in the diet, in the prevention of the growth of human malignancies in the context of biological timing. Melatonin inhibition of tissue-isolated tumor (rat hepatoma 7288CTC) growth in vivo occurs via inhibitory G protein-coupled melatonin receptor-mediated suppression of cAMP and a resultant blockade of tumor linoleic acid (LA) uptake and 13-hydroxyoctadecadienoic acid (13-HODE). This occurs via inhibition of fatty acid transport protein (FATP) function. 13-HODE, which amplifies the epidermal growth factor EGF-mitogenic signaling pathway, is the mitogenic signal responsible for LA-dependent tumor growth. The hypothesis to be tested is: Melatonin, derived from the pineal gland and dietary sources, plays a significant role in the prevention of human tumor development and growth; the mechanism of action is via melatonin receptor-mediated suppression of cAMP-dependent FATP function and/or expression leading to a blockade of tumor LA uptake and production of 13-HODE in the context of circadian time structure. The first aim is to assess the effects of dietary melatonin on tissue-isolated human tumor growth and LA metabolism in vivo. The second aim is to further define the melatonin signal transduction mechanisms involved in the regulation of tissue-isolated tumor LA metabolism and growth in vivo. The third aim is to examine the interactions among FATP function, melatonin inhibitory signaling, and EGF stimulatory signaling in the control of tissue-isolated tumor LA metabolism and growth. The fourth aim is to further define the circadian rhythm regulation of FA metabolism simultaneously in tissue-isolated tumors and contralateral fat pads and the role of melatonin. The proposed studies will help to provide a scientific rationale for the development of new dietary recommendations that consider LA intake, circadian-timed melatonin supplementation and/or photoperiodic alterations for the prevention and treatment of cancer growth and **cachexia.**

Website: http://crisp.cit.nih.gov/crisp/Crisp_Query.Generate_Screen

- **Project Title: PILOT--BIOMARKERS IN EARLY HIV WASTING**

  Principal Investigator & Institution: Koithan, Mary; University of Arizona P O Box 3308 Tucson, Az 857223308

  Timing: Fiscal Year 2002

  Summary: (from applicant's Abstract) While considerable advances have been made in the treatment of the injury of HIV infection and its complications, HIV related wasting continues to be a frequent and devastating biologic response. The currently accepted definition of wasting, the loss of 10 percent body weight, is inadequate to diagnose wasting in a time efficient manner, when intervention may be most effective. There is a growing consensus that wasting would be better defined as a process that is characterized by both early and late biologic phases. Although body composition biomarkers have been identified and tested as late phase indicators, biomarkers consistent with early wasting processes have not been previously identified or tested. Therefore, the purpose of this study is to establish reliable and sensitive clinical biomarkers that signal early HIV wasting, or wasting that occurs prior to the actual loss of body weight and to changes in body composition. Using a retrospective descriptive design, the specific aims are 1) to examine the patterns of variability and sensitivity of early HIV wasting clinical biomarkers and 2) to examine the relationships between early clinical biomarkers of HIV wasting, late wasting biomarkers, age and gender. Subjects who have been diagnosed as wasted will be recruited from four treatment sites in southern Nevada. Early and late serological and body composition biomarkers data will be collected for the 18 months immediately preceding the diagnosis of HIV wasting via a retrospective chart review process. It is anticipated that this feasibility study will provide additional, initial information about early clinical biomarkers of HIV wasting. In addition, this data will also provide valuable information regarding the feasibility and potential of the early ant late wasting syndrome model that is presented, and help identify components of the model that merit further testing. A model that is able to accurately predict both early and late-phase wasting processes using relevant clinical biomarkers would enable health care providers to initiate early diagnosis and treatment of HIV wasting, and subsequently improve quality of life and mortality in persons living with HIV.

  Website: http://crisp.cit.nih.gov/crisp/Crisp_Query.Generate_Screen

- **Project Title: PILOT--IMPACT OF ALCOHOLISM ON AIDS ASOCIATED MUSCLE WASTING**

  Principal Investigator & Institution: Molina, Patricia E.; Associate Professor; Louisiana State Univ Hsc New Orleans New Orleans, La 70112

Timing: Fiscal Year 2002

Summary: Alcohol consumption and HIV infection are frequently co-existent pathologies. Muscle wasting is a common feature of both conditions. The alterations in immune responses resulting from chronic alcohol consumption have been hypothesized to enhance the transmission and acquisition of HIV or the progression from HIV infection to acquired immunodeficiency syndrome (AIDS). Based on available information, it is possible to speculate that these are either related to the direct effects of alcohol on the immune system, or are secondary to the impact of alcohol consumption on the nutritional state of the individual. Excess alcohol consumption is associated with a approximately 50% incidence of skeletal muscle myopathy. Alcohol consumption impairs the nutritional state of the individual either as a result of decreased food consumption or as a result of decreased absorption. affecting micronutrients which in turn have been shown to modulate circulating and tissue levels of growth factors. Hence the effects of alcohol consumption on muscle wasting appear to be multifactorial. Alcohol-induced myopathy appears to be predominantly the result of decreases in muscle protein synthesis, and is characterized by decreased weight, protein, RNA and DNA contents in skeletal muscle. The general hypothesis of the present proposal is that alcohol consumption accelerates and worsens the muscle wasting associated with HIV infection, leading to increased morbidity and mortality. Infection of Rhesus monkeys with simian immunodeficiency virus (SIV) has been established as an excellent model system for studying the pathogenesis of HIV-like infection. The disease is characterized by diarrhea, weight loss, lymphopenia, thrombocytopenia, and lymphadenopathy/lymphoid hyperplasia progressing to immunosuppression with marked reduction in CD4+ cells and in the CD4+/CD8+ cell ratio, and opportunistic infections. The aim of the present proposal is to characterize the time-course and relative contribution of alterations in muscle protein synthesis and proteolysis to the progression of muscle wasting associated with chronic alcohol consumption and SIV infection individually and combined. These studies will allow for the longitudinal investigation of the progression of the alterations in muscle metabolism beginning with a healthy, non-infected animal, throughout the acute infectious period and throughout progression to full blown AIDS. These will provide the preliminary data for a more mechanistic approach to the study of the etiology of alcohol-induced muscle wasting and its impact on a chronic infection.

Website: http://crisp.cit.nih.gov/crisp/Crisp_Query.Generate_Screen

- **Project Title: PUBERTY, IMMUNITY AND MALNUTRITION IN S. JAPONICUM**

  Principal Investigator & Institution: Kurtis, Jonathan D.; Assistant Professor; International Health Institute; Brown University Box 1929 Providence, Ri 02912

  Timing: Fiscal Year 2003; Project Start 01-JUL-2001; Project End 31-MAY-2006

  Summary: The overall objective of this proposal is to prospectively investigate the interrelationships among puberty, protective immune responses, and nutritional status in adolescent Philippine residents of Schistosoma japonicum endemic areas Determining immunologic and developmental predictors of resistance in naturally exposed humans is a fundamental component of the ongoing effort to develop vaccines against schistosomiasis japonicum. Development of protective human immune responses to other schistosomes appears to occur during puberty in endemic communities. A recent hypothesis states that the hormonal changes of puberty, e.g., increasing dehydroepiandrosterone (DHEA), not cumulative exposure, initiate and promote the development of protective immune responses to schistosome infections Schistosomiasis is causally linked to malnutrition leading to the hypothesis that chronic infection results in attenuate growth for age and possibly delayed pubertal development. Animal models of chronic parasitemia have identified TNF-alpha and IL-6 as mediators of malnutrition and **cachexia.** Production of this mediator is significantly attenuated by increasing DHEA levels. These interrelationships suggest that a DHEA-modulated cycle of infection, pubertal delay, and malnutrition may be responsible for the marginal nutritional status of schistosome infected adolescents. This study will employ a longitudinal, treatment-reinfection design of naturally exposed humans to determine the immunologic predictors of resistance to reinfection and their interrelationships with puberty. In addition, the relationships among nutritional status, circulating mediators of inflammation and pubertal hormones will be examined. Information provided by these studies will influence all phases of vaccine development for S. japonicum including the identification of appropriate antigens, protective isotype and cytokine responses and the modulating effects of host pubertal and nutritional development on these responses.

Website: http://crisp.cit.nih.gov/crisp/Crisp_Query.Generate_Screen

- **Project Title: RECOMBINANT HUMAN GROWTH HORMONE FOR HIV-ASSOCIATED CATABOLISM/WASTING**

  Principal Investigator & Institution: Javaly, Kedarnath; New York University School of Medicine 550 1St Ave New York, Ny 10016

  Timing: Fiscal Year 2002

  Summary: This abstract is not available.

  Website: http://crisp.cit.nih.gov/crisp/Crisp_Query.Generate_Screen

- **Project Title: RECYCLING OF UREA NITROGEN IN CANCER**

  Principal Investigator & Institution: Klein, Samuel; Professor of Medicine and Director; Washington University Lindell and Skinker Blvd St. Louis, Mo 63130

  Timing: Fiscal Year 2002

  Summary: Urea nitrogen recycling and the incorporation of orally administered 15N-ammonia into multiple plasma amino acids will be evaluated in (1)normal volunteers, 2) cachectic patients without cancer who have lost more than 10% body weight, 3) patients with stage III or IV orophayrngeal cancer who have been weight stable, 4) patients with stage III or IV orophayrngeal cancer who have lost more than 10% body weight. Stable isotope infusion studies will be performed on inpatients in the CRC after maintenance on a controlled liquid formula diet.

  Website: http://crisp.cit.nih.gov/crisp/Crisp_Query.Generate_Screen

- **Project Title: REGULATION OF FOOD INTAKE AND BODY WEIGHT BY AMYLIN**

  Principal Investigator & Institution: Reidelberger, Roger D.; Biomedical Sciences; Creighton University 2500 California Plaza Omaha, Ne 68178

  Timing: Fiscal Year 2002; Project Start 15-SEP-2001; Project End 31-AUG-2006

  Summary: Amylin (also called Islet Amyloid Polypeptide or IAPP) is a 37 amino acid peptide that is co-produced and secreted with insulin from the pancreas in response to a meal. Amylin is also found in gut endocrine cells, visceral sensory neurons, and hypothalamus. When administered systemically or into the brain of rats amylin potently reduces food intake, body weight and/or adiposity. In contrast, amylin receptor blockade using AC187 has been reported to increase food intake and adiposity. Mice with targeted destruction of the amylin gene develop a 29 percent larger body weight at 4 months of age. Together, these results suggest that amylin plays an essential role in control of food intake and long-term regulation of energy reserves. Thus, it is reasonable to speculate that insufficient amylin production or amylin-insensitivity may contribute to the development of obesity. Amylin may also play a pathophysiological role in the malnutrition associated with pancreatic cancer, because marked elevation of plasma amylin occurs in association with the early, severe **cachexia** in pancreatic cancer patients. Studies are designed to test the hypothesis that pancreatic amylin acts as a hormonal signal to the brain to reduce food intake and to regulate adipose energy reserves. Rat and amylin- null mutant mouse models will be used to test this hypothesis. Specific aims are to: 1. Determine whether amylin acts as an essential hormonal signal (via the bloodstream) to decrease food intake, body weight, and adiposity. 2. Determine whether plasma amylin responses to ingestion (or intragastric infusion) of different nutrients are sufficient to decrease food intake and body weight. 3. Determine whether amylin reduces food intake, body weight, and adiposity through a synergistic interaction with CCK and leptin, peptides known to contribute to the production of satiety and the long-term regulation of energy reserves. 4. Determine whether the source and site of endogenous amylin action to reduce food intake, body weight, and adiposity is in the periphery and/or brain. These studies should advance our understanding of the physiological role of amylin in control of food intake and the long-term regulation of energy reserves. They may also provide direction in the search for pathogenic mechanisms of eating and metabolic disorders and strategies for their treatment.

Website: http://crisp.cit.nih.gov/crisp/Crisp_Query.Generate_Screen

- **Project Title: ROLE OF IL-4 DURING ACUTE SCHISTOSOMIASIS**

  Principal Investigator & Institution: Patton, Elisabeth A.; Comparative Biosciences; University of Wisconsin Madison 750 University Ave Madison, Wi 53706

  Timing: Fiscal Year 2002; Project Start 30-SEP-2001; Project End 21-FEB-2003

  Summary: (adapted from applicant's abstract): Schistosoma mansoni is a parasitic helminth of significant public health concern. Clinical disease is due to the granulomatous response to eggs that become trapped in the liver. In most people and all laboratory wild type mice, S. mansoni leads to the development of a strong Th2 response concurrent with the onset of parasite egg production. Although the granuloma induced by the Th2 response results in liver damage, it is critical for host protection. This is demonstrated in IL- 4-/- mice during S. mansoni infection. These animals are unable to mount a Th2 response and suffer from debilitating **cachexia** and enhanced mortality subsequent to the onset of egg production. One of the aims of this proposal is to address the role of inflammatory mediators in the development of severe **cachexia** and mortality in IL-4-/- mice. During severe disease in schistosome- infected IL-4-/- mice, splenocytes produce increased inflammatory mediators including NO and TNF-alpha, in vitro. TNF-alpha contributes to severe disease as treatment with anti-TNF-alpha antibody prolongs time to death in infected IL-4-/- mice. One hypothesis is that egg excretion results in increased endotoxin translocation across the gut wall and in mice lacking the ability to mount a Th2 response, severe inflammation ensues. This hypothesis will be tested by generating an IL-4-/- mouse strain that is hypo-responsive to LPS, the IL-4/TNF-receptor-1 double knockout strain and by generating an IL-4-/- strain that lacks exposure to LPS, a gnotobiotic IL-4-/- strain. The course of disease and in vitro responses will be followed in these strains; it is anticipated that if endotoxin induces the severe disease in infected IL-4-/- mice, **cachexia** and mortality will be minimized in theses strains. The second aim of this proposal focuses on determining the importance and cause of a defect in splenocyte proliferation that has been observed in infected IL-4-/- mice. Mediators such as TGF-beta and NO are elevated in IL-4-/- mice during infection and are improved in infected IL-4-/- animals. The role of TGF-beta in inhibiting the signal transduction cascade which leads to T-cell proliferation will be evaluated. The level at which proliferation is inhibited by both NO and TGF-beta will be determined through analysis of activation of signaling proteins important in proliferative response and the levels of expression of cdks and cdk inhibitors.

Website: http://crisp.cit.nih.gov/crisp/Crisp_Query.Generate_Screen

- **Project Title: ROLE OF MYOSTATIN IN CACHEXIA**

  Principal Investigator & Institution: Lee, Se-Jins; Molecular Biology and Genetics; Johns Hopkins University 3400 N Charles St Baltimore, Md 21218

  Timing: Fiscal Year 2002; Project Start 01-JAN-2001; Project End 31-DEC-2006

  Summary: Myostatin (GDF-8) is a new TGF-beta family member that is essential for proper regulation of skeletal muscle mass. We have shown that mice lacking myostatin have 2-3 times the amount of muscle present in wild type animals and that this increase in muscle mass results from a combination of hyperplasia and hypertrophy. We have also shown that overexpression of myostatin in nude mice induces a wasting syndrome that resembles the cachectic state often seen in human patients with chronic diseases such as cancer or AIDS. The overall aims of this proposal are to determine the role of the Smad signaling pathway in mediating the effects of myostatin in vivo, to investigate the role of the Smad pathway in regulating muscle growth, and to explore the possibility that inhibition of myostatin activity and/or Smad signaling may have applications in the treatment of **cachexia.** The specific aims of this proposal are: to generate and characterize transgenic mice in which the expression levels of myostatin can be manipulated; to generate and characterize transgenic mice in which a dominant negative form of myostatin or the pro- domain of myostatin is used to block myostatin expression and/or signaling; to generate and characterize transgenic mice in which either dominant negative forms or inhibitors of various TGF-beta signaling components are expressed specifically in skeletal muscle; to determine whether these signaling components are involved in myostatin signaling in mice; to determine whether the activities of these signaling components are essential for the wasting syndrome induced by IL-6, TNF-alpha, and certain tumor cells; and to determine the effects of blocking the activities of these signaling components postnatally in skeletal muscle. These studies will provide key information regarding the signaling molecules involved in the regulation of muscle growth and will be an important first step in investigating the possible benefits of targeting myostatin or the Smad pathway as a strategy for developing novel therapies for the treatment of **cachexia.**

  Website: http://crisp.cit.nih.gov/crisp/Crisp_Query.Generate_Screen

- **Project Title: SKELETAL MUSCLE PROTEIN METABOLISM IN HEART FAILURE**

  Principal Investigator & Institution: Toth, Michael J.; Assistant Professor; Medicine; University of Vermont & St Agric College 340 Waterman Building Burlington, Vt 05405

  Timing: Fiscal Year 2002; Project Start 01-AUG-1999; Project End 31-JUL-2004

  Summary: The PI's short-term goal is to obtain the training required to complete the proposed studies. His long-term goal is to become an independent researcher and to develop his own research program investigating the mechanism of weight loss and skeletal muscle atrophy in healthy and diseased elderly. During this award, the PI will gain experience in several laboratory and clinical research techniques associated with the measurement of skeletal muscle protein metabolism in humans using stable isotopes, arterio-venous balance and skeletal muscle biopsy methodologies. The mentoring team and the facilities available within the College Of Medicine are an ideal environment for the training of junior scientists. Patients with chronic heart failure frequently experience skeletal muscle atrophy which limits functional Capacity by reducing muscular strength and endurance. Moreover, muscle atrophy is associated with increased morbidity and mortality. The primary goal of the proposed studies is to determine the pathophysiological mechanisms underlying the loss of skeletal muscle mass in patients with chronic heart failure. The primary hypothesis is that increased skeletal muscle protein Catabolism in the postabsorptive state and reduced skeletal muscle protein anabolism in the postprandial state promotes skeletal muscle atrophy in heart failure patients. We will measure skeletal muscle protein balance (i.e., difference between synthesis and breakdown) using a combination of arteriovenous balance and stable isotope tracer techniques under postabsorptive (24 hour fast) and simulated-postprandial conditions (euglycemic hyperinsulinemia with concomitant hyperaminoacidemia) in cachectic and noncachectic heart failure patients and healthy controls. We will assess skeletal muscle protein balance during these experimental manipulations to probe for defects in postabsorptive and postprandial muscle protein balance that may contribute to skeletal muscle atrophy. In this design, noncachectic heart failure patients will serve as a diseased control group and healthy controls as a non-diseased control group. The secondary goal is to measure and compare the synthesis rate of skeletal muscle myosin heavy chain between heart failure patients and healthy controls and examine its relationship to reduced muscular strength in heart failure patients. Our secondary hypothesis is that reduced synthesis of myosin heavy chain in heart failure patients will be related to reduced muscular strength. The fractional synthetic rate of myosin heavy chain will be assessed by measuring the incorporation of [1,2- 13C2]leucine into skeletal muscle protein. These experiments will provide new information regarding the pathophysiological mechanisms responsible for the loss of skeletal muscle mass and strength in heart failure patients.

Website: http://crisp.cit.nih.gov/crisp/Crisp_Query.Generate_Screen

- **Project Title: TASTE AND VISCERAL INTEGRATION IN PARABRACHIAL NUCLEUS**

  Principal Investigator & Institution: Baird, John-Paul C.; Oral Biology; Ohio State University 1960 Kenny Road Columbus, Oh 43210

  Timing: Fiscal Year 2002; Project Start 05-MAR-2002; Project End 30-JUN-2002

  Summary: (provided by applicant): Feeding and metabolic disorders such as obesity, anorexia, bulimia, gastroesophageal reflux **cachexia,** dysgeusia, and anosmia contribute to numerous diseases including hypertension, stroke, diabetes, and heart disease, and thus account for a large proportion of health- care costs in North America and other countries. Elucidating the neural mechanisms that control feeding is, therefore, of fundamental clinical significance. Numerous behavioral studies indicate that feeding is regulated by the integration of taste and visceral afferent signals within the central nervous system; however, only a handful of neurophysiological studies have attempted to locate and characterize these mechanisms. This application will evaluate neural interactions between gustatory and visceral afferent signals in the parabrachial nucleus (PBN), a brainstem relay that receives significantly overlapping taste and visceral afferent inputs. The first experiments will use standard neurophysiological recording techniques to test the hypothesis that duodenal nutrient and distension signals are represented in PBN, as they have not been described at this level, and that these signals interact with gastric distension responses. The interaction of duodenal-signals with gastric distension and gustatory responses in PBN will then be neurophysiologically evaluated to test the hypothesis that a concomitant of satiation is expressed in the form of visceral suppression of palatable taste responses in PBN. The final phase of this application will further explore the visceral modulation of PBN taste responses through an attempt to identify whether particular neurotransmitters play a role in mediating the effect. Specifically, neurotransmitter antagonists will be microinjected into the discrete vicinity of single taste cells as they are recorded during visceral and taste stimulation. It is hypothesized that if the suppression of taste responses by visceral stimuli is mediated locally by the neurotransmitter in question, then antagonism of its receptor systems should reverse the taste suppression effect. Identifying the neurotransmitters that participate in the visceral suppression of taste responses in PBN may also provide insight regarding other central mechanisms that participate in feeding control.

Website: http://crisp.cit.nih.gov/crisp/Crisp_Query.Generate_Screen

- **Project Title: TESTOSTERONE AND EXERCISE IN MEN AND WOMEN WITH AIDS**

  Principal Investigator & Institution: Klibanski, Anne; Professor of Medicine; Massachusetts General Hospital 55 Fruit St Boston, Ma 02114

  Timing: Fiscal Year 2002; Project Start 30-SEP-1995; Project End 31-AUG-2005

  Summary: (taken from abstract of application) The presentation and course of HIV-infection have changed significantly in the current era of antiviral therapy. Loss of lean body mass and reduced functional capacity occurs in a substantial number of HIV-infected patients, despite protease inhibitor therapy. For such patients, development of effective anabolic strategies is critical to reverse sarcopenia and increase functional capacity. In this proposal, these investigators build upon preliminary data using testosterone and progressive resistance training (PRT) to increase muscle mass and strength in HIV-infected men. They have previously shown potent independent and maximal combined effects of short-term testosterone and PRT in HIV-infected men with wasting and significant sarcopenia. They will now investigate whether long-term PRT effects are maximized by high dose induction anabolic therapy and are sustainable using sequential low dose maintenance testosterone therapy. The development of novel, combined anabolic and PRT strategies is proposed also for women with AIDS wasting, a population with unique body composition changes for whom there are little data. They have previously shown that androgen administration to such patients is safe and, at high doses, results in increased lean body mass. They will assess whether combined androgen and PRT will maximally increase muscle mass and function in HIV-infected women. In addition to muscle loss, a significant percentage of HIV-infected patients experience fat redistribution, characterized by truncal adiposity, and loss of extremity fat in associate with hyperlipidemia and insulin resistance. In preliminary data they have shown significant truncal and visceral adiposity in such patients, which is highly correlated with hyperinsulinemia. Of concern, is that these changes will result in increased long-term cardiovascular morbidity and mortality. The novel use of combined testosterone and aerobic-resistance raining (men) and training alone (women) is proposed for HIV-infected patients with the lipodystrophy syndrome. No therapy as yet exists for this growing population of patients. In this renewal application, they propose: 1) specific resistance training strategies targeted at muscle accrual for HIV-infected men and women in combination with testosterone administration, and 2) development of novel aerobic/anabolic strategies to reverse lipodystrophy. The strategies outlined in this grant proposal will provide critically needed information to optimize muscle mass and function and redistribution of abnormal regional fat deposition among HIV-infected men and women in the new era of HIV-therapy.

Website: http://crisp.cit.nih.gov/crisp/Crisp_Query.Generate_Screen

- **Project Title: TESTOSTERONE REPLACEMENT AND RESISTANCE EXERCISE IN HIV WASTING SYNDROME**

  Principal Investigator & Institution: Beall, Gildon N.; Harbor-Ucla Research & Educ Inst 1124 W Carson St Torrance, Ca 905022052

  Timing: Fiscal Year 2003

  Summary: This abstract is not available.

  Website: http://crisp.cit.nih.gov/crisp/Crisp_Query.Generate_Screen

- **Project Title: TESTOSTERONE REPLACEMENT, RESISTANCE EXERCISE IN HIV WASTING SYNDROME**

  Principal Investigator & Institution: Bhasin, Shalender; Harbor-Ucla Research & Educ Inst 1124 W Carson St Torrance, Ca 905022052

  Timing: Fiscal Year 2003

  Summary: This abstract is not available.

  Website: http://crisp.cit.nih.gov/crisp/Crisp_Query.Generate_Screen

- **Project Title: TNF ALPHA AND IMPAIRED WOUND HEALING OF CACHEXIA**

  Principal Investigator & Institution: Brenner, David A.; Professor; Medicine; University of North Carolina Chapel Hill Aob 104 Airport Drive Cb#1350 Chapel Hill, Nc 27599

  Timing: Fiscal Year 2002; Project Start 01-APR-1989; Project End 31-MAR-2004

  Summary: Wound healing is a dynamic process characterized by the integrated actions of different cells, cytokines, and the extracellular matrix. Patients with **cachexia,** who frequently require surgery for the underlying illness, have impaired wound healing. The underlying hypothesis of this proposal is that this impaired wound-healing results from effects of excessive tumor necrosis factor alpha (TNFalpha) on extracellular matrix proteins. TNFalpha inhibits fibrillar collagen gene expression and stimulates cytokines and interstitial collagenase (MMP1 and MMP13) gene expression. TNFalpha is a potent activator of the intracellular signaling molecules cJun N-terminal kinase (JNK or SAPK), p38 MAPK, and NF-KB. To gain new insights into the molecular pathogenesis of wound healing, this proposal will focus on specific aspects of the effects of TNFalpha on intracellular signaling which in turn regulate expression of the type I collagen alpha1(I), interstitial collagenase, and cytokines. The specific aims of this proposal are: 1. To identify the regulatory elements in the collagen alpha1(I) gene by which TNFalpha inhibits its transcription. 2. To characterize the role of transforming growth factor beta (TGF-beta) in the inhibition of collagen alpha1(I) by TNFalpha. 3. To investigate the effect of TNFalpha on the stability of mRNAs for collagen alpha1(I), interstitial collagenase, and IL-6. 4. To characterize the signal transduction pathway by which TNFalpha inhibits collagen alpha1(I) gene expression. 5. To study the effect of IL-6 on interstitial collagenase. These studies will use primary cultures of two collagen producing cell lines; fibroblasts and hepatic stellate cells. Our laboratory has developed unique reagents required for in-depth study of the molecular mechanisms of TNFalpha's effects. We are developing novel transgenic mouse lines to study the cis- acting elements in the alpha1(I) collagen gene. We are developing recombinant adenoviruses that will deliver activating or dominant-negative forms of signaling molecules, which will modulate the genetic expression of entire populations of cultured primary cells. Finally, we are combining the above reagents with well validated assays of signaling kinases in order to use the genetics of knockout mice to further assess the role of specific signaling pathways in TNFalpha's down-stream effects.

Website: http://crisp.cit.nih.gov/crisp/Crisp_Query.Generate_Screen

- **Project Title: TNF BLOCKADE IN PANCREATIC CANCER PATIENTS**

  Principal Investigator & Institution: Villalona, Miguel A.; Associate Professor; Internal Medicine; Ohio State University 1960 Kenny Road Columbus, Oh 43210

  Timing: Fiscal Year 2003; Project Start 30-SEP-2003; Project End 31-AUG-2005

  Summary: (provided by applicant): The poor prognosis of patients with advanced pancreatic adenocarcinoma, with a median survival of less than 12 months, indicates an obvious need for more effective treatments. In addition, patients with pancreatic carcinoma are frequently debilitated by **cachexia,** anorexia, nausea/vomiting and abdominal pain. Pro-inflammatory cytokines like tumor necrosis factor (TNF) alpha, interleukin 6 (IL-6) and interleukin 1 (IL-1) have all been found to be elevated in pancreatic cancer patients and have been implicated in causing many of these symptoms, in addition to the possibility of directly promoting tumor progression. One potential target for anticancer therapy is blocking the effects of TNF. We hypothesize that TNF blockade should make chemotherapy more tolerable, should improve quality of life and should retard the time to tumor progression. In the current proposal, we seek to combine standard chemotherapy (gemcitabine) and TNF blockade with soluble TNF receptor molecules (etanercept) in a pilot trial in patients with metastatic or recurrent pancreatic cancer. We will evaluate if TNF blockade can improve the clinical benefit response, quality of life and the rate of cancer progression-free survival at six months obtained with chemotherapy. In addition, serial levels of TNF and other inflammatory cytokines, as well as the transcription factor NF-kappaB, a candidate pathway through which TNF stimulates tumor growth, will be obtained from peripheral blood mononuclear cells lysates. Quality of life and levels of the cytokines and NF-kappaB will also be measured in a control group of 10 patients receiving gemcitabine as a single agent. The observation of benefits in either quality of life or progression-free survival in patients undergoing TNF blockade would encourage evaluation of this novel strategy in properly powered randomized clinical trials.

  Website: http://crisp.cit.nih.gov/crisp/Crisp_Query.Generate_Screen

- **Project Title: TRANSCRIPTION FACTORS IN SKELETAL MUSCLE DURING SEPSIS**

  Principal Investigator & Institution: Mammen, Joshua M.; Surgery; University of Cincinnati 2624 Clifton Ave Cincinnati, Oh 45221

  Timing: Fiscal Year 2002; Project Start 31-AUG-2002

  Summary: (Provided By Applicant) Muscle **cachexia,** mainly reflecting ubiquitin-proteasome-dependent protein breakdown, is one of the metabolic hallmarks of sepsis. Previous studies suggest that gene expression and activity of the ubiquitin-proteasome pathway are upregulated in septic skeletal muscle. Despite the fact that the transcription of several genes in this proteolytic pathway are activated, there is no information regarding the influence of sepsis on the activity of transcription factors in skeletal muscle. The purpose of this project is to study the influence of sepsis in rats on the expression and activity of the "inflammatory" transcription factors, NF-KB, AP-1 and C/EBP. Because glucocorticoids regulate sepsis-induced muscle proteolysis, I will also investigate the role of glucocorticoids in sepsis-induced changes in transcription factor activity in skeletal muscle. In addition, treatment of cultured L6 myotubes with dexamethasone will be used as a "cachectic model" to investigate the expression and activity of NF-KB, AP-1 and C/EBP. The proposed experiments are important because they will further define the molecular regulation of sepsis-induced muscle proteolysis. The experiments in the cultured myotubes will make it possible to test direct effects of glucocorticoids on gene activation by the transcription factors. Knowledge gained from the proposed experiments will make it possible in the future to define genes in the ubiquitin-proteasome-proteolytic pathway that are rate limiting in sepsis/glucocorticoid-induced proteolysis.

Website: http://crisp.cit.nih.gov/crisp/Crisp_Query.Generate_Screen

- **Project Title: TRIAL OF NANDROLONE DECANOATE IN WOMEN WITH HIV CACHEXIA**

  Principal Investigator & Institution: Maenza, Janine; Johns Hopkins University 3400 N Charles St Baltimore, Md 21218

  Timing: Fiscal Year 2002

  Summary: Designed to evaluate the safety of nandrolone decanoate in women with HIV-associated weight loss, and to determine if nandrolone decanoate will increase lean body mass.

  Website: http://crisp.cit.nih.gov/crisp/Crisp_Query.Generate_Screen

- **Project Title: VGF: A NOVEL REGULATOR OF ENERGY BALANCE**

  Principal Investigator & Institution: Salton, Stephen R.; Neurobiology; Mount Sinai School of Medicine of Nyu of New York University New York, Ny 10029

  Timing: Fiscal Year 2002; Project Start 15-DEC-2000; Project End 30-NOV-2004

  Summary: (Adapted from the applicant's abstract) The expression of VGF, a secreted polypeptide that is synthesized by neurons and neuroendocrine cells, is induced rapidly by neurotrophins in vitro and is regulated by electrical activity, injury and the circadian clock in vivo. Although found throughout the adult brain, VGF is particularly abundant in the hypothalamus. To gain insight into the function of VGF in vivo, the applicant has generated mice with a null mutation of the Vgf gene. Mice lacking VGF are indistinguishable at birth from normal littermates, but gain weight very slowly prior to weaning and remain 50-70 percent the size of normal or heterozygous littermates throughout adult life. Ad lib fed adult homozygous mutant mice are hyper metabolic, hyperactive, and relatively infertile with markedly reduced peripheral fat stores. Altered hypothalamic POMC, NPY, and AGRP expression and low peripheral leptin levels suggest that ad lib fed VGF mutant mice have the neuroendocrine profile of a fasted animal. Furthermore, in situ hybridization studies demonstrate induction of VGF mRNA in the hypothalamic arcuate nucleus of fasted normal mice. VGF therefore plays a critical role in the regulation of energy homeostasis, suggesting that study of lean VGF mutant mice may provide insight into wasting disorders and obesity. This proposal seeks support to identify the neuroanatomic distribution of VGF in the hypothalamus (Aim 1), functional mechanisms responsible for resistance to obesity in VGF mutant mice (Aim 2), and mechanisms of regulation of VGF in the hypothalamus (Aim 3). The applicant further propose to determine the results of over expression of VGF in transgenic models and to examine the ability of these mice to rescue the phenotype of VGF mutant mice in genetic cross experiments (Aim 4), to elucidate the contribution of the autonomic nervous system and brown adipose tissue to **cachexia** and the phenotype of VGF mutant mice (Aim 5), and to examine the role that VGF plays in processing and regulated release of co-expressed neurotransmitters (Aim 6).

Website: http://crisp.cit.nih.gov/crisp/Crisp_Query.Generate_Screen

E-Journals: PubMed Central[3]

PubMed Central (PMC) is a digital archive of life sciences journal literature developed and managed by the National Center for Biotechnology Information (NCBI) at the U.S. National Library of Medicine (NLM).[4] Access to this growing archive of e-journals is free and unrestricted.[5] To search, go to **http://www.ncbi.nlm.nih.gov/entrez/query.fcgi?db=Pmc**, and type "cachexia" (or synonyms) into the search box. This search gives you access to full-text articles. The following is a sample of items found for cachexia in the PubMed Central database:

- **Ciliary neurotrophic factor activates leptin-like pathways and reduces body fat, without cachexia or rebound weight gain, even in leptin-resistant obesity.** by Lambert PD, Anderson KD, Sleeman MW, Wong V, Tan J, Hijarunguru A, Corcoran TL, Murray JD, Thabet KE, Yancopoulos GD, Wiegand SJ.; 2001 Apr 10; http://www.pubmedcentral.gov/articlerender.fcgi?tool=pmcentrez&artid=31889
- **Long-term inhibition of tumor growth by tumor necrosis factor in the absence of cachexia or T-cell immunity.** by Teng MN, Park BH, Koeppen HK, Tracey KJ, Fendly BM, Schreiber H.; 1991 May 1; http://www.pubmedcentral.gov/picrender.fcgi?tool=pmcentrez&action=stream&blobtype=pdf&artid=51486
- **The Endogenous Balance of Soluble Tumor Necrosis Factor Receptors and Tumor Necrosis Factor Modulates Cachexia and Mortality in Mice Acutely Infected with Trypanosoma cruzi.** by Truyens C, Torrico F, Lucas R, De Baetselier P, Buurman WA, Carlier Y.; 1999 Nov; http://www.pubmedcentral.gov/articlerender.fcgi?tool=pmcentrez&artid=96929
- **Tumor necrosis factor (cachectin) mediates induction of cachexia by cord factor from mycobacteria.** by Silva CL, Faccioli LH.; 1988 Dec; http://www.pubmedcentral.gov/picrender.fcgi?tool=pmcentrez&action=stream&blobtype=pdf&artid=259702

The National Library of Medicine: PubMed

One of the quickest and most comprehensive ways to find academic studies in both English and other languages is to use PubMed, maintained by the National Library of Medicine.[6] The advantage of PubMed over previously mentioned sources is that it covers a greater

[3] Adapted from the National Library of Medicine: **http://www.pubmedcentral.nih.gov/about/intro.html**.

[4] With PubMed Central, NCBI is taking the lead in preservation and maintenance of open access to electronic literature, just as NLM has done for decades with printed biomedical literature. PubMed Central aims to become a world-class library of the digital age.

[5] The value of PubMed Central, in addition to its role as an archive, lies in the availability of data from diverse sources stored in a common format in a single repository. Many journals already have online publishing operations, and there is a growing tendency to publish material online only, to the exclusion of print.

[6] PubMed was developed by the National Center for Biotechnology Information (NCBI) at the National Library of Medicine (NLM) at the National Institutes of Health (NIH). The PubMed database was developed in conjunction with publishers of biomedical literature as a search tool for accessing literature citations and linking to full-text journal articles at Web sites of participating publishers. Publishers that participate in PubMed supply NLM with their citations electronically prior to or at the time of publication.

number of domestic and foreign references. It is also free to use. If the publisher has a Web site that offers full text of its journals, PubMed will provide links to that site, as well as to sites offering other related data. User registration, a subscription fee, or some other type of fee may be required to access the full text of articles in some journals.

To generate your own bibliography of studies dealing with cachexia, simply go to the PubMed Web site at **http://www.ncbi.nlm.nih.gov/pubmed**. Type "cachexia" (or synonyms) into the search box, and click "Go." The following is the type of output you can expect from PubMed for cachexia (hyperlinks lead to article summaries):

- **A controlled trial of cyproheptadine in cancer patients with anorexia and/or cachexia.**
  Author(s): Kardinal CG, Loprinzi CL, Schaid DJ, Hass AC, Dose AM, Athmann LM, Mailliard JA, McCormack GW, Gerstner JB, Schray MF.
  Source: Cancer. 1990 June 15; 65(12): 2657-62.
  http://www.ncbi.nlm.nih.gov/entrez/query.fcgi?cmd=Retrieve&db=pubmed&dopt=Abstract&list_uids=2187585

- **A double blind placebo controlled trial of medroxyprogesterone acetate (MPA) in cancer cachexia.**
  Author(s): Downer S, Joel S, Allbright A, Plant H, Stubbs L, Talbot D, Slevin M.
  Source: British Journal of Cancer. 1993 May; 67(5): 1102-5.
  http://www.ncbi.nlm.nih.gov/entrez/query.fcgi?cmd=Retrieve&db=pubmed&dopt=Abstract&list_uids=8494706

- **A hypothesis. Cancer cachexia or cachexia in cancer?**
  Author(s): Sudjian AV.
  Source: Acta Chir Scand Suppl. 1980; 498: 155-9. No Abstract Available.
  http://www.ncbi.nlm.nih.gov/entrez/query.fcgi?cmd=Retrieve&db=pubmed&dopt=Abstract&list_uids=6776736

- **A middle-aged woman with dyspnea, cachexia, increased abdominal girth, pericardial effusion, and a continuous murmur.**
  Author(s): Taegtmeyer H, Schroth G, Dickerson CA, Farhood AI.
  Source: Circulation. 1994 January; 89(1): 484-92.
  http://www.ncbi.nlm.nih.gov/entrez/query.fcgi?cmd=Retrieve&db=pubmed&dopt=Abstract&list_uids=8281684

- **A patient with cachexia and ascites.**
  Author(s): Soave R.
  Source: Clin Bull. 1980; 10(3): 114-20. No Abstract Available.
  http://www.ncbi.nlm.nih.gov/entrez/query.fcgi?cmd=Retrieve&db=pubmed&dopt=Abstract&list_uids=7449086

- **A pilot study of megestrol acetate and ibuprofen in the treatment of cachexia in gastrointestinal cancer patients.**
  Author(s): McMillan DC, O'Gorman P, Fearon KC, McArdle CS.
  Source: British Journal of Cancer. 1997; 76(6): 788-90.
  http://www.ncbi.nlm.nih.gov/entrez/query.fcgi?cmd=Retrieve&db=pubmed&dopt=Abstract&list_uids=9310247

- **A review of cancer cachexia and abnormal glucose metabolism in humans with cancer.**
  Author(s): Tayek JA.
  Source: Journal of the American College of Nutrition. 1992 August; 11(4): 445-56. Review.
  http://www.ncbi.nlm.nih.gov/entrez/query.fcgi?cmd=Retrieve&db=pubmed&dopt=Abstract&list_uids=1506607

- **A study of thyroid function in cancer cachexia.**
  Author(s): Tancini G, Barni S, Crispino S, Paolorossi F, Lissoni P.
  Source: Tumori. 1989 April 30; 75(2): 185-8.
  http://www.ncbi.nlm.nih.gov/entrez/query.fcgi?cmd=Retrieve&db=pubmed&dopt=Abstract&list_uids=2741227

- **A systematic review of the evidence on symptom management of cancer-related anorexia and cachexia.**
  Author(s): Brown JK.
  Source: Oncology Nursing Forum. 2002 April; 29(3): 517-32. Review.
  http://www.ncbi.nlm.nih.gov/entrez/query.fcgi?cmd=Retrieve&db=pubmed&dopt=Abstract&list_uids=11979284

- **ABC of palliative care. Anorexia, cachexia, and nutrition.**
  Author(s): Bruera E.
  Source: Bmj (Clinical Research Ed.). 1997 November 8; 315(7117): 1219-22. Review.
  http://www.ncbi.nlm.nih.gov/entrez/query.fcgi?cmd=Retrieve&db=pubmed&dopt=Abstract&list_uids=9393230

- **Abnormal vitamin B6 status in rheumatoid cachexia. Association with spontaneous tumor necrosis factor alpha production and markers of inflammation.**
  Author(s): Roubenoff R, Roubenoff RA, Selhub J, Nadeau MR, Cannon JG, Freeman LM, Dinarello CA, Rosenberg IH.
  Source: Arthritis and Rheumatism. 1995 January; 38(1): 105-9.
  http://www.ncbi.nlm.nih.gov/entrez/query.fcgi?cmd=Retrieve&db=pubmed&dopt=Abstract&list_uids=7818558

- **Acute painful neuropathic cachexia in a young type I diabetic woman. A case report.**
  Author(s): Weintrob N, Josefsberg Z, Galazer A, Vardi P, Karp M.
  Source: Diabetes Care. 1997 March; 20(3): 290-1.
  http://www.ncbi.nlm.nih.gov/entrez/query.fcgi?cmd=Retrieve&db=pubmed&dopt=Abstract&list_uids=9051374

- **Adaptation of the ubiquitin-proteasome proteolytic pathway in cancer cachexia.**
  Author(s): Attaix D, Combaret L, Tilignac T, Taillandier D.
  Source: Molecular Biology Reports. 1999 April; 26(1-2): 77-82. Review.
  http://www.ncbi.nlm.nih.gov/entrez/query.fcgi?cmd=Retrieve&db=pubmed&dopt=Abstract&list_uids=10363651

- **Adenosine triphosphate for cancer cachexia.**
  Author(s): Walsh TD, Rivera NI.
  Source: Current Oncology Reports. 2002 May; 4(3): 231-2.
  http://www.ncbi.nlm.nih.gov/entrez/query.fcgi?cmd=Retrieve&db=pubmed&dopt=Abstract&list_uids=11937013

- **AGA technical review: malnutrition and cachexia, chronic diarrhea, and hepatobiliary disease in patients with human immunodeficiency virus infection.**
  Author(s): Wilcox CM, Rabeneck L, Friedman S.
  Source: Gastroenterology. 1996 December; 111(6): 1724-52. Review.
  http://www.ncbi.nlm.nih.gov/entrez/query.fcgi?cmd=Retrieve&db=pubmed&dopt=Abstract&list_uids=8942756

- **Amino acid metabolism in human cancer cachexia.**
  Author(s): Pisters PW, Brennan MF.
  Source: Annual Review of Nutrition. 1990; 10: 107-32. Review.
  http://www.ncbi.nlm.nih.gov/entrez/query.fcgi?cmd=Retrieve&db=pubmed&dopt=Abstract&list_uids=2200459

- **An experimental model of cachexia induced by a xenografted human tumor.**
  Author(s): Strain AJ, Easty GC, Neville AM.
  Source: Journal of the National Cancer Institute. 1980 February; 64(2): 217-21.
  http://www.ncbi.nlm.nih.gov/entrez/query.fcgi?cmd=Retrieve&db=pubmed&dopt=Abstract&list_uids=6928217

- **Anemia-inducing substance is related to elimination of lipolytic hyperactivity by cyclic plasma perfusion in human cancer cachexia.**
  Author(s): Ishiko O, Sumi T, Yoshida H, Hirai K, Honda K, Matsumoto Y, Ogita S.
  Source: Nutrition and Cancer. 2000; 37(2): 169-72.
  http://www.ncbi.nlm.nih.gov/entrez/query.fcgi?cmd=Retrieve&db=pubmed&dopt=Abstract&list_uids=11142089

- **Anorexia and cachexia in advanced cancer.**
  Author(s): Stepp L, Pakiz TS.
  Source: Nurs Clin North Am. 2001 December; 36(4): 735-44, Vii. Review.
  http://www.ncbi.nlm.nih.gov/entrez/query.fcgi?cmd=Retrieve&db=pubmed&dopt=Abstract&list_uids=11726350

- **Anorexia and cachexia, asthenia, and lethargy.**
  Author(s): Watanabe S, Bruera E.
  Source: Hematology/Oncology Clinics of North America. 1996 February; 10(1): 189-206. Review.
  http://www.ncbi.nlm.nih.gov/entrez/query.fcgi?cmd=Retrieve&db=pubmed&dopt=Abstract&list_uids=8821567

- **Anorexia, cachexia, and dysphagia: the symptom experience.**
  Author(s): Grant MM, Rivera LM.
  Source: Semin Oncol Nurs. 1995 November; 11(4): 266-71. Review.
  http://www.ncbi.nlm.nih.gov/entrez/query.fcgi?cmd=Retrieve&db=pubmed&dopt=Abstract&list_uids=8578034

- **Anorexia/cachexia in patients with HIV: lessons for the oncologist.**
  Author(s): Von Roenn JH, Knopf K.
  Source: Oncology (Huntingt). 1996 July; 10(7): 1049-56; Discussion 1062-4, 1067-8. Review.
  http://www.ncbi.nlm.nih.gov/entrez/query.fcgi?cmd=Retrieve&db=pubmed&dopt=Abstract&list_uids=8837121

- **Another cause of cachexia.**
  Author(s): Rosomoff HL.
  Source: Journal of Pain and Symptom Management. 1989 June; 4(2): 57. Erratum In: J Pain Symptom Manage 1989 September; 4(3): 162.
  http://www.ncbi.nlm.nih.gov/entrez/query.fcgi?cmd=Retrieve&db=pubmed&dopt=Abstract&list_uids=2757692

- **Anthropometric evaluation of cachexia in chronic congestive heart failure: the role of tricuspid regurgitation.**
  Author(s): Ajayi AA, Adigun AQ, Ojofeitimi EO, Yusuph H, Ajayi OE.
  Source: International Journal of Cardiology. 1999 September 30; 71(1): 79-84.
  http://www.ncbi.nlm.nih.gov/entrez/query.fcgi?cmd=Retrieve&db=pubmed&dopt=Abstract&list_uids=10522568

- **Antrochoanal polyp presenting with obstructive sleep apnoea and cachexia.**
  Author(s): Salib RJ, Sadek SA, Dutt SN, Pearman K.
  Source: International Journal of Pediatric Otorhinolaryngology. 2000 August 31; 54(2-3): 163-6.
  http://www.ncbi.nlm.nih.gov/entrez/query.fcgi?cmd=Retrieve&db=pubmed&dopt=Abstract&list_uids=10967389

- **Apoptosis as a potential mechanism of muscle cachexia in chronic obstructive pulmonary disease.**
  Author(s): Lewis MI.
  Source: American Journal of Respiratory and Critical Care Medicine. 2002 August 15; 166(4): 434-6. Review.
  http://www.ncbi.nlm.nih.gov/entrez/query.fcgi?cmd=Retrieve&db=pubmed&dopt=Abstract&list_uids=12186814

- **Are cytokines possible mediators of cancer cachexia?**
  Author(s): Noguchi Y, Yoshikawa T, Matsumoto A, Svaninger G, Gelin J.
  Source: Surgery Today. 1996; 26(7): 467-75. Review.
  http://www.ncbi.nlm.nih.gov/entrez/query.fcgi?cmd=Retrieve&db=pubmed&dopt=Abstract&list_uids=8840426

- **Are preoperative obesity and cachexia risk factors for post heart transplant morbidity and mortality: a multi-institutional study of preoperative weight-height indices. Cardiac Transplant Research Database (CTRD) Group.**
  Author(s): Grady KL, White-Williams C, Naftel D, Costanzo MR, Pitts D, Rayburn B, VanBakel A, Jaski B, Bourge R, Kirklin J.
  Source: The Journal of Heart and Lung Transplantation : the Official Publication of the International Society for Heart Transplantation. 1999 August; 18(8): 750-63.
  http://www.ncbi.nlm.nih.gov/entrez/query.fcgi?cmd=Retrieve&db=pubmed&dopt=Abstract&list_uids=10512521

- **Beneficial response to megoestrol acetate in AIDS-related cachexia and a possible megoestrol withdrawal-associated syndrome?**
  Author(s): Nathwani D, Green ST, Heslop JM, Goldberg DJ, Kennedy DH.
  Source: Acta Dermato-Venereologica. 1990; 70(6): 520-1.
  http://www.ncbi.nlm.nih.gov/entrez/query.fcgi?cmd=Retrieve&db=pubmed&dopt=Abstract&list_uids=1981430

- **Biology of cachexia.**
  Author(s): Tisdale MJ.
  Source: Journal of the National Cancer Institute. 1997 December 3; 89(23): 1763-73. Review.
  http://www.ncbi.nlm.nih.gov/entrez/query.fcgi?cmd=Retrieve&db=pubmed&dopt=Abstract&list_uids=9392617

- **Biomedicine. Protein loss in cancer cachexia.**
  Author(s): Tisdale MJ.
  Source: Science. 2000 September 29; 289(5488): 2293-4.
  http://www.ncbi.nlm.nih.gov/entrez/query.fcgi?cmd=Retrieve&db=pubmed&dopt=Abstract&list_uids=11041796

- **Body composition in cachexia resulting from malignant and non-malignant diseases.**
  Author(s): Watson WS, Sammon AM.
  Source: Cancer. 1980 November 1; 46(9): 2041-6.
  http://www.ncbi.nlm.nih.gov/entrez/query.fcgi?cmd=Retrieve&db=pubmed&dopt=Abstract&list_uids=7427910

- **Body composition in cancer cachexia.**
  Author(s): Fearon KC, Preston T.
  Source: Infusionstherapie. 1990 April; 17 Suppl 3: 63-6. No Abstract Available.
  http://www.ncbi.nlm.nih.gov/entrez/query.fcgi?cmd=Retrieve&db=pubmed&dopt=Abstract&list_uids=2169464

- **Body mass and survival in patients with chronic heart failure without cachexia: the importance of obesity.**
  Author(s): Davos CH, Doehner W, Rauchhaus M, Cicoira M, Francis DP, Coats AJ, Clark AL, Anker SD.
  Source: Journal of Cardiac Failure. 2003 February; 9(1): 29-35.
  http://www.ncbi.nlm.nih.gov/entrez/query.fcgi?cmd=Retrieve&db=pubmed&dopt=Abstract&list_uids=12612870

- **Brain cytokine production and action in anorexia and cachexia.**
  Author(s): Plata-Salaman CR.
  Source: Cytokine. 2001 July 7; 15(1): 1-3.
  http://www.ncbi.nlm.nih.gov/entrez/query.fcgi?cmd=Retrieve&db=pubmed&dopt=Abstract&list_uids=11509002

- **Brain tryptophan and the neoplastic anorexia-cachexia syndrome.**
  Author(s): Krause R, James JH, Ziparo V, Fischer JE.
  Source: Cancer. 1979 September; 44(3): 1003-8.
  http://www.ncbi.nlm.nih.gov/entrez/query.fcgi?cmd=Retrieve&db=pubmed&dopt=Abstract&list_uids=289432

- **Branched chain amino acids as the protein component of parenteral nutrition in cancer cachexia.**
  Author(s): Hunter DC, Weintraub M, Blackburn GL, Bistrian BR.
  Source: The British Journal of Surgery. 1989 February; 76(2): 149-53.
  http://www.ncbi.nlm.nih.gov/entrez/query.fcgi?cmd=Retrieve&db=pubmed&dopt=Abstract&list_uids=2495147

- **Brown adipose tissue in cancer patients: possible cause of cancer-induced cachexia.**
  Author(s): Shellock FG, Riedinger MS, Fishbein MC.
  Source: Journal of Cancer Research and Clinical Oncology. 1986; 111(1): 82-5.
  http://www.ncbi.nlm.nih.gov/entrez/query.fcgi?cmd=Retrieve&db=pubmed&dopt=Abstract&list_uids=3949854

- **Cachexia and anorexia.**
  Author(s): Mantovani G.
  Source: Supportive Care in Cancer : Official Journal of the Multinational Association of Supportive Care in Cancer. 2000 November; 8(6): 506-9.
  http://www.ncbi.nlm.nih.gov/entrez/query.fcgi?cmd=Retrieve&db=pubmed&dopt=Abstract&list_uids=11094998

- **Cachexia and asthenia in cancer patients.**
  Author(s): Bruera E, Sweeney C.
  Source: The Lancet Oncology. 2000 November; 1: 138-47. Review.
  http://www.ncbi.nlm.nih.gov/entrez/query.fcgi?cmd=Retrieve&db=pubmed&dopt=Abstract&list_uids=11905651

- **Cachexia and obesity: two sides of one coin?**
  Author(s): Inui A, Meguid MM.
  Source: Current Opinion in Clinical Nutrition and Metabolic Care. 2003 July; 6(4): 395-9. Review.
  http://www.ncbi.nlm.nih.gov/entrez/query.fcgi?cmd=Retrieve&db=pubmed&dopt=Abstract&list_uids=12806212

- **Cachexia and poor night vision.**
  Author(s): Browning AC, Amoaku WM, Vernon SA, Morgan J, Thirkill CE.
  Source: Lancet. 2004 April 17; 363(9417): 1305.
  http://www.ncbi.nlm.nih.gov/entrez/query.fcgi?cmd=Retrieve&db=pubmed&dopt=Abstract&list_uids=15094277

- **Cachexia in liver cirrhosis.**
  Author(s): Plauth M, Schutz ET.
  Source: International Journal of Cardiology. 2002 September; 85(1): 83-7. Review.
  http://www.ncbi.nlm.nih.gov/entrez/query.fcgi?cmd=Retrieve&db=pubmed&dopt=Abstract&list_uids=12163212

- **Cachexia in patients with advanced cancer.**
  Author(s): Dell DD.
  Source: Clinical Journal of Oncology Nursing. 2002 July-August; 6(4): 235-8.
  http://www.ncbi.nlm.nih.gov/entrez/query.fcgi?cmd=Retrieve&db=pubmed&dopt=Abstract&list_uids=12087622

- **Cachexia in rheumatoid arthritis is not explained by decreased growth hormone secretion.**
  Author(s): Rall LC, Walsmith JM, Snydman L, Reichlin S, Veldhuis JD, Kehayias JJ, Abad LW, Lundgren NT, Roubenoff R.
  Source: Arthritis and Rheumatism. 2002 October; 46(10): 2574-7.
  http://www.ncbi.nlm.nih.gov/entrez/query.fcgi?cmd=Retrieve&db=pubmed&dopt=Abstract&list_uids=12384914

- **Cachexia in rheumatoid arthritis.**
  Author(s): Walsmith J, Roubenoff R.
  Source: International Journal of Cardiology. 2002 September; 85(1): 89-99.
  http://www.ncbi.nlm.nih.gov/entrez/query.fcgi?cmd=Retrieve&db=pubmed&dopt=Abstract&list_uids=12163213

- **Cachexia: a therapeutic approach beyond cytokine antagonism.**
  Author(s): von Haehling S, Genth-Zotz S, Anker SD, Volk HD.
  Source: International Journal of Cardiology. 2002 September; 85(1): 173-83. Review.
  http://www.ncbi.nlm.nih.gov/entrez/query.fcgi?cmd=Retrieve&db=pubmed&dopt=Abstract&list_uids=12163222

- **Cachexia: time to receive more attention.**
  Author(s): Anker SD.
  Source: International Journal of Cardiology. 2002 September; 85(1): 5-6.
  http://www.ncbi.nlm.nih.gov/entrez/query.fcgi?cmd=Retrieve&db=pubmed&dopt=Abstract&list_uids=12163204

- **Cachexia-like symptoms predict a worse prognosis in localized t1 renal cell carcinoma.**
  Author(s): Kim HL, Han KR, Zisman A, Figlin RA, Belldegrun AS.
  Source: The Journal of Urology. 2004 May; 171(5): 1810-3.
  http://www.ncbi.nlm.nih.gov/entrez/query.fcgi?cmd=Retrieve&db=pubmed&dopt=Abstract&list_uids=15076282

- **Cancer anorexia and cachexia.**
  Author(s): Tisdale MJ.
  Source: Nutrition (Burbank, Los Angeles County, Calif.). 2001 May; 17(5): 438-42. Review.
  http://www.ncbi.nlm.nih.gov/entrez/query.fcgi?cmd=Retrieve&db=pubmed&dopt=Abstract&list_uids=11377146

- **Cancer anorexia-cachexia syndrome: current issues in research and management.**
  Author(s): Inui A.
  Source: Ca: a Cancer Journal for Clinicians. 2002 March-April; 52(2): 72-91. Review.
  http://www.ncbi.nlm.nih.gov/entrez/query.fcgi?cmd=Retrieve&db=pubmed&dopt=Abstract&list_uids=11929007

- **Cancer cachexia.**
  Author(s): Fearon KC, Moses AG.
  Source: International Journal of Cardiology. 2002 September; 85(1): 73-81. Review.
  http://www.ncbi.nlm.nih.gov/entrez/query.fcgi?cmd=Retrieve&db=pubmed&dopt=Abstract&list_uids=12163211

- **Cancer cachexia.**
  Author(s): Barber MD, Ross JA, Fearon KC.
  Source: Surgical Oncology. 1999 November; 8(3): 133-41. Review.
  http://www.ncbi.nlm.nih.gov/entrez/query.fcgi?cmd=Retrieve&db=pubmed&dopt=Abstract&list_uids=11113664

- **Cancer cachexia: a therapeutic approach.**
  Author(s): Argiles JM, Meijsing SH, Pallares-Trujillo J, Guirao X, Lopez-Soriano FJ.
  Source: Medicinal Research Reviews. 2001 January; 21(1): 83-101. Review.
  http://www.ncbi.nlm.nih.gov/entrez/query.fcgi?cmd=Retrieve&db=pubmed&dopt=Abstract&list_uids=11135301

- **Cancer cachexia: its correlations and causes.**
  Author(s): Rubin H.
  Source: Proceedings of the National Academy of Sciences of the United States of America. 2003 April 29; 100(9): 5384-9. Epub 2003 Apr 17. Review.
  http://www.ncbi.nlm.nih.gov/entrez/query.fcgi?cmd=Retrieve&db=pubmed&dopt=Abstract&list_uids=12702753

- **Cancer cachexia: the molecular mechanisms.**
  Author(s): Argiles JM, Moore-Carrasco R, Fuster G, Busquets S, Lopez-Soriano FJ.
  Source: The International Journal of Biochemistry & Cell Biology. 2003 April; 35(4): 405-9. Review.
  http://www.ncbi.nlm.nih.gov/entrez/query.fcgi?cmd=Retrieve&db=pubmed&dopt=Abstract&list_uids=12565701

- **Cancer cachexia: what is known about its etiology and what should be the current treatment approach?**
  Author(s): van Halteren HK, Bongaerts GP, Wagener DJ.
  Source: Anticancer Res. 2003 November-December; 23(6D): 5111-5.
  http://www.ncbi.nlm.nih.gov/entrez/query.fcgi?cmd=Retrieve&db=pubmed&dopt=Abstract&list_uids=14981975

- **Cancer-related cachexia and oxidative stress: beyond current therapeutic options.**
  Author(s): Mantovani G, Maccio A, Madeddu C, Massa E.
  Source: Expert Review of Anticancer Therapy. 2003 June; 3(3): 381-92. Review.
  http://www.ncbi.nlm.nih.gov/entrez/query.fcgi?cmd=Retrieve&db=pubmed&dopt=Abstract&list_uids=12820780

- **Cardiac cachexia in early literature: a review of research prior to Medline.**
  Author(s): Doehner W, Anker SD.
  Source: International Journal of Cardiology. 2002 September; 85(1): 7-14.
  http://www.ncbi.nlm.nih.gov/entrez/query.fcgi?cmd=Retrieve&db=pubmed&dopt=Abstract&list_uids=12163205

- **Catabolic mediators as targets for cancer cachexia.**
  Author(s): Argiles JM, Moore-Carrasco R, Busquets S, Lopez-Soriano FJ.
  Source: Drug Discovery Today. 2003 September 15; 8(18): 838-44. Review.
  http://www.ncbi.nlm.nih.gov/entrez/query.fcgi?cmd=Retrieve&db=pubmed&dopt=Abstract&list_uids=12963320

- **Catabolism of skeletal muscle proteins and its reversal in cancer cachexia.**
  Author(s): Tisdale MJ.
  Source: Nestle Nutr Workshop Ser Clin Perform Programme. 2000; 4: 135-43; Discussion 144-6. Review. No Abstract Available.
  http://www.ncbi.nlm.nih.gov/entrez/query.fcgi?cmd=Retrieve&db=pubmed&dopt=Abstract&list_uids=11490570

- **Chronic heart failure: an example of a systemic chronic inflammatory disease resulting in cachexia.**
  Author(s): Conraads VM, Bosmans JM, Vrints CJ.
  Source: International Journal of Cardiology. 2002 September; 85(1): 33-49. Review.
  http://www.ncbi.nlm.nih.gov/entrez/query.fcgi?cmd=Retrieve&db=pubmed&dopt=Abstract&list_uids=12163208

- **Clinical significance of weight loss in cancer patients: rationale for the use of anabolic agents in the treatment of cancer-related cachexia.**
  Author(s): Langer CJ, Hoffman JP, Ottery FD.
  Source: Nutrition (Burbank, Los Angeles County, Calif.). 2001 January; 17(1 Suppl): S1-20. Review.
  http://www.ncbi.nlm.nih.gov/entrez/query.fcgi?cmd=Retrieve&db=pubmed&dopt=Abstract&list_uids=11428126

- **Clinical Trials Update: CAPRICORN, COPERNICUS, MIRACLE, STAF, RITZ-2, RECOVER and RENAISSANCE and cachexia and cholesterol in heart failure. Highlights of the Scientific Sessions of the American College of Cardiology, 2001.**
  Author(s): Louis A, Cleland JG, Crabbe S, Ford S, Thackray S, Houghton T, Clark A.
  Source: European Journal of Heart Failure : Journal of the Working Group on Heart Failure of the European Society of Cardiology. 2001 June; 3(3): 381-7. Review.
  http://www.ncbi.nlm.nih.gov/entrez/query.fcgi?cmd=Retrieve&db=pubmed&dopt=Abstract&list_uids=11378012

- **Cytokines in the pathogenesis of cancer cachexia.**
  Author(s): Argiles JM, Busquets S, Lopez-Soriano FJ.
  Source: Current Opinion in Clinical Nutrition and Metabolic Care. 2003 July; 6(4): 401-6. Review.
  http://www.ncbi.nlm.nih.gov/entrez/query.fcgi?cmd=Retrieve&db=pubmed&dopt=Abstract&list_uids=12806213

- **Cytokines, apoptosis and cachexia: the potential for TNF antagonism.**
  Author(s): Sharma R, Anker SD.
  Source: International Journal of Cardiology. 2002 September; 85(1): 161-71. Review.
  http://www.ncbi.nlm.nih.gov/entrez/query.fcgi?cmd=Retrieve&db=pubmed&dopt=Abstract&list_uids=12163221

- **Death in conditions of cachexia: the price for the dialysis treatment of the elderly?**
  Author(s): Piccoli G, Bonello F, Massara C, Salomone M, Maffei S, Iadarola GM, Stramignoni E, Rosati C, Borca M, Belardi P, et al.
  Source: Kidney International. Supplement. 1993 June; 41: S282-6.
  http://www.ncbi.nlm.nih.gov/entrez/query.fcgi?cmd=Retrieve&db=pubmed&dopt=Abstract&list_uids=8320938

- **Decreased serum tryptophan in patients with cancer cachexia correlates with increased serum neopterin.**
  Author(s): Iwagaki H, Hizuta A, Tanaka N, Orita K.
  Source: Immunological Investigations. 1995 March; 24(3): 467-78.
  http://www.ncbi.nlm.nih.gov/entrez/query.fcgi?cmd=Retrieve&db=pubmed&dopt=Abstract&list_uids=7790043

- **Depressed protein synthesis is the dominant characteristic of muscle wasting and cachexia.**
  Author(s): Rennie MJ, Edwards RH, Emery PW, Halliday D, Lundholm K, Millward DJ.
  Source: Clinical Physiology (Oxford, England). 1983 October; 3(5): 387-98.
  http://www.ncbi.nlm.nih.gov/entrez/query.fcgi?cmd=Retrieve&db=pubmed&dopt=Abstract&list_uids=6357592

- **Diabetes mellitus induced by megestrol acetate in a patient with AIDS and cachexia.**
  Author(s): Henry K, Rathgaber S, Sullivan C, McCabe K.
  Source: Annals of Internal Medicine. 1992 January 1; 116(1): 53-4.
  http://www.ncbi.nlm.nih.gov/entrez/query.fcgi?cmd=Retrieve&db=pubmed&dopt=Abstract&list_uids=1727096

- **Diabetic neuropathic cachexia and acute bilateral cataract formation following rapid glycaemic control in a newly diagnosed type 1 diabetic patient.**
  Author(s): Yuen KC, Day JL, Flannagan DW, Rayman G.
  Source: Diabetic Medicine : a Journal of the British Diabetic Association. 2001 October; 18(10): 854-7.
  http://www.ncbi.nlm.nih.gov/entrez/query.fcgi?cmd=Retrieve&db=pubmed&dopt=Abstract&list_uids=11678979

- **Diabetic neuropathic cachexia and diabetic amyotrophy.**
  Author(s): Massey EW.
  Source: Acta Diabetol Lat. 1982 January-March; 19(1): 91-5. No Abstract Available.
  http://www.ncbi.nlm.nih.gov/entrez/query.fcgi?cmd=Retrieve&db=pubmed&dopt=Abstract&list_uids=7072445

- **Diabetic neuropathic cachexia and hypothyroidism in a woman.**
  Author(s): Wright DL, Shah JH.
  Source: Mo Med. 1987 March; 84(3): 143-5. No Abstract Available.
  http://www.ncbi.nlm.nih.gov/entrez/query.fcgi?cmd=Retrieve&db=pubmed&dopt=Abstract&list_uids=3509122

- **Diabetic neuropathic cachexia associated with malabsorption.**
  Author(s): D'Costa DF, Price DE, Burden AC.
  Source: Diabetic Medicine : a Journal of the British Diabetic Association. 1992 March; 9(2): 203-5.
  http://www.ncbi.nlm.nih.gov/entrez/query.fcgi?cmd=Retrieve&db=pubmed&dopt=Abstract&list_uids=1563256

- **Diabetic neuropathic cachexia.**
  Author(s): Godil A, Berriman D, Knapik S, Norman M, Godil F, Firek AF.
  Source: The Western Journal of Medicine. 1996 December; 165(6): 382-5. Review.
  http://www.ncbi.nlm.nih.gov/entrez/query.fcgi?cmd=Retrieve&db=pubmed&dopt=Abstract&list_uids=9000865

- **Diabetic neuropathic cachexia.**
  Author(s): Chandler PT, Singh RS, Schwetschenau RP.
  Source: Acta Diabetol Lat. 1978 May-August; 15(3-4): 212-6.
  http://www.ncbi.nlm.nih.gov/entrez/query.fcgi?cmd=Retrieve&db=pubmed&dopt=Abstract&list_uids=707003

- **Diabetic neuropathic cachexia.**
  Author(s): Ellenberg M.
  Source: Diabetes. 1974 May; 23(5): 418-23.
  http://www.ncbi.nlm.nih.gov/entrez/query.fcgi?cmd=Retrieve&db=pubmed&dopt=Abstract&list_uids=4364389

- **Diabetic neuropathic cachexia. Beneficial response to combination therapy with amitriptyline and fluphenazine.**
  Author(s): Gade GN, Hofeldt FD, Treece GL.
  Source: Jama : the Journal of the American Medical Association. 1980 March 21; 243(11): 1160-1.
  http://www.ncbi.nlm.nih.gov/entrez/query.fcgi?cmd=Retrieve&db=pubmed&dopt=Abstract&list_uids=7359668

- **Diabetic neuropathic cachexia. Report of a woman with this syndrome and review of the literature.**
  Author(s): Blau RH.
  Source: Archives of Internal Medicine. 1983 October; 143(10): 2011-2.
  http://www.ncbi.nlm.nih.gov/entrez/query.fcgi?cmd=Retrieve&db=pubmed&dopt=Abstract&list_uids=6625793

- **Diabetic neuropathic cachexia: report of a recurrent case.**
  Author(s): Jackson CE, Barohn RJ.
  Source: Journal of Neurology, Neurosurgery, and Psychiatry. 1998 June; 64(6): 785-7.
  http://www.ncbi.nlm.nih.gov/entrez/query.fcgi?cmd=Retrieve&db=pubmed&dopt=Abstract&list_uids=9647310

- **Diabetic neuropathic cachexia: the importance of positive recognition and early nutritional support.**
  Author(s): van Heel DA, Levitt NS, Winter TA.
  Source: Int J Clin Pract. 1998 November-December; 52(8): 591-2.
  http://www.ncbi.nlm.nih.gov/entrez/query.fcgi?cmd=Retrieve&db=pubmed&dopt=Abstract&list_uids=10622062

- **Diencephalic tumor. A cause of infantile nystagmus and cachexia.**
  Author(s): Ciccarelli EC, Huttenlocher PR.
  Source: Archives of Ophthalmology. 1967 September; 78(3): 350-3.
  http://www.ncbi.nlm.nih.gov/entrez/query.fcgi?cmd=Retrieve&db=pubmed&dopt=Abstract&list_uids=5298708

- **Dietary treatment in secondary wasting and cachexia.**
  Author(s): Bistrian BR.
  Source: The Journal of Nutrition. 1999 January; 129(1S Suppl): 290S-294S. Review.
  http://www.ncbi.nlm.nih.gov/entrez/query.fcgi?cmd=Retrieve&db=pubmed&dopt=Abstract&list_uids=9915917

- **Dietetics. Cancer cachexia.**
  Author(s): Sutton A.
  Source: Nurs Times. 1988 January 20-26; 84(3): 65-6. No Abstract Available.
  http://www.ncbi.nlm.nih.gov/entrez/query.fcgi?cmd=Retrieve&db=pubmed&dopt=Abstract&list_uids=3347540

- **Diet-induced thermogenesis in patients with gastrointestinal cancer cachexia.**
Author(s): Weston PM, King RF, Goode AW, Williams NS.
Source: Clinical Science (London, England : 1979). 1989 August; 77(2): 133-8.
http://www.ncbi.nlm.nih.gov/entrez/query.fcgi?cmd=Retrieve&db=pubmed&dopt=Abstract&list_uids=2766653

- **Diminished visceral adipose tissue in cancer cachexia.**
Author(s): Ogiwara H, Takahashi S, Kato Y, Uyama I, Takahara T, Kikuchi K, Iida S.
Source: Journal of Surgical Oncology. 1994 October; 57(2): 129-33.
http://www.ncbi.nlm.nih.gov/entrez/query.fcgi?cmd=Retrieve&db=pubmed&dopt=Abstract&list_uids=7934064

- **Distinguishing starvation from cachexia.**
Author(s): Thomas DR.
Source: Clinics in Geriatric Medicine. 2002 November; 18(4): 883-91. Review.
http://www.ncbi.nlm.nih.gov/entrez/query.fcgi?cmd=Retrieve&db=pubmed&dopt=Abstract&list_uids=12608511

- **DNA fragmentation occurs in skeletal muscle during tumor growth: A link with cancer cachexia?**
Author(s): van Royen M, Carbo N, Busquets S, Alvarez B, Quinn LS, Lopez-Soriano FJ, Argiles JM.
Source: Biochemical and Biophysical Research Communications. 2000 April 13; 270(2): 533-7.
http://www.ncbi.nlm.nih.gov/entrez/query.fcgi?cmd=Retrieve&db=pubmed&dopt=Abstract&list_uids=10753659

- **Editorial: Cachexia and ascites in hemodialysis patients.**
Author(s): Hussey HH.
Source: Jama : the Journal of the American Medical Association. 1974 December 23-30; 230(12): 1680.
http://www.ncbi.nlm.nih.gov/entrez/query.fcgi?cmd=Retrieve&db=pubmed&dopt=Abstract&list_uids=4479868

- **Effect of a fluorinated pyrimidine on cachexia and tumour growth in murine cachexia models: relationship with a proteolysis inducing factor.**
Author(s): Hussey HJ, Todorov PT, Field WN, Inagaki N, Tanaka Y, Ishitsuka H, Tisdale MJ.
Source: British Journal of Cancer. 2000 July; 83(1): 56-62.
http://www.ncbi.nlm.nih.gov/entrez/query.fcgi?cmd=Retrieve&db=pubmed&dopt=Abstract&list_uids=10883668

- **Effect of total parenteral nutrition on the protein kinetics of patients with cancer cachexia.**
Author(s): Bozzetti F, Gavazzi C, Ferrari P, Dworzak F.
Source: Tumori. 2000 September-October; 86(5): 408-11.
http://www.ncbi.nlm.nih.gov/entrez/query.fcgi?cmd=Retrieve&db=pubmed&dopt=Abstract&list_uids=11130571

- **Effects of cachexia due to cancer on whole body and skeletal muscle protein turnover.**
  Author(s): Dworzak F, Ferrari P, Gavazzi C, Maiorana C, Bozzetti F.
  Source: Cancer. 1998 January 1; 82(1): 42-8.
  http://www.ncbi.nlm.nih.gov/entrez/query.fcgi?cmd=Retrieve&db=pubmed&dopt=Abstract&list_uids=9428478

- **Effects of plasmapheresis in a rabbit model of cancer cachexia.**
  Author(s): Hirai K, Ishiko O, Deguchi M, Honda K, Nakata S, Sumi T, Yasui T, Ogita S.
  Source: Osaka City Med J. 1998 June; 44(1): 1-15.
  http://www.ncbi.nlm.nih.gov/entrez/query.fcgi?cmd=Retrieve&db=pubmed&dopt=Abstract&list_uids=9834615

- **Eicosanoid-dependent cancer cachexia and wasting.**
  Author(s): Ross JA, Fearon KC.
  Source: Current Opinion in Clinical Nutrition and Metabolic Care. 2002 May; 5(3): 241-8. Review.
  http://www.ncbi.nlm.nih.gov/entrez/query.fcgi?cmd=Retrieve&db=pubmed&dopt=Abstract&list_uids=11953648

- **Elevated circulating level of ghrelin in cachexia associated with chronic heart failure: relationships between ghrelin and anabolic/catabolic factors.**
  Author(s): Nagaya N, Uematsu M, Kojima M, Date Y, Nakazato M, Okumura H, Hosoda H, Shimizu W, Yamagishi M, Oya H, Koh H, Yutani C, Kangawa K.
  Source: Circulation. 2001 October 23; 104(17): 2034-8.
  http://www.ncbi.nlm.nih.gov/entrez/query.fcgi?cmd=Retrieve&db=pubmed&dopt=Abstract&list_uids=11673342

- **Elevated plasma levels of tumor necrosis factor in chronic heart failure with cachexia.**
  Author(s): Zhao SP, Zeng LH.
  Source: International Journal of Cardiology. 1997 February; 58(3): 257-61.
  http://www.ncbi.nlm.nih.gov/entrez/query.fcgi?cmd=Retrieve&db=pubmed&dopt=Abstract&list_uids=9076551

- **Endogenous cachectin/tumour necrosis factor-alpha production contributes to experimental cancer-associated cachexia.**
  Author(s): Moldawer LL, Sherry B, Lowry SF, Cerami A.
  Source: Cancer Surv. 1989; 8(4): 853-9. Review.
  http://www.ncbi.nlm.nih.gov/entrez/query.fcgi?cmd=Retrieve&db=pubmed&dopt=Abstract&list_uids=2701731

- **Endoscopic treatment of a Zenker's diverticulum using argon plasma coagulation in a patient with massive cachexia and esophageal obstruction: a case report and review of literature.**
  Author(s): Geisler F, Storr M, Fritsch R, Rosch T, Classen M, Allescher HD.
  Source: Diseases of the Esophagus : Official Journal of the International Society for Diseases of the Esophagus / I.S.D.E. 2002; 15(2): 180-5. Review.
  http://www.ncbi.nlm.nih.gov/entrez/query.fcgi?cmd=Retrieve&db=pubmed&dopt=Abstract&list_uids=12220429

- **Energy expenditure and protein metabolism in human immunodeficiency virus infection and cancer cachexia.**
  Author(s): Mulligan K, Bloch AS.
  Source: Seminars in Oncology. 1998 April; 25(2 Suppl 6): 82-91. Review.
  http://www.ncbi.nlm.nih.gov/entrez/query.fcgi?cmd=Retrieve&db=pubmed&dopt=Abstract&list_uids=9625389

- **Enhanced generation of interleukins 1 beta and 6 may contribute to the cachexia of chronic disease.**
  Author(s): Cederholm T, Wretlind B, Hellstrom K, Andersson B, Engstrom L, Brismar K, Scheynius A, Forslid J, Palmblad J.
  Source: The American Journal of Clinical Nutrition. 1997 March; 65(3): 876-82.
  http://www.ncbi.nlm.nih.gov/entrez/query.fcgi?cmd=Retrieve&db=pubmed&dopt=Abstract&list_uids=9062543

- **Evidence that tumor necrosis factor plays a pathogenetic role in the paraneoplastic syndromes of cachexia, hypercalcemia, and leukocytosis in a human tumor in nude mice.**
  Author(s): Yoneda T, Alsina MA, Chavez JB, Bonewald L, Nishimura R, Mundy GR.
  Source: The Journal of Clinical Investigation. 1991 March; 87(3): 977-85.
  http://www.ncbi.nlm.nih.gov/entrez/query.fcgi?cmd=Retrieve&db=pubmed&dopt=Abstract&list_uids=1999505

- **Exercise, cachexia, and cancer therapy: a molecular rationale.**
  Author(s): Ardies CM.
  Source: Nutrition and Cancer. 2002; 42(2): 143-57. Review.
  http://www.ncbi.nlm.nih.gov/entrez/query.fcgi?cmd=Retrieve&db=pubmed&dopt=Abstract&list_uids=12416253

- **Expression of the human cachexia-associated protein (HCAP) in prostate cancer and in a prostate cancer animal model of cachexia.**
  Author(s): Wang Z, Corey E, Hass GM, Higano CS, True LD, Wallace D Jr, Tisdale MJ, Vessella RL.
  Source: International Journal of Cancer. Journal International Du Cancer. 2003 May 20; 105(1): 123-9.
  http://www.ncbi.nlm.nih.gov/entrez/query.fcgi?cmd=Retrieve&db=pubmed&dopt=Abstract&list_uids=12672042

- **Extracts of porcine pancreas prevent progression of hypercalcemia and cachexia and prolong survival in nude mice bearing a human squamous carcinoma.**
  Author(s): Yoneda T, Takaoka Y, Boyce BF, Scott L, Mundy GR.
  Source: Cancer Research. 1994 May 1; 54(9): 2509-13.
  http://www.ncbi.nlm.nih.gov/entrez/query.fcgi?cmd=Retrieve&db=pubmed&dopt=Abstract&list_uids=8162601

- **Factors affecting postoperative ventilatory support in patients with cardiac cachexia.**
  Author(s): Shindo K, Minami C, Yamazaki K, Tsujimoto S, Kato H.
  Source: J Cardiothorac Anesth. 1989 August; 3(4): 455-60.
  http://www.ncbi.nlm.nih.gov/entrez/query.fcgi?cmd=Retrieve&db=pubmed&dopt=Abstract&list_uids=2520918

- **Fat malabsorption in elderly patients with cardiac cachexia.**
  Author(s): King D, Smith ML, Chapman TJ, Stockdale HR, Lye M.
  Source: Age and Ageing. 1996 March; 25(2): 144-9.
  http://www.ncbi.nlm.nih.gov/entrez/query.fcgi?cmd=Retrieve&db=pubmed&dopt=Abstract&list_uids=8670544

- **Fatigue and cachexia in cancer patients.**
  Author(s): Glaus A.
  Source: Supportive Care in Cancer : Official Journal of the Multinational Association of Supportive Care in Cancer. 1998 March; 6(2): 77-8.
  http://www.ncbi.nlm.nih.gov/entrez/query.fcgi?cmd=Retrieve&db=pubmed&dopt=Abstract&list_uids=9540162

- **Fighting cancer cachexia--what about today's armory?**
  Author(s): Delmore G.
  Source: Supportive Care in Cancer : Official Journal of the Multinational Association of Supportive Care in Cancer. 1993 November; 1(6): 283-4.
  http://www.ncbi.nlm.nih.gov/entrez/query.fcgi?cmd=Retrieve&db=pubmed&dopt=Abstract&list_uids=8156243

- **First Cachexia Symposium, Berlin, Germany, 1st-2nd December, 2000.**
  Author(s): Sharma R, Anker S.
  Source: European Journal of Heart Failure : Journal of the Working Group on Heart Failure of the European Society of Cardiology. 2001 December; 3(6): 751-4.
  http://www.ncbi.nlm.nih.gov/entrez/query.fcgi?cmd=Retrieve&db=pubmed&dopt=Abstract&list_uids=11738229

- **Food intake and body composition in cancer cachexia.**
  Author(s): Giacosa A, Frascio F, Sukkar SG, Roncella S.
  Source: Nutrition (Burbank, Los Angeles County, Calif.). 1996 January; 12(1 Suppl): S20-3. Review.
  http://www.ncbi.nlm.nih.gov/entrez/query.fcgi?cmd=Retrieve&db=pubmed&dopt=Abstract&list_uids=8850214

- **Galloway Memorial Lecture. Protein engineering of tumor necrosis factor-beta and its applications in cancer, septicaemia and cachexia.**
  Author(s): Goh CR.
  Source: Ann Acad Med Singapore. 1993 July; 22(4): 651-6.
  http://www.ncbi.nlm.nih.gov/entrez/query.fcgi?cmd=Retrieve&db=pubmed&dopt=Abstract&list_uids=8257076

- **Gastrointestinal absorption studies in cardiac cachexia.**
  Author(s): Buchanan N, Cane RD, Kinsley R, Eyberg CD.
  Source: Intensive Care Medicine. 1977 August; 3(2): 89-91.
  http://www.ncbi.nlm.nih.gov/entrez/query.fcgi?cmd=Retrieve&db=pubmed&dopt=Abstract&list_uids=268356

- **Gastro-intestinal protein loss in elderly patients with cardiac cachexia.**
  Author(s): King D, Smith ML, Lye M.
  Source: Age and Ageing. 1996 May; 25(3): 221-3.
  http://www.ncbi.nlm.nih.gov/entrez/query.fcgi?cmd=Retrieve&db=pubmed&dopt=Abstract&list_uids=8670557

- **Gene therapy for cardiac cachexia?**
  Author(s): Rosenthal N, Musaro A.
  Source: International Journal of Cardiology. 2002 September; 85(1): 185-91. Review.
  http://www.ncbi.nlm.nih.gov/entrez/query.fcgi?cmd=Retrieve&db=pubmed&dopt=Abstract&list_uids=12163223

- **General metabolic abnormalities in cancer patients: anorexia and cachexia.**
  Author(s): Holroyde CP, Reichard GA Jr.
  Source: The Surgical Clinics of North America. 1986 October; 66(5): 947-56. Review.
  http://www.ncbi.nlm.nih.gov/entrez/query.fcgi?cmd=Retrieve&db=pubmed&dopt=Abstract&list_uids=3532380

- **Generalized perturbations in host physiology caused by localized tumors. The anorexia-cachexia syndrome: a new hypothesis.**
  Author(s): Theologides A.
  Source: Annals of the New York Academy of Sciences. 1974; 230: 14-22. Review.
  http://www.ncbi.nlm.nih.gov/entrez/query.fcgi?cmd=Retrieve&db=pubmed&dopt=Abstract&list_uids=4595943

- **Geriatric cachexia: a role for magnesium deficiency as well as for cytokines?**
  Author(s): Caddell JL.
  Source: The American Journal of Clinical Nutrition. 2000 March; 71(3): 851-3.
  http://www.ncbi.nlm.nih.gov/entrez/query.fcgi?cmd=Retrieve&db=pubmed&dopt=Abstract&list_uids=10702192

- **Geriatric cachexia: the role of cytokines.**
  Author(s): Yeh SS, Schuster MW.
  Source: The American Journal of Clinical Nutrition. 1999 August; 70(2): 183-97. Review.
  http://www.ncbi.nlm.nih.gov/entrez/query.fcgi?cmd=Retrieve&db=pubmed&dopt=Abstract&list_uids=10426694

- **Ghrelin and cachexia.**
  Author(s): Inui A, Meguid MM.
  Source: Diabetes, Obesity & Metabolism. 2002 November; 4(6): 431.
  http://www.ncbi.nlm.nih.gov/entrez/query.fcgi?cmd=Retrieve&db=pubmed&dopt=Abstract&list_uids=12406044

- **Ghrelin improves left ventricular dysfunction and cardiac cachexia in heart failure.**
  Author(s): Nagaya N, Kangawa K.
  Source: Current Opinion in Pharmacology. 2003 April; 3(2): 146-51. Review.
  http://www.ncbi.nlm.nih.gov/entrez/query.fcgi?cmd=Retrieve&db=pubmed&dopt=Abstract&list_uids=12681236

- **Growth hormone, insulin, and somatostatin therapy of cancer cachexia.**
  Author(s): Bartlett DL, Charland S, Torosian MH.
  Source: Cancer. 1994 March 1; 73(5): 1499-504.
  http://www.ncbi.nlm.nih.gov/entrez/query.fcgi?cmd=Retrieve&db=pubmed&dopt=Abstract&list_uids=7906609

- **Guarding against cancer's hidden killer: anorexia-cachexia.**
  Author(s): Groer M, Pierce M.
  Source: Nursing. 1981 June; 11(6): 39-43.
  http://www.ncbi.nlm.nih.gov/entrez/query.fcgi?cmd=Retrieve&db=pubmed&dopt=Abstract&list_uids=6941100

- **High-dose megestrol acetate. A possible treatment for cachexia.**
  Author(s): Tchekmedyian NS, Tait N, Moody M, Aisner J.
  Source: Jama : the Journal of the American Medical Association. 1987 March 6; 257(9): 1195-8.
  http://www.ncbi.nlm.nih.gov/entrez/query.fcgi?cmd=Retrieve&db=pubmed&dopt=Abstract&list_uids=3806918

- **High-dose progestins for the treatment of cancer anorexia-cachexia syndrome: a systematic review of randomised clinical trials.**
  Author(s): Maltoni M, Nanni O, Scarpi E, Rossi D, Serra P, Amadori D.
  Source: Annals of Oncology : Official Journal of the European Society for Medical Oncology / Esmo. 2001 March; 12(3): 289-300. Review.
  http://www.ncbi.nlm.nih.gov/entrez/query.fcgi?cmd=Retrieve&db=pubmed&dopt=Abstract&list_uids=11332139

- **HIV-related cachexia: potential mechanisms and treatment.**
  Author(s): Von Roenn JH, Roth EL, Craig R.
  Source: Oncology. 1992; 49 Suppl 2: 50-4. Review.
  http://www.ncbi.nlm.nih.gov/entrez/query.fcgi?cmd=Retrieve&db=pubmed&dopt=Abstract&list_uids=1461629

- **Hormonal changes and catabolic/anabolic imbalance in chronic heart failure and their importance for cardiac cachexia.**
  Author(s): Anker SD, Chua TP, Ponikowski P, Harrington D, Swan JW, Kox WJ, Poole-Wilson PA, Coats AJ.
  Source: Circulation. 1997 July 15; 96(2): 526-34.
  http://www.ncbi.nlm.nih.gov/entrez/query.fcgi?cmd=Retrieve&db=pubmed&dopt=Abstract&list_uids=9244221

- **How the district nurse cares for the terminally ill patient with cachexia.**
  Author(s): Latham D.
  Source: British Journal of Community Nursing. 2001 January; 6(1): 5-10.
  http://www.ncbi.nlm.nih.gov/entrez/query.fcgi?cmd=Retrieve&db=pubmed&dopt=Abstract&list_uids=11972110

- **Human immunodeficiency virus-associated wasting and mechanisms of cachexia associated with inflammation.**
Author(s): Moldawer LL, Sattler FR.
Source: Seminars in Oncology. 1998 February; 25(1 Suppl 1): 73-81. Review.
http://www.ncbi.nlm.nih.gov/entrez/query.fcgi?cmd=Retrieve&db=pubmed&dopt=Abstract&list_uids=9482543

- **Hypothalamic melanocortin signaling in cachexia.**
Author(s): Lechan RM, Tatro JB.
Source: Endocrinology. 2001 August; 142(8): 3288-91. Review.
http://www.ncbi.nlm.nih.gov/entrez/query.fcgi?cmd=Retrieve&db=pubmed&dopt=Abstract&list_uids=11459769

- **II--Cancer cachexia: treatments strategies.**
Author(s): Gough DB, Heys SD, Eremin O.
Source: European Journal of Surgical Oncology : the Journal of the European Society of Surgical Oncology and the British Association of Surgical Oncology. 1996 June; 22(3): 286-92.
http://www.ncbi.nlm.nih.gov/entrez/query.fcgi?cmd=Retrieve&db=pubmed&dopt=Abstract&list_uids=8654614

- **IL-6-like cytokines and cancer cachexia: consequences of chronic inflammation.**
Author(s): Barton BE.
Source: Immunologic Research. 2001; 23(1): 41-58. Review.
http://www.ncbi.nlm.nih.gov/entrez/query.fcgi?cmd=Retrieve&db=pubmed&dopt=Abstract&list_uids=11417859

- **Immunohistochemical expression of cyclin T1 in a case of AIDS-related cachexia.**
Author(s): Esposito V, Visciano ML, De Luca L, Cavallotti I, Loiacono L, Rossiello L, Chirianni A, Baldi F, De Luca B.
Source: In Vivo. 2001 September-October; 15(5): 391-5.
http://www.ncbi.nlm.nih.gov/entrez/query.fcgi?cmd=Retrieve&db=pubmed&dopt=Abstract&list_uids=11695235

- **Immunohistochemical study of apelin, the natural ligand of receptor APJ, in a case of AIDS-related cachexia.**
Author(s): Esposito V, De Falco M, De Luca L, Acanfora F, Onori N, Loiacono L, Montesarchio V, Rossi M, De Luca B, Chirianni A.
Source: In Vivo. 2002 September-October; 16(5): 337-40.
http://www.ncbi.nlm.nih.gov/entrez/query.fcgi?cmd=Retrieve&db=pubmed&dopt=Abstract&list_uids=12494874

- **Improvement in quality-of-life measures and stimulation of weight gain after treatment with megestrol acetate oral suspension in geriatric cachexia: results of a double-blind, placebo-controlled study.**
Author(s): Yeh SS, Wu SY, Lee TP, Olson JS, Stevens MR, Dixon T, Porcelli RJ, Schuster MW.
Source: Journal of the American Geriatrics Society. 2000 May; 48(5): 485-92.
http://www.ncbi.nlm.nih.gov/entrez/query.fcgi?cmd=Retrieve&db=pubmed&dopt=Abstract&list_uids=10811540

- **Inappropriately low plasma leptin concentration in the cachexia associated with chronic heart failure.**
  Author(s): Murdoch DR, Rooney E, Dargie HJ, Shapiro D, Morton JJ, McMurray JJ.
  Source: Heart (British Cardiac Society). 1999 September; 82(3): 352-6.
  http://www.ncbi.nlm.nih.gov/entrez/query.fcgi?cmd=Retrieve&db=pubmed&dopt=Abstract&list_uids=10455089

- **Increased plasma ghrelin level in lung cancer cachexia.**
  Author(s): Shimizu Y, Nagaya N, Isobe T, Imazu M, Okumura H, Hosoda H, Kojima M, Kangawa K, Kohno N.
  Source: Clinical Cancer Research : an Official Journal of the American Association for Cancer Research. 2003 February; 9(2): 774-8.
  http://www.ncbi.nlm.nih.gov/entrez/query.fcgi?cmd=Retrieve&db=pubmed&dopt=Abstract&list_uids=12576449

- **Induction of cachexia in mice by a product isolated from the urine of cachectic cancer patients.**
  Author(s): Cariuk P, Lorite MJ, Todorov PT, Field WN, Wigmore SJ, Tisdale MJ.
  Source: British Journal of Cancer. 1997; 76(5): 606-13.
  http://www.ncbi.nlm.nih.gov/entrez/query.fcgi?cmd=Retrieve&db=pubmed&dopt=Abstract&list_uids=9303359

- **Induction of cachexia in mice.**
  Author(s): Gullu I, Marangoz S.
  Source: British Journal of Cancer. 1999 March; 79(9-10): 1620-1.
  http://www.ncbi.nlm.nih.gov/entrez/query.fcgi?cmd=Retrieve&db=pubmed&dopt=Abstract&list_uids=10188916

- **Inflammatory and hormonal mediators of cachexia.**
  Author(s): Roubenoff R.
  Source: The Journal of Nutrition. 1997 May; 127(5 Suppl): 1014S-1016S. Review.
  http://www.ncbi.nlm.nih.gov/entrez/query.fcgi?cmd=Retrieve&db=pubmed&dopt=Abstract&list_uids=9164287

- **Inhibition of experimental cancer cachexia by anti-cytokine and anti-cytokine-receptor therapy.**
  Author(s): Strassmann G, Kambayashi T.
  Source: Cytokines Mol Ther. 1995 June; 1(2): 107-13. Review.
  http://www.ncbi.nlm.nih.gov/entrez/query.fcgi?cmd=Retrieve&db=pubmed&dopt=Abstract&list_uids=9384667

- **Insights into the pathogenesis of chronic heart failure: immune activation and cachexia.**
  Author(s): Anker SD, Rauchhaus M.
  Source: Current Opinion in Cardiology. 1999 May; 14(3): 211-6. Review.
  http://www.ncbi.nlm.nih.gov/entrez/query.fcgi?cmd=Retrieve&db=pubmed&dopt=Abstract&list_uids=10358792

- **Insulin action on glucose and branched-chain amino acid metabolism in cancer cachexia: differential effects of insulin.**
  Author(s): Pisters PW, Cersosimo E, Rogatko A, Brennan MF.
  Source: Surgery. 1992 March; 111(3): 301-10.
  http://www.ncbi.nlm.nih.gov/entrez/query.fcgi?cmd=Retrieve&db=pubmed&dopt=Abstract&list_uids=1542855

- **Interaction between dactinomycin and tumor necrosis factor in mesothelioma. Cachexia without oncolysis.**
  Author(s): Bowman RV, Whitaker D, Manning LS, Davis MR, Robinson BW.
  Source: Cancer. 1991 May 15; 67(10): 2495-500.
  http://www.ncbi.nlm.nih.gov/entrez/query.fcgi?cmd=Retrieve&db=pubmed&dopt=Abstract&list_uids=2015549

- **Interleukin-1 alpha promotes tumor growth and cachexia in MCF-7 xenograft model of breast cancer.**
  Author(s): Kumar S, Kishimoto H, Chua HL, Badve S, Miller KD, Bigsby RM, Nakshatri H.
  Source: American Journal of Pathology. 2003 December; 163(6): 2531-41.
  http://www.ncbi.nlm.nih.gov/entrez/query.fcgi?cmd=Retrieve&db=pubmed&dopt=Abstract&list_uids=14633625

- **Investigation of the potential of capillary electrophoresis with off-line matrix-assisted laser desorption/ionization time-of-flight mass spectrometry for clinical analysis: examination of a glycoprotein factor associated with cancer cachexia.**
  Author(s): Choudhary G, Chakel J, Hancock W, Torres-Duarte A, McMahon G, Wainer I.
  Source: Analytical Chemistry. 1999 February 15; 71(4): 855-9.
  http://www.ncbi.nlm.nih.gov/entrez/query.fcgi?cmd=Retrieve&db=pubmed&dopt=Abstract&list_uids=10051848

- **Is there a role for melatonin in the treatment of neoplastic cachexia?**
  Author(s): Lissoni P, Paolorossi F, Tancini G, Barni S, Ardizzoia A, Brivio F, Zubelewicz B, Chatikhine V.
  Source: European Journal of Cancer (Oxford, England : 1990). 1996 July; 32A(8): 1340-3.
  http://www.ncbi.nlm.nih.gov/entrez/query.fcgi?cmd=Retrieve&db=pubmed&dopt=Abstract&list_uids=8869096

- **Is TNF really involved in cachexia?**
  Author(s): Garcia-Martinez C, Costelli P, Lopez-Soriano FJ, Argiles JM.
  Source: Cancer Investigation. 1997; 15(1): 47-54. Review.
  http://www.ncbi.nlm.nih.gov/entrez/query.fcgi?cmd=Retrieve&db=pubmed&dopt=Abstract&list_uids=9028389

- **Journey from cachexia to obesity by TNF.**
  Author(s): Argiles JM, Lopez-Soriano J, Busquets S, Lopez-Soriano FJ.
  Source: The Faseb Journal : Official Publication of the Federation of American Societies for Experimental Biology. 1997 August; 11(10): 743-51. Review.
  http://www.ncbi.nlm.nih.gov/entrez/query.fcgi?cmd=Retrieve&db=pubmed&dopt=Abstract&list_uids=9271359

- **Juvenile polyps with cachexia. Report of an infant and comparison with Cronkhite-Canada syndrome in adults.**
  Author(s): Ruymann FB.
  Source: Gastroenterology. 1969 October; 57(4): 431-8.
  http://www.ncbi.nlm.nih.gov/entrez/query.fcgi?cmd=Retrieve&db=pubmed&dopt=Abstract&list_uids=4378049

- **Lateral hypothalamic demyelination and cachexia in a case of "malignant" multiple sclerosis.**
  Author(s): Kamalian N, Keesey RE, ZuRhein GM.
  Source: Neurology. 1975 January; 25(1): 25-30.
  http://www.ncbi.nlm.nih.gov/entrez/query.fcgi?cmd=Retrieve&db=pubmed&dopt=Abstract&list_uids=803304

- **Leptin and cardiac cachexia: marker or mediator?**
  Author(s): Cleland JG, Clark AL.
  Source: European Heart Journal. 1998 October; 19(10): 1421-2. Review.
  http://www.ncbi.nlm.nih.gov/entrez/query.fcgi?cmd=Retrieve&db=pubmed&dopt=Abstract&list_uids=9820983

- **Leptin, insulin sensitivity and growth hormone binding protein in chronic heart failure with and without cardiac cachexia.**
  Author(s): Doehner W, Pflaum CD, Rauchhaus M, Godsland IF, Egerer K, Cicoira M, Florea VG, Sharma R, Bolger AP, Coats AJ, Anker SD, Strasburger CJ.
  Source: European Journal of Endocrinology / European Federation of Endocrine Societies. 2001 December; 145(6): 727-35.
  http://www.ncbi.nlm.nih.gov/entrez/query.fcgi?cmd=Retrieve&db=pubmed&dopt=Abstract&list_uids=11720897

- **Leucine kinetics in patients with benign disease, non-weight-losing cancer, and cancer cachexia: studies at the whole-body and tissue level and the response to nutritional support.**
  Author(s): Shaw JH, Humberstone DA, Douglas RG, Koea J.
  Source: Surgery. 1991 January; 109(1): 37-50.
  http://www.ncbi.nlm.nih.gov/entrez/query.fcgi?cmd=Retrieve&db=pubmed&dopt=Abstract&list_uids=1984636

- **Lipid mobilising factors specifically associated with cancer cachexia.**
  Author(s): Beck SA, Tisdale MJ.
  Source: British Journal of Cancer. 1991 June; 63(6): 846-50.
  http://www.ncbi.nlm.nih.gov/entrez/query.fcgi?cmd=Retrieve&db=pubmed&dopt=Abstract&list_uids=2069843

- **Lipolytic and lipoprotein lipase (LPL)-inhibiting activities produced by a human lung cancer cell line responsible for cachexia induction.**
  Author(s): Nara-Ashizawa N, Akiyama Y, Maruyama K, Tsukada T, Yamaguchi K.
  Source: Anticancer Res. 2001 September-October; 21(5): 3381-7.
  http://www.ncbi.nlm.nih.gov/entrez/query.fcgi?cmd=Retrieve&db=pubmed&dopt=Abstract&list_uids=11848498

- **Lipolytic factors associated with murine and human cancer cachexia.**
  Author(s): Beck SA, Mulligan HD, Tisdale MJ.
  Source: Journal of the National Cancer Institute. 1990 December 19; 82(24): 1922-6.
  http://www.ncbi.nlm.nih.gov/entrez/query.fcgi?cmd=Retrieve&db=pubmed&dopt=Abstract&list_uids=2250313

- **Lipoprotein lipase expression exclusively in liver. A mouse model for metabolism in the neonatal period and during cachexia.**
  Author(s): Merkel M, Weinstock PH, Chajek-Shaul T, Radner H, Yin B, Breslow JL, Goldberg IJ.
  Source: The Journal of Clinical Investigation. 1998 September 1; 102(5): 893-901.
  http://www.ncbi.nlm.nih.gov/entrez/query.fcgi?cmd=Retrieve&db=pubmed&dopt=Abstract&list_uids=9727057

- **Liver protein and glutamine metabolism during cachexia.**
  Author(s): Hulsewe KW, Deutz NE, de Blaauw I, van der Hulst RR, von Meyenfeldt MM, Soeters PB.
  Source: The Proceedings of the Nutrition Society. 1997 July; 56(2): 801-6. Review.
  http://www.ncbi.nlm.nih.gov/entrez/query.fcgi?cmd=Retrieve&db=pubmed&dopt=Abstract&list_uids=9264131

- **Loss of bone mineral in patients with cachexia due to chronic heart failure.**
  Author(s): Anker SD, Clark AL, Teixeira MM, Hellewell PG, Coats AJ.
  Source: The American Journal of Cardiology. 1999 February 15; 83(4): 612-5, A10.
  http://www.ncbi.nlm.nih.gov/entrez/query.fcgi?cmd=Retrieve&db=pubmed&dopt=Abstract&list_uids=10073875

- **Low dose megestrol acetate can abrogate cachexia in advanced tumor patients receiving systemic interferon-alpha and/or interleukin-2 based antineoplastic therapy.**
  Author(s): Ackermann M, Kirchner H, Atzpodien J.
  Source: Anti-Cancer Drugs. 1993 October; 4(5): 585-7.
  http://www.ncbi.nlm.nih.gov/entrez/query.fcgi?cmd=Retrieve&db=pubmed&dopt=Abstract&list_uids=8292817

- **Malignant appearing cachexia in an older patient with Bruns-Garland syndrome.**
  Author(s): Derk CT, Cynwyd B.
  Source: Journal of the American Geriatrics Society. 2000 December; 48(12): 1741.
  http://www.ncbi.nlm.nih.gov/entrez/query.fcgi?cmd=Retrieve&db=pubmed&dopt=Abstract&list_uids=11129775

- **Management of cancer cachexia.**
  Author(s): Finley JP.
  Source: Aacn Clinical Issues. 2000 November; 11(4): 590-603. Review.
  http://www.ncbi.nlm.nih.gov/entrez/query.fcgi?cmd=Retrieve&db=pubmed&dopt=Abstract&list_uids=11288421

- **Management of common symptoms in terminally ill patients: Part I. Fatigue, anorexia, cachexia, nausea and vomiting.**
  Author(s): Ross DD, Alexander CS.
  Source: American Family Physician. 2001 September 1; 64(5): 807-14. Review.
  http://www.ncbi.nlm.nih.gov/entrez/query.fcgi?cmd=Retrieve&db=pubmed&dopt=Abstract&list_uids=11563572

- **Management of muscle wasting in cancer-associated cachexia: understanding gained from experimental studies.**
  Author(s): Baracos VE.
  Source: Cancer. 2001 September 15; 92(6 Suppl): 1669-77. Review.
  http://www.ncbi.nlm.nih.gov/entrez/query.fcgi?cmd=Retrieve&db=pubmed&dopt=Abstract&list_uids=11598885

- **Managing cancer-related anorexia/cachexia.**
  Author(s): Mantovani G, Maccio A, Massa E, Madeddu C.
  Source: Drugs. 2001; 61(4): 499-514. Review.
  http://www.ncbi.nlm.nih.gov/entrez/query.fcgi?cmd=Retrieve&db=pubmed&dopt=Abstract&list_uids=11324680

- **Mechanism of transient adrenal insufficiency with megestrol acetate treatment of cachexia in children with cancer.**
  Author(s): Meacham LR, Mazewski C, Krawiecki N.
  Source: Journal of Pediatric Hematology/Oncology : Official Journal of the American Society of Pediatric Hematology/Oncology. 2003 May; 25(5): 414-7.
  http://www.ncbi.nlm.nih.gov/entrez/query.fcgi?cmd=Retrieve&db=pubmed&dopt=Abstract&list_uids=12759631

- **Mechanisms mediating cancer cachexia.**
  Author(s): Toomey D, Redmond HP, Bouchier-Hayes D.
  Source: Cancer. 1995 December 15; 76(12): 2418-26. Review.
  http://www.ncbi.nlm.nih.gov/entrez/query.fcgi?cmd=Retrieve&db=pubmed&dopt=Abstract&list_uids=8625066

- **Medroxyprogesterone acetate reduces the in vitro production of cytokines and serotonin involved in anorexia/cachexia and emesis by peripheral blood mononuclear cells of cancer patients.**
  Author(s): Mantovani G, Maccio A, Esu S, Lai P, Santona MC, Massa E, Dessi D, Melis GB, Del Giacco GS.
  Source: European Journal of Cancer (Oxford, England : 1990). 1997 April; 33(4): 602-7.
  http://www.ncbi.nlm.nih.gov/entrez/query.fcgi?cmd=Retrieve&db=pubmed&dopt=Abstract&list_uids=9274442

- **Medroxyprogesterone acetate reduces the production of cytokines and serotonin involved in anorexia/cachexia and emesis by peripheral blood mononuclear cells of cancer patients.**
  Author(s): Mantovani G, Maccio A, Esu S, Lai P, Santona MC, Massa E, Dessi D, Melis G, Del Giacco S.
  Source: Biochemical Society Transactions. 1997 May; 25(2): 296S.
  http://www.ncbi.nlm.nih.gov/entrez/query.fcgi?cmd=Retrieve&db=pubmed&dopt=Abstract&list_uids=9191340

- **Megestrol acetate for cachexia and anorexia in advanced non-small cell lung cancer: a randomized study comparing two different doses.**
  Author(s): Ulutin HC, Arpaci F, Pak Y.
  Source: Tumori. 2002 July-August; 88(4): 277-80.
  http://www.ncbi.nlm.nih.gov/entrez/query.fcgi?cmd=Retrieve&db=pubmed&dopt=Abstract&list_uids=12400976

- **Megestrol acetate in patients with AIDS-related cachexia.**
  Author(s): Bell SJ, Hestnes JC, Wanke C, Forse RA.
  Source: Jpen. Journal of Parenteral and Enteral Nutrition. 1996 March-April; 20(2): 165-6.
  http://www.ncbi.nlm.nih.gov/entrez/query.fcgi?cmd=Retrieve&db=pubmed&dopt=Abstract&list_uids=8676538

- **Metabolic and nutritional disorders in cardiac cachexia.**
  Author(s): Mustafa I, Leverve X.
  Source: Nutrition (Burbank, Los Angeles County, Calif.). 2001 September; 17(9): 756-60. Review.
  http://www.ncbi.nlm.nih.gov/entrez/query.fcgi?cmd=Retrieve&db=pubmed&dopt=Abstract&list_uids=11527673

- **Modern management of the cancer anorexia-cachexia syndrome.**
  Author(s): Nelson KA.
  Source: Current Pain and Headache Reports. 2001 June; 5(3): 250-6. Review.
  http://www.ncbi.nlm.nih.gov/entrez/query.fcgi?cmd=Retrieve&db=pubmed&dopt=Abstract&list_uids=11309213

- **Modern management of the cancer anorexia-cachexia syndrome.**
  Author(s): Nelson KA.
  Source: Current Oncology Reports. 2000 July; 2(4): 362-8. Review.
  http://www.ncbi.nlm.nih.gov/entrez/query.fcgi?cmd=Retrieve&db=pubmed&dopt=Abstract&list_uids=11122866

- **Molecular regulation of muscle cachexia: it may be more than the proteasome.**
  Author(s): Hasselgren PO, Wray C, Mammen J.
  Source: Biochemical and Biophysical Research Communications. 2002 January 11; 290(1): 1-10. Review.
  http://www.ncbi.nlm.nih.gov/entrez/query.fcgi?cmd=Retrieve&db=pubmed&dopt=Abstract&list_uids=11779124

- **Molecular-based therapeutic approaches in treatment of anorexia of aging and cancer cachexia.**
  Author(s): Hamerman D.
  Source: The Journals of Gerontology. Series A, Biological Sciences and Medical Sciences. 2002 August; 57(8): M511-8. Review.
  http://www.ncbi.nlm.nih.gov/entrez/query.fcgi?cmd=Retrieve&db=pubmed&dopt=Abstract&list_uids=12145364

- **Muscle cachexia: current concepts of intracellular mechanisms and molecular regulation.**
  Author(s): Hasselgren PO, Fischer JE.
  Source: Annals of Surgery. 2001 January; 233(1): 9-17. Review.
  http://www.ncbi.nlm.nih.gov/entrez/query.fcgi?cmd=Retrieve&db=pubmed&dopt=Abstract&list_uids=11141219

- **Muscle wasting and dedifferentiation induced by oxidative stress in a murine model of cachexia is prevented by inhibitors of nitric oxide synthesis and antioxidants.**
  Author(s): Buck M, Chojkier M.
  Source: The Embo Journal. 1996 April 15; 15(8): 1753-65.
  http://www.ncbi.nlm.nih.gov/entrez/query.fcgi?cmd=Retrieve&db=pubmed&dopt=Abstract&list_uids=8617220

- **Neurohormonal factors in the development of catabolic/anabolic imbalance and cachexia.**
  Author(s): Brink M, Anwar A, Delafontaine P.
  Source: International Journal of Cardiology. 2002 September; 85(1): 111-21, Discussion 121-4. Review.
  http://www.ncbi.nlm.nih.gov/entrez/query.fcgi?cmd=Retrieve&db=pubmed&dopt=Abstract&list_uids=12163215

- **Neuroleptic-withdrawal cachexia.**
  Author(s): Mikkelsen EJ, Albert LG, Upadhyaya A.
  Source: The New England Journal of Medicine. 1988 April 7; 318(14): 929.
  http://www.ncbi.nlm.nih.gov/entrez/query.fcgi?cmd=Retrieve&db=pubmed&dopt=Abstract&list_uids=2895425

- **Neuropeptide Y: a key molecule in anorexia and cachexia in wasting disorders?**
  Author(s): Inui A.
  Source: Molecular Medicine Today. 1999 February; 5(2): 79-85. Review.
  http://www.ncbi.nlm.nih.gov/entrez/query.fcgi?cmd=Retrieve&db=pubmed&dopt=Abstract&list_uids=10200949

- **New drugs for the anorexia-cachexia syndrome.**
  Author(s): Davis MP.
  Source: Current Oncology Reports. 2002 May; 4(3): 264-74. Review.
  http://www.ncbi.nlm.nih.gov/entrez/query.fcgi?cmd=Retrieve&db=pubmed&dopt=Abstract&list_uids=11937018

- **New mediators in cancer cachexia.**
  Author(s): Argiles JM, Lopez-Soriano FJ.
  Source: Nestle Nutr Workshop Ser Clin Perform Programme. 2000; 4: 147-62; Discussion 163-5. Review. No Abstract Available.
  http://www.ncbi.nlm.nih.gov/entrez/query.fcgi?cmd=Retrieve&db=pubmed&dopt=Abstract&list_uids=11490571

- **New treatment available for AIDS cachexia.**
  Author(s): Hoyt G.
  Source: Surviv News (Atlanta Ga). 2003 September-October; : 7. No Abstract Available.
  http://www.ncbi.nlm.nih.gov/entrez/query.fcgi?cmd=Retrieve&db=pubmed&dopt=Abstract&list_uids=14666919

- **Newly identified factors that alter host metabolism in cancer cachexia.**
  Author(s): Tisdale MJ.
  Source: Trends in Pharmacological Sciences. 1990 December; 11(12): 473-5. Review.
  http://www.ncbi.nlm.nih.gov/entrez/query.fcgi?cmd=Retrieve&db=pubmed&dopt=Abstract&list_uids=2080549

- **Nutrition, cancer, and aging: an annotated review. II. Cancer cachexia and aging.**
  Author(s): Hardy C, Wallace C, Khansur T, Vance RB, Thigpen JT, Balducci L.
  Source: Journal of the American Geriatrics Society. 1986 March; 34(3): 219-28. Review.
  http://www.ncbi.nlm.nih.gov/entrez/query.fcgi?cmd=Retrieve&db=pubmed&dopt=Abstract&list_uids=3081618

- **Nutritional abnormalities contributing to cachexia in chronic illness.**
  Author(s): Witte KK, Clark AL.
  Source: International Journal of Cardiology. 2002 September; 85(1): 23-31. Review.
  http://www.ncbi.nlm.nih.gov/entrez/query.fcgi?cmd=Retrieve&db=pubmed&dopt=Abstract&list_uids=12163207

- **Nutritional assessment in cancer cachexia.**
  Author(s): Edelstein S.
  Source: Pediatric Nursing. 1991 May-June; 17(3): 237-40.
  http://www.ncbi.nlm.nih.gov/entrez/query.fcgi?cmd=Retrieve&db=pubmed&dopt=Abstract&list_uids=2062582

- **Nutritional support and cancer cachexia. Evolving concepts of mechanisms and adjunctive therapies.**
  Author(s): Ng EH, Lowry SF.
  Source: Hematology/Oncology Clinics of North America. 1991 February; 5(1): 161-84. Review.
  http://www.ncbi.nlm.nih.gov/entrez/query.fcgi?cmd=Retrieve&db=pubmed&dopt=Abstract&list_uids=1902829

- **Nutritional support in advanced lung disease. The pulmonary cachexia syndrome.**
  Author(s): Donahoe M.
  Source: Clinics in Chest Medicine. 1997 September; 18(3): 547-61. Review.
  http://www.ncbi.nlm.nih.gov/entrez/query.fcgi?cmd=Retrieve&db=pubmed&dopt=Abstract&list_uids=9329876

- **Nutritional support in cardiac cachexia.**
  Author(s): Blackburn GL, Gibbons GW, Bothe A, Benotti PN, Harken DE, McEnany TM.
  Source: The Journal of Thoracic and Cardiovascular Surgery. 1977 April; 73(4): 489-96.
  http://www.ncbi.nlm.nih.gov/entrez/query.fcgi?cmd=Retrieve&db=pubmed&dopt=Abstract&list_uids=402509

- **Occurrence of hypercalcemia and leukocytosis with cachexia in a human squamous cell carcinoma of the maxilla in athymic nude mice: a novel experimental model of three concomitant paraneoplastic syndromes.**
  Author(s): Yoneda T, Aufdemorte TB, Nishimura R, Nishikawa N, Sakuda M, Alsina MM, Chavez JB, Mundy GR.
  Source: Journal of Clinical Oncology : Official Journal of the American Society of Clinical Oncology. 1991 March; 9(3): 468-77.
  http://www.ncbi.nlm.nih.gov/entrez/query.fcgi?cmd=Retrieve&db=pubmed&dopt=Abstract&list_uids=1999718

- **Oesophageal cancer and cachexia: the effect of short-term treatment with thalidomide on weight loss and lean body mass.**
  Author(s): Khan ZH, Simpson EJ, Cole AT, Holt M, MacDonald I, Pye D, Austin A, Freeman JG.
  Source: Alimentary Pharmacology & Therapeutics. 2003 March 1; 17(5): 677-82.
  http://www.ncbi.nlm.nih.gov/entrez/query.fcgi?cmd=Retrieve&db=pubmed&dopt=Abstract&list_uids=12641516

- **Origin of symptoms in patients with cachexia with special reference to weakness and shortness of breath.**
  Author(s): Coats AJ.
  Source: International Journal of Cardiology. 2002 September; 85(1): 133-9. Review.
  http://www.ncbi.nlm.nih.gov/entrez/query.fcgi?cmd=Retrieve&db=pubmed&dopt=Abstract&list_uids=12163218

- **Ovarian cancer cachexia--surgical interactions.**
  Author(s): Fuller AF Jr, Griffiths CT.
  Source: Gynecologic Oncology. 1979 December; 8(3): 301-10.
  http://www.ncbi.nlm.nih.gov/entrez/query.fcgi?cmd=Retrieve&db=pubmed&dopt=Abstract&list_uids=116914

- **Overexpression of mutant ras in human melanoma increases invasiveness, proliferation and anchorage-independent growth in vitro and induces tumour formation and cachexia in vivo.**
  Author(s): Fujita M, Norris DA, Yagi H, Walsh P, Morelli JG, Weston WL, Terada N, Bennion SD, Robinson W, Lemon M, Maxwell IH, Yohn JJ.
  Source: Melanoma Research. 1999 June; 9(3): 279-91.
  http://www.ncbi.nlm.nih.gov/entrez/query.fcgi?cmd=Retrieve&db=pubmed&dopt=Abstract&list_uids=10465584

- **Oxidation and metabolic interconversion in malignant cachexia.**
Author(s): Waterhouse C.
Source: Cancer Treat Rep. 1981; 65 Suppl 5: 61-6.
http://www.ncbi.nlm.nih.gov/entrez/query.fcgi?cmd=Retrieve&db=pubmed&dopt=Abstract&list_uids=7346162

- **Pancreatic cancer as a model: inflammatory mediators, acute-phase response, and cancer cachexia.**
Author(s): Fearon KC, Barber MD, Falconer JS, McMillan DC, Ross JA, Preston T.
Source: World Journal of Surgery. 1999 June; 23(6): 584-8. Review.
http://www.ncbi.nlm.nih.gov/entrez/query.fcgi?cmd=Retrieve&db=pubmed&dopt=Abstract&list_uids=10227928

- **Partial reversal of cachexia by beta-adrenergic receptor blocker therapy in patients with chronic heart failure.**
Author(s): Hryniewicz K, Androne AS, Hudaihed A, Katz SD.
Source: Journal of Cardiac Failure. 2003 December; 9(6): 464-8.
http://www.ncbi.nlm.nih.gov/entrez/query.fcgi?cmd=Retrieve&db=pubmed&dopt=Abstract&list_uids=14966787

- **Pathophysiology of cancer cachexia.**
Author(s): Younes RN, Noguchi Y.
Source: Revista Do Hospital Das Clinicas. 2000 September-October; 55(5): 181-93.
http://www.ncbi.nlm.nih.gov/entrez/query.fcgi?cmd=Retrieve&db=pubmed&dopt=Abstract&list_uids=11175579

- **Pathophysiology of cancer cachexia.**
Author(s): Keller U.
Source: Supportive Care in Cancer : Official Journal of the Multinational Association of Supportive Care in Cancer. 1993 November; 1(6): 290-4. Review.
http://www.ncbi.nlm.nih.gov/entrez/query.fcgi?cmd=Retrieve&db=pubmed&dopt=Abstract&list_uids=8156245

- **Pentoxifylline for treatment of cancer anorexia and cachexia? A randomized, double-blind, placebo-controlled trial.**
Author(s): Goldberg RM, Loprinzi CL, Mailliard JA, O'Fallon JR, Krook JE, Ghosh C, Hestorff RD, Chong SF, Reuter NF, Shanahan TG.
Source: Journal of Clinical Oncology : Official Journal of the American Society of Clinical Oncology. 1995 November; 13(11): 2856-9.
http://www.ncbi.nlm.nih.gov/entrez/query.fcgi?cmd=Retrieve&db=pubmed&dopt=Abstract&list_uids=7595749

- **Pharmacological treatment of cachexia: any progress?**
Author(s): Bruera E.
Source: Supportive Care in Cancer : Official Journal of the Multinational Association of Supportive Care in Cancer. 1998 March; 6(2): 109-13. Review.
http://www.ncbi.nlm.nih.gov/entrez/query.fcgi?cmd=Retrieve&db=pubmed&dopt=Abstract&list_uids=9540168

- **Phase III evaluation of 4 doses of megestrol acetate as therapy for patients with cancer anorexia and/or cachexia.**
  Author(s): Loprinzi CL, Bernath AM, Schaid DJ, Malliard JA, Athmann LM, Michalak JC, Tschetter LK, Hatfield AK, Morton RF.
  Source: Oncology. 1994 October; 51 Suppl 1: 2-7.
  http://www.ncbi.nlm.nih.gov/entrez/query.fcgi?cmd=Retrieve&db=pubmed&dopt=Abstract&list_uids=7970505

- **Phase III evaluation of four doses of megestrol acetate as therapy for patients with cancer anorexia and/or cachexia.**
  Author(s): Loprinzi CL, Michalak JC, Schaid DJ, Mailliard JA, Athmann LM, Goldberg RM, Tschetter LK, Hatfield AK, Morton RF.
  Source: Journal of Clinical Oncology : Official Journal of the American Society of Clinical Oncology. 1993 April; 11(4): 762-7.
  http://www.ncbi.nlm.nih.gov/entrez/query.fcgi?cmd=Retrieve&db=pubmed&dopt=Abstract&list_uids=8478668

- **Plasma concentration of total leptin and human lung-cancer-associated cachexia.**
  Author(s): Simons JP, Schols AM, Campfield LA, Wouters EF, Saris WH.
  Source: Clinical Science (London, England : 1979). 1997 September; 93(3): 273-7.
  http://www.ncbi.nlm.nih.gov/entrez/query.fcgi?cmd=Retrieve&db=pubmed&dopt=Abstract&list_uids=9337643

- **Plasma neopterin/C-reactive protein ratio as an adjunct to the assessment of infection and cancer cachexia.**
  Author(s): Iwagaki H, Hizuta A, Tanaka N, Orita K.
  Source: Immunological Investigations. 1995 March; 24(3): 479-87.
  http://www.ncbi.nlm.nih.gov/entrez/query.fcgi?cmd=Retrieve&db=pubmed&dopt=Abstract&list_uids=7790044

- **Plasma protein (albumin) catabolism by the tumor itself--implications for tumor metabolism and the genesis of cachexia.**
  Author(s): Stehle G, Sinn H, Wunder A, Schrenk HH, Stewart JC, Hartung G, Maier-Borst W, Heene DL.
  Source: Critical Reviews in Oncology/Hematology. 1997 July; 26(2): 77-100. Review.
  http://www.ncbi.nlm.nih.gov/entrez/query.fcgi?cmd=Retrieve&db=pubmed&dopt=Abstract&list_uids=9298326

- **Polynitroxylated starch/TPL attenuates cachexia and increased epithelial permeability associated with TNBS colitis.**
  Author(s): Park JH, Ma L, Oshima T, Carter P, Coe L, Ma JW, Specian R, Grisham MB, Trimble CE, Hsia CJ, Liu JE, Alexander JS.
  Source: Inflammation. 2002 February; 26(1): 1-11.
  http://www.ncbi.nlm.nih.gov/entrez/query.fcgi?cmd=Retrieve&db=pubmed&dopt=Abstract&list_uids=11936750

- **Pretransplant cachexia and morbid obesity are predictors of increased mortality after heart transplantation.**
Author(s): Lietz K, John R, Burke EA, Ankersmit JH, McCue JD, Naka Y, Oz MC, Mancini DM, Edwards NM.
Source: Transplantation. 2001 July 27; 72(2): 277-83.
http://www.ncbi.nlm.nih.gov/entrez/query.fcgi?cmd=Retrieve&db=pubmed&dopt=Abstract&list_uids=11477353

- **Prevention of runting and cachexia by a chimeric TNF receptor-Fc protein.**
Author(s): Teng MN, Turksen K, Jacobs CA, Fuchs E, Schreiber H.
Source: Clinical Immunology and Immunopathology. 1993 November; 69(2): 215-22.
http://www.ncbi.nlm.nih.gov/entrez/query.fcgi?cmd=Retrieve&db=pubmed&dopt=Abstract&list_uids=8403559

- **Production of multiple cytokines and induction of cachexia in athymic nude mice by a new anaplastic thyroid carcinoma cell line.**
Author(s): Chang JW, Yeh KY, Shen YC, Hsieh JJ, Chuang CK, Liao SK, Tsai LH, Wang CH.
Source: The Journal of Endocrinology. 2003 December; 179(3): 387-94.
http://www.ncbi.nlm.nih.gov/entrez/query.fcgi?cmd=Retrieve&db=pubmed&dopt=Abstract&list_uids=14656208

- **Proinflammatory cytokines, nutritional support, and the cachexia syndrome: interactions and therapeutic options.**
Author(s): Moldawer LL, Copeland EM 3rd.
Source: Cancer. 1997 May 1; 79(9): 1828-39. Review.
http://www.ncbi.nlm.nih.gov/entrez/query.fcgi?cmd=Retrieve&db=pubmed&dopt=Abstract&list_uids=9129003

- **Prospective randomised trial of two dose levels of megestrol acetate in the management of anorexia-cachexia syndrome in patients with metastatic cancer.**
Author(s): Gebbia V, Testa A, Gebbia N.
Source: British Journal of Cancer. 1996 June; 73(12): 1576-80.
http://www.ncbi.nlm.nih.gov/entrez/query.fcgi?cmd=Retrieve&db=pubmed&dopt=Abstract&list_uids=8664133

- **Pulmonary cachexia.**
Author(s): Schols AM.
Source: International Journal of Cardiology. 2002 September; 85(1): 101-10. Review.
http://www.ncbi.nlm.nih.gov/entrez/query.fcgi?cmd=Retrieve&db=pubmed&dopt=Abstract&list_uids=12163214

- **Purification and characterization of a lipid-mobilizing factor associated with cachexia-inducing tumors in mice and humans.**
Author(s): McDevitt TM, Todorov PT, Beck SA, Khan SH, Tisdale MJ.
Source: Cancer Research. 1995 April 1; 55(7): 1458-63.
http://www.ncbi.nlm.nih.gov/entrez/query.fcgi?cmd=Retrieve&db=pubmed&dopt=Abstract&list_uids=7882353

- **Randomized comparison of megestrol acetate versus dexamethasone versus fluoxymesterone for the treatment of cancer anorexia/cachexia.**
Author(s): Loprinzi CL, Kugler JW, Sloan JA, Mailliard JA, Krook JE, Wilwerding MB, Rowland KM Jr, Camoriano JK, Novotny PJ, Christensen BJ.
Source: Journal of Clinical Oncology : Official Journal of the American Society of Clinical Oncology. 1999 October; 17(10): 3299-306.
http://www.ncbi.nlm.nih.gov/entrez/query.fcgi?cmd=Retrieve&db=pubmed&dopt=Abstract&list_uids=10506633

- **Randomized trials of megestrol acetate for AIDS-associated anorexia and cachexia.**
Author(s): Von Roenn JH.
Source: Oncology. 1994 October; 51 Suppl 1: 19-24.
http://www.ncbi.nlm.nih.gov/entrez/query.fcgi?cmd=Retrieve&db=pubmed&dopt=Abstract&list_uids=7970504

- **Rapid progression of advanced "hormone-resistant" prostate cancer during palliative treatment with progestins for cancer cachexia.**
Author(s): Tassinari D, Fochessati F, Panzini I, Poggi B, Sartori S, Ravaioli A.
Source: Journal of Pain and Symptom Management. 2003 May; 25(5): 481-4.
http://www.ncbi.nlm.nih.gov/entrez/query.fcgi?cmd=Retrieve&db=pubmed&dopt=Abstract&list_uids=12727047

- **Reducing cardiac cachexia before cardiac valve replacement.**
Author(s): Georges JM, Stotts NA.
Source: Dimensions of Critical Care Nursing : Dccn. 1985 November-December; 4(6): 349-53.
http://www.ncbi.nlm.nih.gov/entrez/query.fcgi?cmd=Retrieve&db=pubmed&dopt=Abstract&list_uids=3851737

- **Regulation of lipolysis: natriuretic peptides and the development of cachexia.**
Author(s): Kalra PR, Tigas S.
Source: International Journal of Cardiology. 2002 September; 85(1): 125-32. Review.
http://www.ncbi.nlm.nih.gov/entrez/query.fcgi?cmd=Retrieve&db=pubmed&dopt=Abstract&list_uids=12163217

- **Regulation of skeletal-muscle-protein turnover in cancer-associated cachexia.**
Author(s): Baracos VE.
Source: Nutrition (Burbank, Los Angeles County, Calif.). 2000 October; 16(10): 1015-8. Review.
http://www.ncbi.nlm.nih.gov/entrez/query.fcgi?cmd=Retrieve&db=pubmed&dopt=Abstract&list_uids=11054610

- **Regulatory climate for therapeutic nutritional claims regarding cachexia.**
Author(s): McCamish MA, Geraghty ME, Abbruzzese BC.
Source: Nutrition (Burbank, Los Angeles County, Calif.). 1996 January; 12(1 Suppl): S63-5. Review.
http://www.ncbi.nlm.nih.gov/entrez/query.fcgi?cmd=Retrieve&db=pubmed&dopt=Abstract&list_uids=8850224

- **Re-validation and shortening of the Functional Assessment of Anorexia/Cachexia Therapy (FAACT) questionnaire.**
  Author(s): Ribaudo JM, Cella D, Hahn EA, Lloyd SR, Tchekmedyian NS, Von Roenn J, Leslie WT.
  Source: Quality of Life Research : an International Journal of Quality of Life Aspects of Treatment, Care and Rehabilitation. 2000; 9(10): 1137-46.
  http://www.ncbi.nlm.nih.gov/entrez/query.fcgi?cmd=Retrieve&db=pubmed&dopt=Abstract&list_uids=11401046

- **Reversal of cachexia in patients treated with potent antiretroviral therapy.**
  Author(s): Scevola D, Di Matteo A, Uberti F, Minoia G, Poletti F, Faga A.
  Source: Aids Read. 2000 June; 10(6): 365-9, 371-5. Review.
  http://www.ncbi.nlm.nih.gov/entrez/query.fcgi?cmd=Retrieve&db=pubmed&dopt=Abstract&list_uids=10881368

- **Revisiting: Biology of cachexia.**
  Author(s): Gold J.
  Source: Journal of the National Cancer Institute. 1998 November 18; 90(22): 1749-50.
  http://www.ncbi.nlm.nih.gov/entrez/query.fcgi?cmd=Retrieve&db=pubmed&dopt=Abstract&list_uids=9827533

- **Rheumatoid cachexia: cytokine-driven hypermetabolism accompanying reduced body cell mass in chronic inflammation.**
  Author(s): Roubenoff R, Roubenoff RA, Cannon JG, Kehayias JJ, Zhuang H, Dawson-Hughes B, Dinarello CA, Rosenberg IH.
  Source: The Journal of Clinical Investigation. 1994 June; 93(6): 2379-86.
  http://www.ncbi.nlm.nih.gov/entrez/query.fcgi?cmd=Retrieve&db=pubmed&dopt=Abstract&list_uids=8200971

- **Rheumatoid cachexia: depletion of lean body mass in rheumatoid arthritis. Possible association with tumor necrosis factor.**
  Author(s): Roubenoff R, Roubenoff RA, Ward LM, Holland SM, Hellmann DB.
  Source: The Journal of Rheumatology. 1992 October; 19(10): 1505-10.
  http://www.ncbi.nlm.nih.gov/entrez/query.fcgi?cmd=Retrieve&db=pubmed&dopt=Abstract&list_uids=1464859

- **Role of a proteolysis-inducing factor (PIF) in cachexia induced by a human melanoma (G361).**
  Author(s): Todorov PT, Field WN, Tisdale MJ.
  Source: British Journal of Cancer. 1999 August; 80(11): 1734-7.
  http://www.ncbi.nlm.nih.gov/entrez/query.fcgi?cmd=Retrieve&db=pubmed&dopt=Abstract&list_uids=10468289

- **Role of cysteine and glutathione in HIV infection and cancer cachexia: therapeutic intervention with N-acetylcysteine.**
  Author(s): Droge W, Gross A, Hack V, Kinscherf R, Schykowski M, Bockstette M, Mihm S, Galter D.
  Source: Adv Pharmacol. 1997; 38: 581-600. Review. No Abstract Available.
  http://www.ncbi.nlm.nih.gov/entrez/query.fcgi?cmd=Retrieve&db=pubmed&dopt=Abstract&list_uids=8895825

- **Role of cysteine and glutathione in signal transduction, immunopathology and cachexia.**
Author(s): Droge W, Hack V, Breitkreutz R, Holm E, Shubinsky G, Schmid E, Galter D.
Source: Biofactors (Oxford, England). 1998; 8(1-2): 97-102. Review.
http://www.ncbi.nlm.nih.gov/entrez/query.fcgi?cmd=Retrieve&db=pubmed&dopt=Abstract&list_uids=9699016

- **Role of cytokines in cancer cachexia in a murine model of intracerebral injection of human tumours.**
Author(s): Negri DR, Mezzanzanica D, Sacco S, Gadina M, Benigni F, Cajola L, Finocchiaro G, Ghezzi P, Canevari S.
Source: Cytokine. 2001 July 7; 15(1): 27-38.
http://www.ncbi.nlm.nih.gov/entrez/query.fcgi?cmd=Retrieve&db=pubmed&dopt=Abstract&list_uids=11509006

- **Role of whole-body lipids and nitrogen as limiting factors for survival in tumor-bearing mice with anorexia and cachexia.**
Author(s): Eden E, Lindmark L, Karlberg I, Lundholm K.
Source: Cancer Research. 1983 August; 43(8): 3707-11.
http://www.ncbi.nlm.nih.gov/entrez/query.fcgi?cmd=Retrieve&db=pubmed&dopt=Abstract&list_uids=6574817

- **Secondary diabetes induced by megestrol acetate therapy in a patient with AIDS-associated cachexia.**
Author(s): Salinas I, Lucas A, Clotet B.
Source: Aids (London, England). 1993 June; 7(6): 894.
http://www.ncbi.nlm.nih.gov/entrez/query.fcgi?cmd=Retrieve&db=pubmed&dopt=Abstract&list_uids=8363766

- **Selective IL-1-mediated pancreatic islet beta-cell damage in tumour cachexia: a hypothesis.**
Author(s): Di Guardo G.
Source: Ann Inst Pasteur Immunol. 1988 September-October; 139(5): 587-8. No Abstract Available.
http://www.ncbi.nlm.nih.gov/entrez/query.fcgi?cmd=Retrieve&db=pubmed&dopt=Abstract&list_uids=3061397

- **Serotonergic blockade in the treatment of the cancer anorexia-cachexia syndrome.**
Author(s): Edelman MJ, Gandara DR, Meyers FJ, Ishii R, O'Mahony M, Uhrich M, Lauder I, Houston J, Gietzen DW.
Source: Cancer. 1999 August 15; 86(4): 684-8.
http://www.ncbi.nlm.nih.gov/entrez/query.fcgi?cmd=Retrieve&db=pubmed&dopt=Abstract&list_uids=10440697

- **Skeletal muscle and whole body protein turnover in cardiac cachexia: influence of branched-chain amino acid administration.**
Author(s): Morrison WL, Gibson JN, Rennie MJ.
Source: European Journal of Clinical Investigation. 1988 December; 18(6): 648-54.
http://www.ncbi.nlm.nih.gov/entrez/query.fcgi?cmd=Retrieve&db=pubmed&dopt=Abstract&list_uids=3147192

- **Sodium and the cachexia and hypophagia of tumor growth.**
Author(s): Morrison SD.
Source: Journal of the National Cancer Institute. 1974 March; 52(3): 869-74.
http://www.ncbi.nlm.nih.gov/entrez/query.fcgi?cmd=Retrieve&db=pubmed&dopt=Abstract&list_uids=4524118

- **Studies of cachexia in parasitic infection.**
Author(s): Tracey KJ, Cerami A.
Source: Annals of the New York Academy of Sciences. 1989; 569: 211-8. Review.
http://www.ncbi.nlm.nih.gov/entrez/query.fcgi?cmd=Retrieve&db=pubmed&dopt=Abstract&list_uids=2698089

- **Studies of high-dose megestrol acetate: potential applications in cachexia.**
Author(s): Aisner J, Tchekmedyian NS, Tait N, Parnes H, Novak M.
Source: Seminars in Oncology. 1988 April; 15(2 Suppl 1): 68-75. Review.
http://www.ncbi.nlm.nih.gov/entrez/query.fcgi?cmd=Retrieve&db=pubmed&dopt=Abstract&list_uids=3285486

- **Studies on apoptosis and fibrosis in skeletal musculature: a comparison of heart failure patients with and without cardiac cachexia.**
Author(s): Filippatos GS, Kanatselos C, Manolatos DD, Vougas B, Sideris A, Kardara D, Anker SD, Kardaras F, Uhal B.
Source: International Journal of Cardiology. 2003 July; 90(1): 107-13.
http://www.ncbi.nlm.nih.gov/entrez/query.fcgi?cmd=Retrieve&db=pubmed&dopt=Abstract&list_uids=12821225

- **Suffering and dying in cancer patients. Research frontiers in controlling confusion, cachexia, and dyspnea.**
Author(s): MacDonald N.
Source: The Western Journal of Medicine. 1995 September; 163(3): 278-86.
http://www.ncbi.nlm.nih.gov/entrez/query.fcgi?cmd=Retrieve&db=pubmed&dopt=Abstract&list_uids=7571592

- **Supportive nutrition to prevent cachexia and improve quality of life.**
Author(s): Ottery FD.
Source: Seminars in Oncology. 1995 April; 22(2 Suppl 3): 98-111. Review.
http://www.ncbi.nlm.nih.gov/entrez/query.fcgi?cmd=Retrieve&db=pubmed&dopt=Abstract&list_uids=7740324

- **Suppression of lipoprotein lipase in 3T3-L1 cells by a mediator produced by SEKI melanoma, a cachexia-inducing human melanoma cell line.**
  Author(s): Kawakami M, Kondo Y, Imai Y, Hashiguchi M, Ogawa H, Hiragun A, Aotsuka S, Shibata S, Oda T, Murase T, et al.
  Source: Journal of Biochemistry. 1991 January; 109(1): 78-82.
  http://www.ncbi.nlm.nih.gov/entrez/query.fcgi?cmd=Retrieve&db=pubmed&dopt=Abstract&list_uids=2016276

- **Suramin interferes with interleukin-6 receptor binding in vitro and inhibits colon-26-mediated experimental cancer cachexia in vivo.**
  Author(s): Strassmann G, Fong M, Freter CE, Windsor S, D'Alessandro F, Nordan RP.
  Source: The Journal of Clinical Investigation. 1993 November; 92(5): 2152-9.
  http://www.ncbi.nlm.nih.gov/entrez/query.fcgi?cmd=Retrieve&db=pubmed&dopt=Abstract&list_uids=8227330

- **Surgical treatment of patients with cardiac cachexia. An analysis of factors affecting operative mortality.**
  Author(s): Otaki M.
  Source: Chest. 1994 May; 105(5): 1347-51.
  http://www.ncbi.nlm.nih.gov/entrez/query.fcgi?cmd=Retrieve&db=pubmed&dopt=Abstract&list_uids=8181317

- **Syndromes of cardiac cachexia and the cachectic heart: current perspective.**
  Author(s): Ansari A.
  Source: Progress in Cardiovascular Diseases. 1987 July-August; 30(1): 45-60. Review.
  http://www.ncbi.nlm.nih.gov/entrez/query.fcgi?cmd=Retrieve&db=pubmed&dopt=Abstract&list_uids=3299491

- **Synthesis rates of albumin and fibrinogen in patients with cardiac and pulmonary cachexia.**
  Author(s): Mayer G, Schomerus H.
  Source: Acta Hepatogastroenterol (Stuttg). 1977 April; 24(2): 82-5.
  http://www.ncbi.nlm.nih.gov/entrez/query.fcgi?cmd=Retrieve&db=pubmed&dopt=Abstract&list_uids=855627

- **Systematic review of megestrol acetate in the treatment of anorexia-cachexia syndrome.**
  Author(s): Pascual Lopez A, Roque i Figuls M, Urrutia Cuchi G, Berenstein EG, Almenar Pasies B, Balcells Alegre M, Herdman M.
  Source: Journal of Pain and Symptom Management. 2004 April; 27(4): 360-9. Review.
  http://www.ncbi.nlm.nih.gov/entrez/query.fcgi?cmd=Retrieve&db=pubmed&dopt=Abstract&list_uids=15050664

- **Thalidomide in patients with cachexia due to terminal cancer: preliminary report.**
  Author(s): Bruera E, Neumann CM, Pituskin E, Calder K, Ball G, Hanson J.
  Source: Annals of Oncology : Official Journal of the European Society for Medical Oncology / Esmo. 1999 July; 10(7): 857-9.
  http://www.ncbi.nlm.nih.gov/entrez/query.fcgi?cmd=Retrieve&db=pubmed&dopt=Abstract&list_uids=10470435

- **The cancer anorexia-cachexia syndrome: a survey of the Prognostic Inflammatory and Nutritional Index (PINI) in advanced disease.**
Author(s): Nelson KA, Walsh D.
Source: Journal of Pain and Symptom Management. 2002 October; 24(4): 424-8.
http://www.ncbi.nlm.nih.gov/entrez/query.fcgi?cmd=Retrieve&db=pubmed&dopt=Abstract&list_uids=12505211

- **The cancer cachexia syndrome.**
Author(s): Fearon KC, Barber MD, Moses AG.
Source: Surg Oncol Clin N Am. 2001 January; 10(1): 109-26. Review.
http://www.ncbi.nlm.nih.gov/entrez/query.fcgi?cmd=Retrieve&db=pubmed&dopt=Abstract&list_uids=11406454

- **The cancer cachexia syndrome.**
Author(s): Puccio M, Nathanson L.
Source: Seminars in Oncology. 1997 June; 24(3): 277-87. Review.
http://www.ncbi.nlm.nih.gov/entrez/query.fcgi?cmd=Retrieve&db=pubmed&dopt=Abstract&list_uids=9208884

- **The cardiac component of cardiac cachexia.**
Author(s): Florea VG, Henein MY, Rauchhaus M, Koloczek V, Sharma R, Doehner W, Poole-Wilson PA, Coats AJ, Anker SD.
Source: American Heart Journal. 2002 July; 144(1): 45-50.
http://www.ncbi.nlm.nih.gov/entrez/query.fcgi?cmd=Retrieve&db=pubmed&dopt=Abstract&list_uids=12094187

- **The effects of enalapril-digoxin-diuretic combination therapy on nutritional and anthropometric indices in chronic congestive heart failure: preliminary findings in cardiac cachexia.**
Author(s): Adigun AQ, Ajayi AA.
Source: European Journal of Heart Failure : Journal of the Working Group on Heart Failure of the European Society of Cardiology. 2001 June; 3(3): 359-63.
http://www.ncbi.nlm.nih.gov/entrez/query.fcgi?cmd=Retrieve&db=pubmed&dopt=Abstract&list_uids=11378008

- **The importance of cachexia in the syndrome of heart failure.**
Author(s): Ferrari R.
Source: European Heart Journal. 1997 February; 18(2): 187-9.
http://www.ncbi.nlm.nih.gov/entrez/query.fcgi?cmd=Retrieve&db=pubmed&dopt=Abstract&list_uids=9043833

- **The melanocortin system and its role in obesity and cachexia.**
Author(s): Goodfellow VS, Saunders J.
Source: Current Topics in Medicinal Chemistry. 2003; 3(8): 855-83. Review.
http://www.ncbi.nlm.nih.gov/entrez/query.fcgi?cmd=Retrieve&db=pubmed&dopt=Abstract&list_uids=12678837

- **The metabolic basis of cancer cachexia.**
  Author(s): Argiles JM, Alvarez B, Lopez-Soriano FJ.
  Source: Medicinal Research Reviews. 1997 September; 17(5): 477-98. Review.
  http://www.ncbi.nlm.nih.gov/entrez/query.fcgi?cmd=Retrieve&db=pubmed&dopt=Abstract&list_uids=9276862

- **The pulmonary cachexia syndrome: aspects of energy balance.**
  Author(s): Congleton J.
  Source: The Proceedings of the Nutrition Society. 1999 May; 58(2): 321-8. Review.
  http://www.ncbi.nlm.nih.gov/entrez/query.fcgi?cmd=Retrieve&db=pubmed&dopt=Abstract&list_uids=10466173

- **The role of cytokines in cancer cachexia.**
  Author(s): Argiles JM, Lopez-Soriano FJ.
  Source: Medicinal Research Reviews. 1999 May; 19(3): 223-48. Review.
  http://www.ncbi.nlm.nih.gov/entrez/query.fcgi?cmd=Retrieve&db=pubmed&dopt=Abstract&list_uids=10232651

- **The role of the melanocortin-3 receptor in cachexia.**
  Author(s): Marks DL, Cone RD.
  Source: Annals of the New York Academy of Sciences. 2003 June; 994: 258-66. Review.
  http://www.ncbi.nlm.nih.gov/entrez/query.fcgi?cmd=Retrieve&db=pubmed&dopt=Abstract&list_uids=12851324

- **The syndrome of anorexia-cachexia.**
  Author(s): Body JJ.
  Source: Current Opinion in Oncology. 1999 July; 11(4): 255-60. Review.
  http://www.ncbi.nlm.nih.gov/entrez/query.fcgi?cmd=Retrieve&db=pubmed&dopt=Abstract&list_uids=10416877

- **The syndrome of cardiac cachexia.**
  Author(s): Anker SD, Sharma R.
  Source: International Journal of Cardiology. 2002 September; 85(1): 51-66. Review.
  http://www.ncbi.nlm.nih.gov/entrez/query.fcgi?cmd=Retrieve&db=pubmed&dopt=Abstract&list_uids=12163209

- **Thrombotic events associated with megestrol acetate in patients with AIDS cachexia.**
  Author(s): Koller E, Gibert C, Green L, Mann M, Bernstein B.
  Source: Nutrition (Burbank, Los Angeles County, Calif.). 1999 April; 15(4): 294-8.
  http://www.ncbi.nlm.nih.gov/entrez/query.fcgi?cmd=Retrieve&db=pubmed&dopt=Abstract&list_uids=10319362

- **Transcription factors and muscle cachexia: is there a therapeutic target?**
  Author(s): Mitch WE, Price SR.
  Source: Lancet. 2001 March 10; 357(9258): 734-5.
  http://www.ncbi.nlm.nih.gov/entrez/query.fcgi?cmd=Retrieve&db=pubmed&dopt=Abstract&list_uids=11253960

- **Treatment of cachexia with recombinant growth hormone in a patient before lung transplantation: a case report.**
  Author(s): Pichard C, Kyle UG, Jolliet P, Slosman DO, Rochat T, Nicod L, Romand J, Mensi N, Chevrolet JC.
  Source: Critical Care Medicine. 1999 August; 27(8): 1639-42.
  http://www.ncbi.nlm.nih.gov/entrez/query.fcgi?cmd=Retrieve&db=pubmed&dopt=Abstract&list_uids=10470777

- **Treatment of malignancy-associated hypercalcemia and cachexia with humanized anti-parathyroid hormone-related protein antibody.**
  Author(s): Sato K, Onuma E, Yocum RC, Ogata E.
  Source: Seminars in Oncology. 2003 October; 30(5 Suppl 16): 167-73. Review.
  http://www.ncbi.nlm.nih.gov/entrez/query.fcgi?cmd=Retrieve&db=pubmed&dopt=Abstract&list_uids=14613038

- **Treatment of the cancer anorexia-cachexia syndrome: a critical reappraisal.**
  Author(s): Lelli G, Montanari M, Gilli G, Scapoli D, Antonietti C, Scapoli D.
  Source: J Chemother. 2003 June; 15(3): 220-5. Review.
  http://www.ncbi.nlm.nih.gov/entrez/query.fcgi?cmd=Retrieve&db=pubmed&dopt=Abstract&list_uids=12868546

- **Uncomplicated starvation versus cancer cachexia.**
  Author(s): Brennan MF.
  Source: Cancer Research. 1977 July; 37(7 Pt 2): 2359-64.
  http://www.ncbi.nlm.nih.gov/entrez/query.fcgi?cmd=Retrieve&db=pubmed&dopt=Abstract&list_uids=861953

- **Understanding and managing cancer cachexia.**
  Author(s): MacDonald N, Easson AM, Mazurak VC, Dunn GP, Baracos VE.
  Source: Journal of the American College of Surgeons. 2003 July; 197(1): 143-61. Review.
  http://www.ncbi.nlm.nih.gov/entrez/query.fcgi?cmd=Retrieve&db=pubmed&dopt=Abstract&list_uids=12831935

- **Update on anorexia and cachexia.**
  Author(s): Strasser F, Bruera ED.
  Source: Hematology/Oncology Clinics of North America. 2002 June; 16(3): 589-617. Review.
  http://www.ncbi.nlm.nih.gov/entrez/query.fcgi?cmd=Retrieve&db=pubmed&dopt=Abstract&list_uids=12170570

- **Usefulness of megestrol acetate in cancer cachexia and anorexia. A placebo-controlled study.**
  Author(s): Feliu J, Gonzalez-Baron M, Berrocal A, Artal A, Ordonez A, Garrido P, Zamora P, Garcia de Paredes ML, Montero JM.
  Source: American Journal of Clinical Oncology : the Official Publication of the American Radium Society. 1992 October; 15(5): 436-40.
  http://www.ncbi.nlm.nih.gov/entrez/query.fcgi?cmd=Retrieve&db=pubmed&dopt=Abstract&list_uids=1524045

- **Ventilator-induced cachexia.**
  Author(s): Hussain SN, Vassilakopoulos T.
  Source: American Journal of Respiratory and Critical Care Medicine. 2002 November 15; 166(10): 1307-8.
  http://www.ncbi.nlm.nih.gov/entrez/query.fcgi?cmd=Retrieve&db=pubmed&dopt=Abstract&list_uids=12421738

- **Visceral leishmaniasis: a model for infection-induced cachexia.**
  Author(s): Pearson RD, Cox G, Jeronimo SM, Castracane J, Drew JS, Evans T, de Alencar JE.
  Source: The American Journal of Tropical Medicine and Hygiene. 1992 July; 47(1 Pt 2): 8-15. Review.
  http://www.ncbi.nlm.nih.gov/entrez/query.fcgi?cmd=Retrieve&db=pubmed&dopt=Abstract&list_uids=1632476

- **Walker carcinoma 256: a model for studies on tumor-induced anorexia and cachexia.**
  Author(s): Guaitani A, Recchia M, Carli M, Rocchetti M, Bartosek I, Garattini S.
  Source: Oncology. 1982; 39(3): 173-8.
  http://www.ncbi.nlm.nih.gov/entrez/query.fcgi?cmd=Retrieve&db=pubmed&dopt=Abstract&list_uids=6952138

- **Wasting and cachexia in patients with HIV.**
  Author(s): Cianfrocca M, Von Roenn JH.
  Source: Aids Patient Care and Stds. 1997 August; 11(4): 259-67. Review.
  http://www.ncbi.nlm.nih.gov/entrez/query.fcgi?cmd=Retrieve&db=pubmed&dopt=Abstract&list_uids=11361840

- **Wasting away: cancer cachexia.**
  Author(s): Blackburn G.
  Source: Health News. 1998 March 31; 4(4): 4. Review. No Abstract Available.
  http://www.ncbi.nlm.nih.gov/entrez/query.fcgi?cmd=Retrieve&db=pubmed&dopt=Abstract&list_uids=9553605

- **Weight gain in patients with AIDS-related cachexia: is bigger better?**
  Author(s): Haller DG.
  Source: Annals of Internal Medicine. 1994 September 15; 121(6): 462-3.
  http://www.ncbi.nlm.nih.gov/entrez/query.fcgi?cmd=Retrieve&db=pubmed&dopt=Abstract&list_uids=8053621

- **What is the role of the insulin-like growth factor system in the pathophysiology of cancer cachexia, and how is it regulated?**
  Author(s): Crown AL, Cottle K, Lightman SL, Falk S, Mohamed-Ali V, Armstrong L, Millar AB, Holly JM.
  Source: Clinical Endocrinology. 2002 June; 56(6): 723-33.
  http://www.ncbi.nlm.nih.gov/entrez/query.fcgi?cmd=Retrieve&db=pubmed&dopt=Abstract&list_uids=12072041

- **What we have learned about cachexia in gastrointestinal cancer.**
Author(s): Palesty JA, Dudrick SJ.
Source: Digestive Diseases (Basel, Switzerland). 2003; 21(3): 198-213. Review.
http://www.ncbi.nlm.nih.gov/entrez/query.fcgi?cmd=Retrieve&db=pubmed&dopt=Abstract&list_uids=14571093

- **Working conference on anorexia and cachexia of neoplastic disease.**
Author(s): De Wys W.
Source: Cancer Research. 1970 November; 30(11): 2816-8.
http://www.ncbi.nlm.nih.gov/entrez/query.fcgi?cmd=Retrieve&db=pubmed&dopt=Abstract&list_uids=5274947

- **Zinc-alpha2-glycoprotein, a lipid mobilizing factor, is expressed in adipocytes and is up-regulated in mice with cancer cachexia.**
Author(s): Bing C, Bao Y, Jenkins J, Sanders P, Manieri M, Cinti S, Tisdale MJ, Trayhurn P.
Source: Proceedings of the National Academy of Sciences of the United States of America. 2004 February 24; 101(8): 2500-5.
http://www.ncbi.nlm.nih.gov/entrez/query.fcgi?cmd=Retrieve&db=pubmed&dopt=Abstract&list_uids=14983038

Chapter 2. Nutrition and Cachexia

Overview

In this chapter, we will show you how to find studies dedicated specifically to nutrition and cachexia.

Finding Nutrition Studies on Cachexia

The National Institutes of Health's Office of Dietary Supplements (ODS) offers a searchable bibliographic database called the IBIDS (International Bibliographic Information on Dietary Supplements; National Institutes of Health, Building 31, Room 1B29, 31 Center Drive, MSC 2086, Bethesda, Maryland 20892-2086, Tel: 301-435-2920, Fax: 301-480-1845, E-mail: ods@nih.gov). The IBIDS contains over 460,000 scientific citations and summaries about dietary supplements and nutrition as well as references to published international, scientific literature on dietary supplements such as vitamins, minerals, and botanicals.[7] The IBIDS includes references and citations to both human and animal research studies.

As a service of the ODS, access to the IBIDS database is available free of charge at the following Web address: **http://ods.od.nih.gov/databases/ibids.html**. After entering the search area, you have three choices: (1) IBIDS Consumer Database, (2) Full IBIDS Database, or (3) Peer Reviewed Citations Only.

Now that you have selected a database, click on the "Advanced" tab. An advanced search allows you to retrieve up to 100 fully explained references in a comprehensive format. Type "cachexia" (or synonyms) into the search box, and click "Go." To narrow the search, you can also select the "Title" field.

---

[7] Adapted from **http://ods.od.nih.gov**. IBIDS is produced by the Office of Dietary Supplements (ODS) at the National Institutes of Health to assist the public, healthcare providers, educators, and researchers in locating credible, scientific information on dietary supplements. IBIDS was developed and will be maintained through an interagency partnership with the Food and Nutrition Information Center of the National Agricultural Library, U.S. Department of Agriculture.

The following information is typical of that found when using the "Full IBIDS Database" to search for "cachexia" (or a synonym):

- **A comparison of long-chain triglycerides and medium-chain triglycerides on weight loss and tumour size in a cachexia model.**
  Author(s): Pharmaceutical Sciences Institute, Aston University, Birmingham, UK.
  Source: Tisdale, M J Brennan, R A Br-J-Cancer. 1988 November; 58(5): 580-3 0007-0920
- **Cancer cachexia and cannabinoids.**
  Author(s): Europaisches Institut fur onkologische und immunologische Forschung, Berlin, Germany.
  Source: Gorter, R W Forsch-Komplementarmed. 1999 October; 6 Suppl 321-2 1021-7096
- **Effect of insulin on weight loss and tumour growth in a cachexia model.**
  Author(s): Pharmaceutical Sciences Institute, Aston University, Birmingham, UK.
  Source: Beck, S A Tisdale, M J Br-J-Cancer. 1989 May; 59(5): 677-81 0007-0920
- **Effects of L-carnitine on serum triglyceride and cytokine levels in rat models of cachexia and septic shock.**
  Author(s): Department of Biochemistry and Molecular Biology, George Washington University Medical Center, Washington, DC 20037, USA.
  Source: Winter, B K Fiskum, G Gallo, L L Br-J-Cancer. 1995 November; 72(5): 1173-9 0007-0920
- **Is the pharmacological treatment of cancer cachexia possible?**
  Author(s): Palliative Care Program, Edmonton General Hospital, Alberta, Canada.
  Source: Bruera, E Support-Care-Cancer. 1993 November; 1(6): 298-304 0941-4355
- **Modulation of adipocyte G-protein expression in cancer cachexia by a lipid-mobilizing factor (LMF).**
  Author(s): Pharmaceutical Sciences Research Institute, Aston University, Birmingham, B4 7ET, UK.
  Source: Islam Ali, B Khan, S Price, S A Tisdale, M J Br-J-Cancer. 2001 September 1; 85(5): 758-63 0007-0920
- **Prevention of adjuvant-induced cachexia in rats by cyclosporin A.**
  Source: Rofe, A.M. Whitehouse, M.W. Bourgeois, C.S. Haynes, D.R. Vernon Roberts, B. Immunol-Cell-Biol. Carlton, Aust. : Blackwell Scientific Publishers & University of Adelaide. February 1990. volume 68 (pt.1) page 63-69. 0818-9641
- **Reduction of weight loss and tumour size in a cachexia model by a high fat diet.**
  Source: Tisdale, M J Brennan, R A Fearon, K C Br-J-Cancer. 1987 July; 56(1): 39-43 0007-0920
- **Reversal of cancer cachexia in rats by cimaterol and supplemental nutrition.**
  Author(s): Department of Surgery, University of Cincinnati Medical Center, OH 45267-0558.
  Source: Stallion, A Zhang, F S Chance, W T Foley Nelson, T Fischer, J E Surgery. 1991 October; 110(4): 678-84 0039-6060
- **The RXR agonist LG100268 causes hepatomegaly, improves glycaemic control and decreases cardiovascular risk and cachexia in diabetic mice suffering from pancreatic beta-cell dysfunction.**
  Author(s): Department of Metabolic Diseases, Glaxo Wellcome Inc., Research Triangle Park, North Carolina 27709, USA.
  Source: Lenhard, J M Lancaster, M E Paulik, M A Weiel, J E Binz, J G Sundseth, S S Gaskill, B A Lightfoot, R M Brown, H R Diabetologia. 1999 May; 42(5): 545-54 0012-186X

Federal Resources on Nutrition

In addition to the IBIDS, the United States Department of Health and Human Services (HHS) and the United States Department of Agriculture (USDA) provide many sources of information on general nutrition and health. Recommended resources include:

- healthfinder®, HHS's gateway to health information, including diet and nutrition: **http://www.healthfinder.gov/scripts/SearchContext.asp?topic=238&page=0**
- The United States Department of Agriculture's Web site dedicated to nutrition information: **www.nutrition.gov**
- The Food and Drug Administration's Web site for federal food safety information: **www.foodsafety.gov**
- The National Action Plan on Overweight and Obesity sponsored by the United States Surgeon General: **http://www.surgeongeneral.gov/topics/obesity/**
- The Center for Food Safety and Applied Nutrition has an Internet site sponsored by the Food and Drug Administration and the Department of Health and Human Services: **http://vm.cfsan.fda.gov/**
- Center for Nutrition Policy and Promotion sponsored by the United States Department of Agriculture: **http://www.usda.gov/cnpp/**
- Food and Nutrition Information Center, National Agricultural Library sponsored by the United States Department of Agriculture: **http://www.nal.usda.gov/fnic/**
- Food and Nutrition Service sponsored by the United States Department of Agriculture: **http://www.fns.usda.gov/fns/**

Additional Web Resources

A number of additional Web sites offer encyclopedic information covering food and nutrition. The following is a representative sample:

- AOL: **http://search.aol.com/cat.adp?id=174&layer=&from=subcats**
- Family Village: **http://www.familyvillage.wisc.edu/med_nutrition.html**
- Google: **http://directory.google.com/Top/Health/Nutrition/**
- Healthnotes: **http://www.healthnotes.com/**
- Open Directory Project: **http://dmoz.org/Health/Nutrition/**
- Yahoo.com: **http://dir.yahoo.com/Health/Nutrition/**
- WebMD®Health: **http://my.webmd.com/nutrition**
- WholeHealthMD.com: **http://www.wholehealthmd.com/reflib/0,1529,00.html**

Chapter 3. Alternative Medicine and Cachexia

Overview

In this chapter, we will begin by introducing you to official information sources on complementary and alternative medicine (CAM) relating to cachexia. At the conclusion of this chapter, we will provide additional sources.

National Center for Complementary and Alternative Medicine

The National Center for Complementary and Alternative Medicine (NCCAM) of the National Institutes of Health (**http://nccam.nih.gov/**) has created a link to the National Library of Medicine's databases to facilitate research for articles that specifically relate to cachexia and complementary medicine. To search the database, go to the following Web site: **http://www.nlm.nih.gov/nccam/camonpubmed.html**. Select "CAM on PubMed." Enter "cachexia" (or synonyms) into the search box. Click "Go." The following references provide information on particular aspects of complementary and alternative medicine that are related to cachexia:

- **A review of the drug treatment of cachexia associated with cancer.**
  Author(s): Gagnon B, Bruera E.
  Source: Drugs. 1998 May; 55(5): 675-88. Review.
  http://www.ncbi.nlm.nih.gov/entrez/query.fcgi?cmd=Retrieve&db=pubmed&dopt=Abstract&list_uids=9585863

- **Adjuvant arthritis as a model of inflammatory cachexia.**
  Author(s): Roubenoff R, Freeman LM, Smith DE, Abad LW, Dinarello CA, Kehayias JJ.
  Source: Arthritis and Rheumatism. 1997 March; 40(3): 534-9.
  http://www.ncbi.nlm.nih.gov/entrez/query.fcgi?cmd=Retrieve&db=pubmed&dopt=Abstract&list_uids=9082942

- **Alleviation of cancer anorexia and cachexia: studies of the Mayo Clinic and the North Central Cancer Treatment Group.**
  Author(s): Loprinzi CL, Ellison NM, Goldberg RM, Michalak JC, Burch PA.

Source: Seminars in Oncology. 1990 December; 17(6 Suppl 9): 8-12. Review.
http://www.ncbi.nlm.nih.gov/entrez/query.fcgi?cmd=Retrieve&db=pubmed&dopt=Abstract&list_uids=2259930

- **Anorexia and cachexia in advanced cancer patients.**
  Author(s): Vigano A, Watanabe S, Bruera E.
  Source: Cancer Surv. 1994; 21: 99-115. Review.
  http://www.ncbi.nlm.nih.gov/entrez/query.fcgi?cmd=Retrieve&db=pubmed&dopt=Abstract&list_uids=8565002

- **Cachexia in cancer patients.**
  Author(s): Tisdale MJ.
  Source: Nature Reviews. Cancer. 2002 November; 2(11): 862-71. Review.
  http://www.ncbi.nlm.nih.gov/entrez/query.fcgi?cmd=Retrieve&db=pubmed&dopt=Abstract&list_uids=12415256

- **Cachexia of malignancy: potential role of insulin in nutritional management.**
  Author(s): Schein PS, Kisner D, Haller D, Blecher M, Hamosh M.
  Source: Cancer. 1979 May; 43(5 Suppl): 2070-6.
  http://www.ncbi.nlm.nih.gov/entrez/query.fcgi?cmd=Retrieve&db=pubmed&dopt=Abstract&list_uids=445387

- **Cancer cachexia and cannabinoids.**
  Author(s): Gorter RW.
  Source: Forschende Komplementarmedizin. 1999 October; 6 Suppl 3: 21-2. Review.
  http://www.ncbi.nlm.nih.gov/entrez/query.fcgi?cmd=Retrieve&db=pubmed&dopt=Abstract&list_uids=10575285

- **Cancer cachexia and its treatment with fish-oil-enriched nutritional supplementation.**
  Author(s): Barber MD.
  Source: Nutrition (Burbank, Los Angeles County, Calif.). 2001 September; 17(9): 751-5. Review.
  http://www.ncbi.nlm.nih.gov/entrez/query.fcgi?cmd=Retrieve&db=pubmed&dopt=Abstract&list_uids=11527672

- **Cancer cachexia and tumor growth reduction in Walker 256 tumor-bearing rats supplemented with N-3 polyunsaturated fatty acids for one generation.**
  Author(s): Togni V, Ota CC, Folador A, Junior OT, Aikawa J, Yamazaki RK, Freitas FA, Longo R, Martins EF, Calder PC, Curi R, Fernandes LC.
  Source: Nutrition and Cancer. 2003; 46(1): 52-8.
  http://www.ncbi.nlm.nih.gov/entrez/query.fcgi?cmd=Retrieve&db=pubmed&dopt=Abstract&list_uids=12925304

- **Cancer cachexia: influence of systemic ketosis on substrate levels and nitrogen metabolism.**
  Author(s): Fearon KC, Borland W, Preston T, Tisdale MJ, Shenkin A, Calman KC.
  Source: The American Journal of Clinical Nutrition. 1988 January; 47(1): 42-8.
  http://www.ncbi.nlm.nih.gov/entrez/query.fcgi?cmd=Retrieve&db=pubmed&dopt=Abstract&list_uids=3122552

- **Cancer-associated anorexia and cachexia. Implications for drug therapy.**
  Author(s): Loprinzi CL, Goldberg RM, Burnham NL.
  Source: Drugs. 1992 April; 43(4): 499-506. Review.
  http://www.ncbi.nlm.nih.gov/entrez/query.fcgi?cmd=Retrieve&db=pubmed&dopt=Abstract&list_uids=1377116

- **Clinical management of anorexia and cachexia in patients with advanced cancer.**
  Author(s): Bruera E.
  Source: Oncology. 1992; 49 Suppl 2: 35-42. Review.
  http://www.ncbi.nlm.nih.gov/entrez/query.fcgi?cmd=Retrieve&db=pubmed&dopt=Abstract&list_uids=1461626

- **Continuing: Biology of cachexia.**
  Author(s): Gold J.
  Source: Journal of the National Cancer Institute. 1999 June 16; 91(12): 1077; Author Reply 1077-8.
  http://www.ncbi.nlm.nih.gov/entrez/query.fcgi?cmd=Retrieve&db=pubmed&dopt=Abstract&list_uids=10379973

- **Continuing: Biology of cachexia.**
  Author(s): Bozzetti F.
  Source: Journal of the National Cancer Institute. 1999 June 16; 91(12): 1077; Author Reply 1077-8.
  http://www.ncbi.nlm.nih.gov/entrez/query.fcgi?cmd=Retrieve&db=pubmed&dopt=Abstract&list_uids=10379972

- **Dietary conjugated linoleic acid decreased cachexia, macrophage tumor necrosis factor-alpha production, and modifies splenocyte cytokines production.**
  Author(s): Yang M, Cook ME.
  Source: Experimental Biology and Medicine (Maywood, N.J.). 2003 January; 228(1): 51-8.
  http://www.ncbi.nlm.nih.gov/entrez/query.fcgi?cmd=Retrieve&db=pubmed&dopt=Abstract&list_uids=12524473

- **Down-regulation of the acute-phase response in patients with pancreatic cancer cachexia receiving oral eicosapentaenoic acid is mediated via suppression of interleukin-6.**
  Author(s): Wigmore SJ, Fearon KC, Maingay JP, Ross JA.
  Source: Clinical Science (London, England : 1979). 1997 February; 92(2): 215-21.
  http://www.ncbi.nlm.nih.gov/entrez/query.fcgi?cmd=Retrieve&db=pubmed&dopt=Abstract&list_uids=9059324

- **Effect of a fish oil-enriched nutritional supplement on metabolic mediators in patients with pancreatic cancer cachexia.**
  Author(s): Barber MD, Fearon KC, Tisdale MJ, McMillan DC, Ross JA.
  Source: Nutrition and Cancer. 2001; 40(2): 118-24.
  http://www.ncbi.nlm.nih.gov/entrez/query.fcgi?cmd=Retrieve&db=pubmed&dopt=Abstract&list_uids=11962246

- **Effect of a protein and energy dense N-3 fatty acid enriched oral supplement on loss of weight and lean tissue in cancer cachexia: a randomised double blind trial.**

Author(s): Fearon KC, Von Meyenfeldt MF, Moses AG, Van Geenen R, Roy A, Gouma DJ, Giacosa A, Van Gossum A, Bauer J, Barber MD, Aaronson NK, Voss AC, Tisdale MJ.
Source: Gut. 2003 October; 52(10): 1479-86.
http://www.ncbi.nlm.nih.gov/entrez/query.fcgi?cmd=Retrieve&db=pubmed&dopt=Abstract&list_uids=12970142

- **Effect of fish oil on appetite and other symptoms in patients with advanced cancer and anorexia/cachexia: a double-blind, placebo-controlled study.**
  Author(s): Bruera E, Strasser F, Palmer JL, Willey J, Calder K, Amyotte G, Baracos V.
  Source: Journal of Clinical Oncology : Official Journal of the American Society of Clinical Oncology. 2003 January 1; 21(1): 129-34.
  http://www.ncbi.nlm.nih.gov/entrez/query.fcgi?cmd=Retrieve&db=pubmed&dopt=Abstract&list_uids=12506181

- **Effect of fish oil on cancer cachexia and host liver metabolism in rats with prostate tumors.**
  Author(s): Dagnelie PC, Bell JD, Williams SC, Bates TE, Abel PD, Foster CS.
  Source: Lipids. 1994 March; 29(3): 195-203.
  http://www.ncbi.nlm.nih.gov/entrez/query.fcgi?cmd=Retrieve&db=pubmed&dopt=Abstract&list_uids=8170289

- **Effect of insulin on weight loss and tumour growth in a cachexia model.**
  Author(s): Beck SA, Tisdale MJ.
  Source: British Journal of Cancer. 1989 May; 59(5): 677-81.
  http://www.ncbi.nlm.nih.gov/entrez/query.fcgi?cmd=Retrieve&db=pubmed&dopt=Abstract&list_uids=2736199

- **Effects of eicosapentaenoic acid on tumour growth and cachexia in mouse colon cancer.**
  Author(s): Tisdale MJ, Beck SA, Hudson EA.
  Source: World Review of Nutrition and Dietetics. 1994; 76: 86-8. Review.
  http://www.ncbi.nlm.nih.gov/entrez/query.fcgi?cmd=Retrieve&db=pubmed&dopt=Abstract&list_uids=7856243

- **Eicosapentaenoic acid as a targeted therapy for cancer cachexia.**
  Author(s): Belda-Iniesta C, de Castro Carpeno J, Fresno Vara JA, Cejas Guerrero P, Casado Saenz E, Espinosa Arranz E, Redondo Sanchez A, Feliu Battle J, Gonzalez Baron M.
  Source: Journal of Clinical Oncology : Official Journal of the American Society of Clinical Oncology. 2003 December 15; 21(24): 4657-8; Author Reply 4658.
  http://www.ncbi.nlm.nih.gov/entrez/query.fcgi?cmd=Retrieve&db=pubmed&dopt=Abstract&list_uids=14673061

- **Eicosapentaenoic acid supplementation reduces tumor volume and attenuates cachexia in a rat model of progressive non-metastasizing malignancy.**
  Author(s): Jho DH, Babcock TA, Tevar R, Helton WS, Espat NJ.

Source: Jpen. Journal of Parenteral and Enteral Nutrition. 2002 September-October; 26(5): 291-7.
http://www.ncbi.nlm.nih.gov/entrez/query.fcgi?cmd=Retrieve&db=pubmed&dopt=Abstract&list_uids=12216709

- **Fish oil supplementation in F1 generation associated with naproxen, clenbuterol, and insulin administration reduce tumor growth and cachexia in Walker 256 tumor-bearing rats.**
Author(s): Pinto JA Jr, Folador A, Bonato SJ, Aikawa J, Yamazaki RK, Pizato N, Facin M, Grohs H, de Oliveira HH, Naliwaiko K, Ferraz AC, Nishiyama A, Fernandez R, Curi R, Fernandes LC.
Source: The Journal of Nutritional Biochemistry. 2004 June; 15(6): 358-65.
http://www.ncbi.nlm.nih.gov/entrez/query.fcgi?cmd=Retrieve&db=pubmed&dopt=Abstract&list_uids=15157942

- **Fish oil supplementation in patients with cancer cachexia undergoing chemotherapy and radiotherapy. What is the effect and how well do patients comply?**
Author(s): Keville MM, Grimble G, Howard N.
Source: Clinical Nutrition (Edinburgh, Lothian). 2003 August; 22(S1): S66.
http://www.ncbi.nlm.nih.gov/entrez/query.fcgi?cmd=Retrieve&db=pubmed&dopt=Abstract&list_uids=14683995

- **Historical perspective and potential use of n-3 fatty acids in therapy of cancer cachexia.**
Author(s): Karmali RA.
Source: Nutrition (Burbank, Los Angeles County, Calif.). 1996 January; 12(1 Suppl): S2-4. Review.
http://www.ncbi.nlm.nih.gov/entrez/query.fcgi?cmd=Retrieve&db=pubmed&dopt=Abstract&list_uids=8850210

- **Improvement by eicosanoids in cancer cachexia induced by LLC-IL6 transplantation.**
Author(s): Ohira T, Nishio K, Ohe Y, Arioka H, Nishio M, Funayama Y, Ogasawara H, Fukuda M, Yazawa K, Kato H, Saijo N.
Source: Journal of Cancer Research and Clinical Oncology. 1996; 122(12): 711-5.
http://www.ncbi.nlm.nih.gov/entrez/query.fcgi?cmd=Retrieve&db=pubmed&dopt=Abstract&list_uids=8954167

- **Inhibition of lipolysis and muscle protein degradation by EPA in cancer cachexia.**
Author(s): Tisdale MJ.
Source: Nutrition (Burbank, Los Angeles County, Calif.). 1996 January; 12(1 Suppl): S31-3.
http://www.ncbi.nlm.nih.gov/entrez/query.fcgi?cmd=Retrieve&db=pubmed&dopt=Abstract&list_uids=8850217

- **Inhibition of tumour-induced lipolysis in vitro and cachexia and tumour growth in vivo by eicosapentaenoic acid.**
Author(s): Tisdale MJ, Beck SA.

Source: Biochemical Pharmacology. 1991 January 1; 41(1): 103-7.
http://www.ncbi.nlm.nih.gov/entrez/query.fcgi?cmd=Retrieve&db=pubmed&dopt=Abstract&list_uids=1846070

- **Inhibition of weight loss by omega-3 fatty acids in an experimental cachexia model.**
Author(s): Tisdale MJ, Dhesi JK.
Source: Cancer Research. 1990 August 15; 50(16): 5022-6.
http://www.ncbi.nlm.nih.gov/entrez/query.fcgi?cmd=Retrieve&db=pubmed&dopt=Abstract&list_uids=2379167

- **Is the pharmacological treatment of cancer cachexia possible?**
Author(s): Bruera E.
Source: Supportive Care in Cancer : Official Journal of the Multinational Association of Supportive Care in Cancer. 1993 November; 1(6): 298-304. Review.
http://www.ncbi.nlm.nih.gov/entrez/query.fcgi?cmd=Retrieve&db=pubmed&dopt=Abstract&list_uids=8156247

- **Lack of effect of eicosapentaenoic acid in preventing cancer cachexia and inhibiting tumor growth.**
Author(s): Costelli P, Llovera M, Lopez-Soriano J, Carbo N, Tessitore L, Lopez-Soriano FJ, Baccino FM, Argiles JM.
Source: Cancer Letters. 1995 October 20; 97(1): 25-32.
http://www.ncbi.nlm.nih.gov/entrez/query.fcgi?cmd=Retrieve&db=pubmed&dopt=Abstract&list_uids=7585474

- **Malnutrition and cachexia in ovarian cancer patients: pathophysiology and management.**
Author(s): Gadducci A, Cosio S, Fanucchi A, Genazzani AR.
Source: Anticancer Res. 2001 July-August; 21(4B): 2941-7. Review.
http://www.ncbi.nlm.nih.gov/entrez/query.fcgi?cmd=Retrieve&db=pubmed&dopt=Abstract&list_uids=11712791

- **Malnutrition, muscle wasting and cachexia in chronic heart failure: the nutritional approach.**
Author(s): Pasini E, Aquilani R, Gheorghiade M, Dioguardi FS.
Source: Ital Heart J. 2003 April; 4(4): 232-5. Review.
http://www.ncbi.nlm.nih.gov/entrez/query.fcgi?cmd=Retrieve&db=pubmed&dopt=Abstract&list_uids=12784775

- **Management of anorexia-cachexia associated with cancer and HIV infection.**
Author(s): Gorter R.
Source: Oncology (Huntingt). 1991 September; 5(9 Suppl): 13-7. Review.
http://www.ncbi.nlm.nih.gov/entrez/query.fcgi?cmd=Retrieve&db=pubmed&dopt=Abstract&list_uids=1721521

- **Management of cancer anorexia/cachexia.**
Author(s): Loprinzi CL.

Source: Supportive Care in Cancer : Official Journal of the Multinational Association of Supportive Care in Cancer. 1995 March; 3(2): 120-2. Review.
http://www.ncbi.nlm.nih.gov/entrez/query.fcgi?cmd=Retrieve&db=pubmed&dopt=Abstract&list_uids=7773579

- **Mechanism of attenuation of skeletal muscle protein catabolism in cancer cachexia by eicosapentaenoic acid.**
  Author(s): Whitehouse AS, Smith HJ, Drake JL, Tisdale MJ.
  Source: Cancer Research. 2001 May 1; 61(9): 3604-9.
  http://www.ncbi.nlm.nih.gov/entrez/query.fcgi?cmd=Retrieve&db=pubmed&dopt=Abstract&list_uids=11325828

- **Mechanism of lipid mobilization associated with cancer cachexia: interaction between the polyunsaturated fatty acid, eicosapentaenoic acid, and inhibitory guanine nucleotide-regulatory protein.**
  Author(s): Tisdale MJ.
  Source: Prostaglandins, Leukotrienes, and Essential Fatty Acids. 1993 January; 48(1): 105-9. Review.
  http://www.ncbi.nlm.nih.gov/entrez/query.fcgi?cmd=Retrieve&db=pubmed&dopt=Abstract&list_uids=8380931

- **Mechanism of muscle protein degradation in cancer cachexia.**
  Author(s): Smith KL, Tisdale MJ.
  Source: British Journal of Cancer. 1993 August; 68(2): 314-8.
  http://www.ncbi.nlm.nih.gov/entrez/query.fcgi?cmd=Retrieve&db=pubmed&dopt=Abstract&list_uids=8347486

- **Modulation of adipocyte G-protein expression in cancer cachexia by a lipid-mobilizing factor (LMF).**
  Author(s): Islam-Ali B, Khan S, Price SA, Tisdale MJ.
  Source: British Journal of Cancer. 2001 September 1; 85(5): 758-63.
  http://www.ncbi.nlm.nih.gov/entrez/query.fcgi?cmd=Retrieve&db=pubmed&dopt=Abstract&list_uids=11531264

- **More about: biology of cachexia.**
  Author(s): Gold J.
  Source: Journal of the National Cancer Institute. 1998 July 15; 90(14): 1101-2.
  http://www.ncbi.nlm.nih.gov/entrez/query.fcgi?cmd=Retrieve&db=pubmed&dopt=Abstract&list_uids=9672260

- **Neopterin is decreased in patients with cancer cachexia receiving fish oil supplementation.**
  Author(s): Keville MM, Grimble G, Beaney R.
  Source: Clinical Nutrition (Edinburgh, Lothian). 2003 August; 22(S1): S65.
  http://www.ncbi.nlm.nih.gov/entrez/query.fcgi?cmd=Retrieve&db=pubmed&dopt=Abstract&list_uids=14683993

- **Nutritional therapy for cancer cachexia.**
  Author(s): Grimble RF.

Source: Gut. 2003 October; 52(10): 1391-2.
http://www.ncbi.nlm.nih.gov/entrez/query.fcgi?cmd=Retrieve&db=pubmed&dopt=Abstract&list_uids=12970126

- **Phase I clinical study of fish oil fatty acid capsules for patients with cancer cachexia: cancer and leukemia group B study 9473.**
  Author(s): Burns CP, Halabi S, Clamon GH, Hars V, Wagner BA, Hohl RJ, Lester E, Kirshner JJ, Vinciguerra V, Paskett E.
  Source: Clinical Cancer Research : an Official Journal of the American Association for Cancer Research. 1999 December; 5(12): 3942-7.
  http://www.ncbi.nlm.nih.gov/entrez/query.fcgi?cmd=Retrieve&db=pubmed&dopt=Abstract&list_uids=10632323

- **Proinflammatory cytokines, nutritional support, and the cachexia syndrome: interactions and therapeutic options.**
  Author(s): Barber MD, Wigmore SJ, Ross JA, Fearon KC, Tisdale MJ.
  Source: Cancer. 1998 March 1; 82(5): 1000.
  http://www.ncbi.nlm.nih.gov/entrez/query.fcgi?cmd=Retrieve&db=pubmed&dopt=Abstract&list_uids=9486598

- **Protein and amino acid metabolism in cancer cachexia: investigative techniques and therapeutic interventions.**
  Author(s): Pisters PW, Pearlstone DB.
  Source: Critical Reviews in Clinical Laboratory Sciences. 1993; 30(3): 223-72. Review.
  http://www.ncbi.nlm.nih.gov/entrez/query.fcgi?cmd=Retrieve&db=pubmed&dopt=Abstract&list_uids=8260072

- **Re: Biology of cachexia.**
  Author(s): Wheeler BM.
  Source: Journal of the National Cancer Institute. 1998 April 15; 90(8): 628.
  http://www.ncbi.nlm.nih.gov/entrez/query.fcgi?cmd=Retrieve&db=pubmed&dopt=Abstract&list_uids=9554447

- **Rethinking nutritional support for persons with cancer cachexia.**
  Author(s): McCarthy DO.
  Source: Biological Research for Nursing. 2003 July; 5(1): 3-17. Review.
  http://www.ncbi.nlm.nih.gov/entrez/query.fcgi?cmd=Retrieve&db=pubmed&dopt=Abstract&list_uids=12886666

- **The effect of adrenaline and Walker-256 tumour-induced cachexia upon Kupffer cell metabolism.**
  Author(s): Seelaender MC, Kazantzis M, Costa Rosa LF.
  Source: Cell Biochemistry and Function. 1999 September; 17(3): 151-6.
  http://www.ncbi.nlm.nih.gov/entrez/query.fcgi?cmd=Retrieve&db=pubmed&dopt=Abstract&list_uids=10451535

- **The effect of polyunsaturated fatty acids on the progress of cachexia in patients with pancreatic cancer.**
  Author(s): Wigmore SJ, Ross JA, Falconer JS, Plester CE, Tisdale MJ, Carter DC, Fearon KC.

Source: Nutrition (Burbank, Los Angeles County, Calif.). 1996 January; 12(1 Suppl): S27-30.
http://www.ncbi.nlm.nih.gov/entrez/query.fcgi?cmd=Retrieve&db=pubmed&dopt=Abstract&list_uids=8850216

- **Tolerance and incorporation of a high-dose eicosapentaenoic acid diester emulsion by patients with pancreatic cancer cachexia.**
  Author(s): Barber MD, Fearon KC.
  Source: Lipids. 2001 April; 36(4): 347-51.
  http://www.ncbi.nlm.nih.gov/entrez/query.fcgi?cmd=Retrieve&db=pubmed&dopt=Abstract&list_uids=11383684

Additional Web Resources

A number of additional Web sites offer encyclopedic information covering CAM and related topics. The following is a representative sample:

- Alternative Medicine Foundation, Inc.: **http://www.herbmed.org/**
- AOL: **http://search.aol.com/cat.adp?id=169&layer=&from=subcats**
- Chinese Medicine: **http://www.newcenturynutrition.com/**
- drkoop.com®: **http://www.drkoop.com/InteractiveMedicine/IndexC.html**
- Family Village: **http://www.familyvillage.wisc.edu/med_altn.htm**
- Google: **http://directory.google.com/Top/Health/Alternative/**
- Healthnotes: **http://www.healthnotes.com/**
- MedWebPlus: **http://medwebplus.com/subject/Alternative_and_Complementary_Medicine**
- Open Directory Project: **http://dmoz.org/Health/Alternative/**
- HealthGate: **http://www.tnp.com/**
- WebMD®Health: **http://my.webmd.com/drugs_and_herbs**
- WholeHealthMD.com: **http://www.wholehealthmd.com/reflib/0,1529,00.html**
- Yahoo.com: **http://dir.yahoo.com/Health/Alternative_Medicine/**

The following is a specific Web list relating to cachexia; please note that any particular subject below may indicate either a therapeutic use, or a contraindication (potential danger), and does not reflect an official recommendation:

- **General Overview**

  Breast Cancer
  Source: Healthnotes, Inc.; www.healthnotes.com

  Colon Cancer
  Source: Healthnotes, Inc.; www.healthnotes.com

Colorectal Cancer
Source: Integrative Medicine Communications; www.drkoop.com

Lung Cancer
Source: Healthnotes, Inc.; www.healthnotes.com

Prostate Cancer
Source: Healthnotes, Inc.; www.healthnotes.com

Shock
Source: Integrative Medicine Communications; www.drkoop.com

General References

A good place to find general background information on CAM is the National Library of Medicine. It has prepared within the MEDLINEplus system an information topic page dedicated to complementary and alternative medicine. To access this page, go to the MEDLINEplus site at **http://www.nlm.nih.gov/medlineplus/alternativemedicine.html**. This Web site provides a general overview of various topics and can lead to a number of general sources.

CHAPTER 4. PATENTS ON CACHEXIA

Overview

Patents can be physical innovations (e.g. chemicals, pharmaceuticals, medical equipment) or processes (e.g. treatments or diagnostic procedures). The United States Patent and Trademark Office defines a patent as a grant of a property right to the inventor, issued by the Patent and Trademark Office.[8] Patents, therefore, are intellectual property. For the United States, the term of a new patent is 20 years from the date when the patent application was filed. If the inventor wishes to receive economic benefits, it is likely that the invention will become commercially available within 20 years of the initial filing. It is important to understand, therefore, that an inventor's patent does not indicate that a product or service is or will be commercially available. The patent implies only that the inventor has "the right to exclude others from making, using, offering for sale, or selling" the invention in the United States. While this relates to U.S. patents, similar rules govern foreign patents.

In this chapter, we show you how to locate information on patents and their inventors. If you find a patent that is particularly interesting to you, contact the inventor or the assignee for further information. **IMPORTANT NOTE:** When following the search strategy described below, you may discover non-medical patents that use the generic term "cachexia" (or a synonym) in their titles. To accurately reflect the results that you might find while conducting research on cachexia, we have not necessarily excluded non-medical patents in this bibliography.

Patents on Cachexia

By performing a patent search focusing on cachexia, you can obtain information such as the title of the invention, the names of the inventor(s), the assignee(s) or the company that owns or controls the patent, a short abstract that summarizes the patent, and a few excerpts from the description of the patent. The abstract of a patent tends to be more technical in nature, while the description is often written for the public. Full patent descriptions contain much more information than is presented here (e.g. claims, references, figures, diagrams, etc.). We

---

[8] Adapted from the United States Patent and Trademark Office:
http://www.uspto.gov/web/offices/pac/doc/general/whatis.htm.

will tell you how to obtain this information later in the chapter. The following is an example of the type of information that you can expect to obtain from a patent search on cachexia:

- **DNA encoding a novel homolog of CSBP/p38 MAP kinase**

  Inventor(s): Kumar; Sanjay (King of Prussia, PA)

  Assignee(s): SmithKline Beecham Corporation (Philadelphia, PA)

  Patent Number: 6,376,214

  Date filed: February 18, 1997

  Abstract: p38beta2 polypeptides and polynucleotides and methods for producing such polypeptides by recombinant techniques are disclosed. Also disclosed are methods for utilizing p38beta2 polypeptides and polynucleotides in the design of protocols for the treatment of central nervous system disorder such as senile dementia of the Alzheimer's type (SDAT), mutiple sclerosis, cerebral malaria, stroke, head trauma and spinal cord injury; cardiovascular diseases such as restenosis and atherosclerosis; inflammatory diseases such as Adult Respiratory Disease Syndrome (ARDS), Rheumatoid arthritis, Osteoarthritis, Inflammatory Bowel Disease (IBD), psoriasis, derratitis, asthma; and other such diseases or conditions associated with dysregulated or excess cytokines such as osteoporosis, sepsis due to surgical or traumatic incident, chronic renal failure, AIDs, **cachexia** and autoimmune conditions such as lupus erthyromatosis, host graft rejection and graft verus host disease, among others, and diagnostic assays for such conditions.

  Excerpt(s): This invention relates to newly identified polynucleotides, polypeptides encoded by them and to the use of such polynucleotides and polypeptides, and to their production. More particularly, the polynucleotides and polypeptides of the present invention relate to CSBP/p38 MAP Kinases family, hereinafter referred to as p38beta2. The invention also relates to inhibiting or activating the action of such polynucleotides and polypeptides. Cytokines play an important role in regulating the cellular response during inflammation and other immune functions. Of particular interest are the cytokines interleukin-1 (IL-1,.alpha. and.beta.) and tumor necrosis factor (TNF,.alpha. and.beta.), which are the intercellular proteins involved in the initial step of the inflammatory response cascade (Arai, et al., Ann. Rev. Biochem 59: 783-836 (1990)). Thus, there has been a substantial amount of research recently devoted to interfering with the production of IL-1 and TNF in response to an inflammatory stimulus. One therapeutic approach involves suppressing the production of IL-1 and TNF at the level of transcription and/or translation and/or secretion. The activities associated with certain of pyridinyl imidazoles led to a class of compounds referred to as "CSAIDs", or Cytokine Suppressing Anti-Inflammatory Drugs. These compounds appear to arrest the expression of IL-1 and TNF predominantly at the translational level, although a lesser effect on transcription has also been observed but effects on other steps cannot be ruled out.

  Web site: http://www.delphion.com/details?pn=US06376214__

- **Method for the prevention and treatment of cachexia and anorexia**

  Inventor(s): Abbruzzese; Bonnie Chandler (Dublin, OH), Cope; Frederick Oliver (Worthington, OH), DeMichele; Stephen Joseph (Dublin, OH), McCamish; Mark Anthony (Worthington, OH)

  Assignee(s): Abbott Laboratories (Abbott Park, IL)

  Patent Number: 6,387,883

  Date filed: August 18, 2000

  Abstract: The present invention relates to methods and nutritional compositions for the prevention and treatment of **cachexia** and anorexia. The methods of the invention comprise administering a composition comprising effective amounts of.omega.-3 fatty acids such as alpha-linolenic acid, stearidonic acid, eicosapentaenoic acid, docosapentaenoic acid, docosahexaenoic acid or mixtures thereof; of branched-chain amino acids valine, leucine, isoleucine or mixtures thereof; with or without reduced levels of tryptophan and 5-hydroxytryptophan; and of antioxidant system selected from the group comprising beta-carotene, vitamin C, vitamin E, selenium, or mixtures thereof.

  Excerpt(s): The present invention relates to methods and nutritional compositions for the prevention and treatment of cancer **cachexia** and anorexia. In the practice of the present invention patients are enterally administered.omega.-3 fatty acids including, but not limited to alpha-linolenic (18:3.omega.-3), stearidonic (18:4.omega.-3), eicosapentaenoic (20:5.omega.-3) docosapentaenoic: (22:5.omega.-3), and docosahexaenoic (22:6.omega.-3), in combination with antioxidants including, but not limited to, beta-carotene, vitamin C, vitamin E, selenium, or mixtures thereof; a source of amino-nitrogen with high levels of branched-chain amino acids including valine, leucine, isoleucine, and with or without reduced levels of tryptophan and 5-hydroxytryptophan. Cancer **cachexia** is a syndrome characterized by anorexia, weight loss, premature satiety, asthenia, loss of lean body mass, and multiple organ dysfunction. The majority of patients with cancer whose disease progresses to metastatic disease develop **cachexia** during their treatment program and the **cachexia** contributes to their deaths. The frequency of weight loss in cancer patients ranges from 40% for patients with breast cancer, acute myelocytic leukemia, and sarcoma to more than 80% in patients with carcinoma of the pancreas and stomach. About 60% of patients with carcinomas of the lung, colon or prostate have experienced weight loss prior to beginning chemotherapy. Although the relationship between pretreatment malnutrition (weightless) and adverse outcome is established, no consistent relationship has been demonstrated between the development of **cachexia** and tumor size, disease stage, and type or duration of the malignancy. Development of **cachexia** in the cancer patient is not caused simply by increased energy expenditure by the host or by the tumor. The malignant **cachexia** is partially related to reduced caloric intake. Cancer **cachexia** is not simply a local effect of the tumor. Alterations in protein, fat, and carbohyrate metabolism occur commonly. For example, abnormalities in carbohydrate metabolism include increased rates of total glucose turnover, increased hepatic gluconeogenesis, glucose intolerance and elevated glucose levels. Increased lipolysis, increased free fatty acid and glycerol turnover, hyperlipidemia, and reduced lipoprotein lipase activity pre frequently noted. The weight loss associated with cancer **cachexia** is caused not only by a reduction in body fat stores but also by a reduction in total body protein mass, with extensive skeletal muscle wasting. Increased protein turnover and poorly regulated amino acid oxidation may also be important. Presence of host-derived factors produced in response to the cancer have been implicated as causative agents of **cachexia,** e.g., tumor necrosis factor-.alpha. (TNF) or cachectin, interleukin-1 (IL-1), IL-6, gamma-interferon (IFN), and prostaglandins (PGs) (e.g., PGE.sub.2).

Web site: http://www.delphion.com/details?pn=US06387883__

- **Methods and composition for the diagnosis and treatment of body weight disorders, including obesity**

  Inventor(s): Moore; Karen (Maynard, MA), Nagle; Deborah Lynn (Watertown, MA)

  Assignee(s): Millennium Pharmaceuticals, Inc. (Cambridge, MA)

  Patent Number: 6,713,277

  Date filed: July 21, 1999

  Excerpt(s): The present invention relates to mammalian mahogany genes, including the human mahogany gene, which are novel genes involved in the control of mammalian body weight. The invention encompasses nucleotide sequences of the mahogany gene, host cell expression systems of the mahogany gene, and hosts which have been transformed by these expression systems, including transgenic animals. The invention also encompasses novel mahogany gene products, including mahogany proteins, polypeptides and peptides containing amino acid sequences mahogany proteins, fusion proteins of mahogany proteins polypeptides and peptides, and antibodies directed against such mahogany gene products. The present invention also relates to methods and compositions for the diagnosis and treatment of mammalian body weight disorders, including obesity, **cachexia,** and anorexia, and for the identification of subjects susceptible to such disorders. Further, the invention relates to methods of using the mahogany gene and gene products of the invention for the identification of compounds which modulate the expression of the mahogany gene and/or the activity of the mahogany gene product. Such compounds can be useful as therapeutic agents in the treatment of mammalian body weight disorders, including obesity, **cachexia,** and anorexia. Obesity represents the most prevalent of body weight disorders, and it is the most important nutritional disorder in the western world, with estimates of its prevalence ranging from 30% to 50% within the middle-aged population. Other body weight disorders, such as anorexia nervosa and bulimia nervosa, which together affect approximately 0.2% of the female population of the western world, also pose serious health threats. Further, such disorders as anorexia and **cachexia** (wasting) are also prominent features of other diseases such as cancer, cystic fibrosis, and AIDS.

  Web site: http://www.delphion.com/details?pn=US06713277__

- **Methods of increasing body weight in a subject by administering TGF-.alpha.**

  Inventor(s): Felker; Thomas S. (Vashon, WA), Paskell; Stefan (Bainbridge Island, WA), Twardzik; Daniel R. (Bainbridge Island, WA)

  Assignee(s): Stem Cell Pharmaceuticals, Inc. (Seattle, WA)

  Patent Number: 6,486,122

  Date filed: April 26, 2000

  Abstract: Disclosed are peptides related to human TGF-.alpha., having TGF-.alpha. biological activity, which are useful for many of the indications that full-length TGF-.alpha. polypeptide is useful. Also provided are methods of use of such peptides, as well as human TGF-.alpha. and biologically related polypeptides. For example, methods for treating or preventing **cachexia** in subjects are provided as well as methods for stimulating hematopoiesis in patients undergoing cytotoxic chemotherapy. In addition, the use of TGF-.alpha. related peptides to related neurodengenerative diseases is also provided. Methods of the invention also provide protection for patients undergoing cytotoxic therapy from side effects such as gastrointestinal (GI) mucositis.

Excerpt(s): The invention relates generally to transforming growth factor alpha ( ) and more specifically to methods of using TGF-.alpha. for stimulating hematopoiesis, for suppressing immune function associated with autoimmune diseases, for suppressing inflammatory responses mediated by excessive histamine release and by expression of TNF-receptors and associated pro-inflammatory cytokines, and for treating **cachexia** or for treating or preventing mucositis and gastrointestinal-associated disorders. There are several disease treatments that could significantly benefit by having cells regenerate after injury or lesion formation, particularly in the CNS, in the immune system and in the gastrointestinal tract. In some instances, a particular treatment for a disease often detrimentally affects the subject being treated. For example, administration of chemotherapeutic agents to subjects results in destruction of healthy cells, for example, cells of the gastrointestinal tract. A number treatment-related disorders are related to the choice of chemotherapeutic agent. Such agents include carmustine (BCNU), chlorambucil (LEUKERAN), cisplatin (PLATINOL), Cytarabine, doxorubicin (ADRIAMYCIN), fluorouracil (5-FU), methoxetrate (MEXATE), taxol, CPT111, etoposide, and plicamycin (MITHRACIN) which are known for their direct stomatotoxic potential (Sonis, 1993, "Oral Complications in Cancer Therapy," In: Principles and Practice of Oncology, pp. 2385-2394, DeVitta et al., Eds., J. B. Lippincott, Philadelphia) and hence incidence of mucositis. Oral mucositis can be initiated by the cytotoxic effects of chemotherapy and/or radiotherapy on the rapidly dividing epithelial cells of the oropharyngeal mucosa, and is exacerbated by infection with both endogenous oral flora and opportunistic bacterial and fungal pathogens. Complications related to oral mucositis vary in the different patient populations affected, but typically include pain, poor oral intake with consequent dehydration and weight loss, and systemic infection with organisms originating in the oral cavity. The pain associated with oral mucositis may be severe requiring narcotic analgesics, and the difficulty in eating can result in patients receiving total parenteral nutrition.

Web site: http://www.delphion.com/details?pn=US06486122__

- **Nucleic acid molecules encoding the cytoplasmic domain of human Ob receptor**

  Inventor(s): Culpepper; Janice A. (Brookline, MA), Tartaglia; Louis Anthony (Cambridge, MA), Tepper; Robert I. (Weston, MA)

  Assignee(s): Millennium Pharmaceuticals, Inc. (Cambridge, MA)

  Patent Number: 6,509,189

  Date filed: December 11, 1995

  Abstract: The presention invention relates to the discovery, identification and characterization of nucleotides that encode Ob receptor (ObR), a receptor protein that participates in mammalian body weight regulation. The invention encompasses obR nucleotides, host cell expression systems, ObR proteins, fusion proteins, polypeptides and peptides, antibodies to the receptor, transgenic animals that express an obR transgene, or recombinant knock-out animals that do not express the ObR, antagonists and agonists of the receptor, and other compounds that modulate obR gene expression or ObR activity that can be used for diagnosis, drug screening, clinical trial monitoring, and/or the treatment of body weight disorders, including but not limited to obesity, **cachexia** and anorexia.

Excerpt(s): The present invention relates to the discovery, identification and characterization of nucleotides that encode Ob receptor (ObR), a receptor protein that participates in mammalian body weight regulation. The invention encompasses obR nucleotides, host cell expression systems, ObR proteins, fusion proteins, polypeptides and peptides, antibodies to the receptor, transgenic animals that express an obR transgene, or recombinant knock-out animals that do not express the ObR, antagonists and agonists of the receptor, and other compounds that modulate obR gene expression or ObR activity that can be used for diagnosis, drug screening, clinical trial monitoring, and/or the treatment of body weight disorders, including but not limited to obesity, **cachexia** and anorexia. Obesity represents the most prevalent of body weight disorders, and it is the most important nutritional disorder in the western world, with estimates of its prevalence ranging from 30% to 50% within the middle-aged population. Other body weight disorders, such as anorexia nervosa and bulimia nervosa which together affect approximately 0.2% of the female population of the western world, also pose serious health threats. Further, such disorders as anorexia and **cachexia** (wasting) are also prominent features of other diseases such as cancer, cystic fibrosis, and AIDS. Obesity, defined as an excess of body fat relative to lean body mass, also contributes to other diseases. For example, this disorder is responsible for increased incidences of diseases such as coronary artery disease, stroke, and diabetes. (See, e.g., Nishina, P. M. et al., 1994, Metab. 43:554-558.) Obesity is not merely a behavioral problem, i.e., the result of voluntary hyperphagia. Rather, the differential body composition observed between obese and normal subjects results from differences in both metabolism and neurologic/metabolic interactions. These differences seem to be, to some extent, due to differences in gene expression, and/or level of gene products or activity (Friedman, J. M. et al., 1991, Mammalian Gene 1:130-144).

Web site: http://www.delphion.com/details?pn=US06509189__

- **Pharmaceutical compositions for inhibition of cytokine production and secretion**

  Inventor(s): Bencherif; Merouane (Winston-Salem, NC), Caldwell; William Scott (Winston-Salem, NC), Dobson; Grayland Page (Winston-Salem, NC), Dull; Gary Maurice (Lewisville, NC)

  Assignee(s): Targacept, Inc. (Winston-Salem, NC)

  Patent Number: 6,489,349

  Date filed: September 6, 2000

  Abstract: Pharmaceutical compositions incorporate compounds that affect cytokine production and/or secretion. Such compounds include aryl substituted olefinic amine compounds, pyridyloxylalkylamines and phenoxyalkylamines, and aryl substituted amine compounds, such as 3-aminophenyl amine compounds. Such pharmaceutical compositions can be used for treating a wide variety of conditions, diseases and disorders, and particularly those associated with dysfunction of cytokine production and/or secretion. Of particular interest are pharmaceutical compositions useful for preventing and treating conditions, diseases and disorders associated with undesirably high levels of cytokine production and/or secretion. Such pharmaceutical compositions are useful for treating the effects of inflammatory bowel disease, inflammation, arthritis, **cachexia** in neoplastics diseases or associated with AIDS, and autoimmune diseases.

Excerpt(s): The present invention relates to pharmaceutical compositions, and particularly pharmaceutical compositions incorporating compounds that affect cytokine production and/or secretion. The present invention also relates to methods for treating a wide variety of conditions, diseases and disorders, and particularly those associated with dysfunction of cytokine production and/or secretion. Of particular interest are pharmaceutical compositions useful for preventing and treating conditions, diseases and disorders associated with undesirably high levels of cytokine production and/or secretion. Cytokines are polypeptides that affect cell function and modulate interactions between cells associated with immune, inflammatory or hematopoietic responses. Cytokines include monokines (which are generally produced and secreted by mononuclear cells, such as macrophages and monocytes) and lymphokines (which are generally produced and secreted by lymphocytes). Examples of cytokines include interleukin-1 (IL-1), interleukin-6 (IL-6), interleukin-8 (IL-8) and tumor necrosis factor (TNF, which includes TNF-alpha and TNF-beta). Cytokines have been recognized as having numerous functions, particularly with regards to immune system and inflammatory responses. See, Ebadi et al., Neurochem. Int., 30(4-5): 347-374 (1997). However, excessive or unregulated cytokine production and secretion has been implicated in mediating or exacerbating various diseases and disorders, particularly those associated with deficiencies in immunoregulation and physiological conditions (e.g., inflammation). See, for example, Tamaka, Jap. J. Clin. Med., 56(1): 97-101 (1998); Dinarello, J. Biol. Regul. Homeostat. Ag., 11(3): 91-103 (1997); Moldawer et al., Sem. Oncol., 25(1): 73-81 (1998); Balkwill, J. Viral Hepat., 4(2): 6-15 (1997); Martin et al., Eur. Resp. J., 10(9): 2139-2146 (1997) and PCT WO 98/25619. For example, pro-inflammatory cytokines are produced by a variety of cell types, play major roles in the regulation of host immune responses, and have been implicated in diverse pathologies. Exemplary pro-inflammatory cytokines include interleukin species, prostaglandin species, colony stimulating factor and tumor necrosis factor.

Web site: http://www.delphion.com/details?pn=US06489349__

- **Substituted imides**

Inventor(s): Muller; George W. (Bridgewater, NJ), Shire; Mary (North Plainfield, NJ), Stirling; David I. (Branchburg, NJ)

Assignee(s): Celgene Corporation (Warren, NJ)

Patent Number: 6,429,221

Date filed: December 30, 1994

Abstract: Novel imides are inhibitors of tumor necrosis factor.alpha. and can be used to combat **cachexia,** endotoxic shock, and retrovirus replication. A typical embodiment is 2-Phthalimido-3-(3',4'-dimethoxyphenyl)propane.

Excerpt(s): The present invention relates a method of reducing levels of TNF.alpha. in a mammal and to compounds and compositions useful therein. Excessive or unregulated TNF.alpha. production has been implicated in a number of disease conditions. These include endotoxemia and/or toxic shock syndrome {Tracey et al., Nature 330, 662-664 (1987) and Hinshaw et al., Circ. Shock 30, 279-292 (1990)}; **cachexia** {Dezube et al., Lancet, 335(8690), 662 (1990)}; and Adult Respiratory Distress Syndrome where TNF.alpha. concentration in excess of 12,000 pg/milliliters have been detected in pulmonary aspirates from ARDS patients {Millar et al., Lancet 2(8665), 712-714 (1989)}. Systemic infusion of recombinant TNF.alpha. also resulted in changes typically seen in ARDS {Ferrai-Baliviera et al., Arch Surg. 124(12), 1400-1405 (1989)}. Cerebral malaria is a lethal hyperacute neurological syndrome associated with high blood levels of TNF.alpha. and the most severe complication occurring in malaria patients. Levels of serum TNF.alpha. correlated directly with the severity of disease and the prognosis in patients with acute malaria attacks {Grau et al., N. Engl. J. Med, 320(24), 1586-1591 (1989)}.

Web site: http://www.delphion.com/details?pn=US06429221__

- **Therapeutic nutrient regimen for alleviating mucositis, stomatitis and cachexia in oncology patients**

  Inventor(s): Sherratt; J. Dale (Sherborn, MA), Somerville; Joann (Reading, MA)

  Assignee(s): Baxter International Inc. (Deerfield, IL)

  Patent Number: 6,479,068

  Date filed: June 30, 2000

  Abstract: The present invention relates to a daily regimen for oncology patient suffering from mucositis, stomatis, and **cachexia** wherein the daily regimen involves administering to the patient at least one dose of an oral composition in unit dosage form which comprises L-glutamine, vitamin A, vitamin C, vitamin E, and selenium; and at least four glutamine lozenges throughout the day which comprises about 2 grams of glutamine each, beginning 4-7 days prior to said treatment and continuing through said treatment.

  Excerpt(s): The present invention relates to the use of the amino acid glutamine in combination with additional nutrients in a composition for alleviating side effects of oncology treatment in a cancer patient comprising administering to the patient a daily regimen which comprises administering (a) at least one dose of an oral composition in unit dosage form which comprises L-glutamine, vitamin A, vitamin C, vitamin E, and selenium twice daily; and (b) at least four glutamine lozenges throughout the day which comprise about 2 grams of glutamine each, beginning 4-7 days prior to said treatment and continuing through said treatment. The daily regimen allows for physical contact of mucosal membranes with glutamine as well as systemic administration for alleviating the side effects of oncology therapy. Skubitz et al. in U.S. Pat. Nos. 5,438,075 and 5,545,668 disclose an oral glutamine composition which is used to treat oropharyngeal mucositis in patients undergoing chemotherapy or radiotherapy. The patents disclose a method of alleviating stomatitis or esophagitis originating from treatment with chemotherapy and/or radiotherapy by administering the glutamine composition described in the patent. Anderson et al. disclose a patient study involving administration of a glutamine suspension to swish and swallow on days of chemotherapy administration and for at least 14 additional days. Anderson et al. conclude that low dose oral glutamine supplementation during and after chemotherapy significantly reduced both the duration and severity of chemotherapy-associated stomatitis and decreased the chance of patients developing mouth sores as a consequence of intensive cancer chemotherapy. See Anderson et al., Cancer, vol. 83 pages 1433-9 (1998).

  Web site: http://www.delphion.com/details?pn=US06479068__

- **TNF-.alpha. production inhibitor comprising kavalactone as an active ingredient**

  Inventor(s): Asakawa; Yoshinori (Tokushima, JP), Murata; Natsuko (Odawara, JP), Okabe; Sachiko (Ageo, JP), Suma; Yukie (Tokyo, JP), Suzuki; Hiroto (Tokyo, JP), Uchida; Masayuki (Odawara, JP), Yamada; Masashi (Tokyo, JP)

  Assignee(s): Meiji Dairies Corporation (Tokyo, JP)

  Patent Number: 6,608,105

  Date filed: August 30, 2001

  Abstract: The present invention provides a TNF-.alpha. production inhibitor containing a kavalactone as an active ingredient, which inhibitor has high safety, exerts an excellent effect of inhibiting TNF-.alpha. production, and is useful as a drug or an animal drug for preventing, ameliorating, or treating diseases such as **cachexia** attributed to cancer or infectious diseases, chronic rheumatoid arthritis, inflammatory diseases, osteoarthritis, systemic lupus erythematosus (SLE), rejection during bone marrow transplantation, multiple organ failure, AIDS, meningitis, hepatitis, and type-II diabetes. The present invention also provides a preventive, ameliorating, or therapeutic agent for diseases caused by abnormal production of TNF-.alpha., the agent containing a kavalactone as an active ingredient.

  Excerpt(s): The present invention relates to a TNF-.alpha. production inhibitor containing a kavalactone as an active ingredient, and to a preventive, ameliorating, or therapeutic agent for diseases caused by abnormal production of TNF-.alpha. Recent studies have shown that excessive production of TNF-.alpha. induces onset of a variety of diseases, including **cachexia** attributed to cancer or infectious diseases (Nature, 316: 552, 1985), septic shock (J. Immunol., 145: 4185, 1990; Science, 229: 869, 1985; Shock, 30: 1990), chronic rheumatoid arthritis (Ann. Rheum. Dis., 49: 665, 1990; Lancet, 344: 1105, 1994; Lancet, 344: 1125, 1994; British J. Rheum., 34: 334, 1995), inflammatory diseases such: as ulcerative colitis and Crohn disease (Arch. Dis. Child, 66: 561, 1991; Gastroenterology), osteoarthritis (Arthritis Rheum., 36: 819, 1993), Kawasaki's disease (Clin. Immunol. Immunopathol., 56: 29, 1990), multiple sclerosis (N. Engl. J. Med., 325(7): 467, 1991), Behchet's disease (J. Rheumatol., 17: 1107, 1990), systemic lupus erythematosus (SLE) (Arthritis Rheum., 32: 146, 1989), rejection during bone marrow transplantation (J. Exp. Med., 175: 405, 1992), multiple organ failure (Rinshoi, 17(20), 2006, 1991), malaria (Science, 237: 1210, 1987), AIDS (J. Acquir. Immune Defic. Syndr., 5: 1099, 1992), meningitis (Lancet, 1: 355,1987), hepatitis (Kozo Kanno, Kanzo, 33: 213, 1992), and type-II diabetes (Science, 259: 87, 1993). The aforementioned diseases caused by excessive production of TNF-.alpha. have hitherto been treated from a mere palliative approach by use of steroid agents, anti-inflammatory agents, antibiotics, etc., and drugs for fundamentally treating the diseases have not yet been developed.

  Web site: http://www.delphion.com/details?pn=US06608105__

- **Tumor necrosis factor alpha (TNF-.alpha.) inhibiting pharmaceuticals**

  Inventor(s): Gallily; Ruth (Jerusalem, IL), Mechoulam; Raphael (Jerusalem, IL), Shohami; Esther (Jerusalem, IL)

  Assignee(s): Yessum Research Development Co. of the Hebrew University of Jerusalem (Jerusalem, IL)

  Patent Number: 6,545,041

  Date filed: October 4, 2001

Abstract: Pharmaceutical compositions are described for preventing TNF toxicity, comprising as active ingredient the stereospecific (+) enantiomer, having (3S,4S) configuration of.DELTA.sup.6 tetrahydrocannabinol type compounds. The compositions are particularly effective in alleviating and even preventing neurotoxicity due to elevated levels of TNF, including septic shock, **cachexia** and trauma. They are also effective in the treatment of certain chronic degenerative diseases characterized by TNF production, including autoimmune diseases such as AIDS.

Excerpt(s): Tumor necrosis factor alpha (TNF-.alpha.) is a pleiotropic cytokine, which has been implicated in inflammatory and immunological responses, as well as in pathogenesis of endotoxic and septic shock (reviewed by Tracey and Cerami, Ann. Rev. Med. 45, 491-503, 1994; Glauser et al. Clin. Infect Dis. 18, suppl. 2, 205-216, 1994). TNF is one of several cytokines released mainly by mononuclear phagocytic cells in response to various stimuli. Though the role of cytokines in pathophysiological states has not been fully elucidated, it appears that TNF-.alpha. is a major mediator in the cascade of injury and morbidity. Among the serious disease states related to the production of TNF-.alpha., a partial list includes the following: septic shock; endotoxic shock; **cachexia** syndromes associated with bacterial infections (e.g., tuberculosis, meningitis), viral infections (e.g., AIDS), parasite infections (e.g., malaria), and neoplastic disease; autoimmune disease, including some forms of arthritis (especially rheumatoid and degenerative forms); and adverse effects associated with treatment for the prevention of graft rejection. Septic shock is an often lethal syndrome associated with the massive release of host cytokines due to stimuli present on, or released by, invasive micro-organisms. These invasive stimuli induce polyclonal stimulation of the infected host immune system, and include both lipopolysaccharide (LPS), an endotoxin that stimulates B-cells and macrophages, and superantigens which are exotoxins that stimulate T-cells.

Web site: http://www.delphion.com/details?pn=US06545041__

- **Use of L-acetylcarnitine, L-isovalerylcarnitine, L-propionylcarnitine for increasing the levels of IGF-1**

  Inventor(s): De Simone; Claudio (Ardrea, IT)

  Assignee(s): Mendes S.R.L. (Ardea, IT), Sigma-Tau Industrie Farmaceutiche Riunite S.p.A. (Rome, IT)

  Patent Number: 6,380,252

  Date filed: February 22, 2000

  Abstract: A method is provided for increasing the levels of IGF-1 for the therapeutic treatment or prophylaxis of cytological disorders or diseases related to IGF-1 selected from the group including neuropathies of the optic nerve and of the olfactory nerve, neuralgia of the trigmeninal nerve, Bell's paralysis, amyotrophic lateral sclerosis, osteoporosis, anthropathy, arthritis, cervical spondylosis and hernia of the intervertebral discs clinical syndromes of reduced height, **cachexia** and acute or chronic hepatic necrosis, Turner's syndrome, sarcopoenia, growth hormone insensitivity syndromes, obesity, asthenia, myasthenia and heart asthenia, immunodeficiences and reperfusion injuries, and for the cicatrization of wounds, the healing of ulcers, the treatment of burns, tissue regeneration, cutaneous, intestinal and hepatic tissue regeneration and the formation of dentine, that includes administering, to a patient in need thereof, at least one selected from the group including L-acetylcarnitine, L-isovalerylcarnitine, and L-propionylcarnitine or pharmacologically acceptable salts thereof. The present invention also relates to a method and composition for treating HCV and/or increasing the levels of IGF-1 of a patient in need thereof, the composition including at least one selected from the group including L-acetylcarnitine, L-isovalerylcarnitine, L-propionylcarnitine and pharmacologically acceptable salts thereof and mixtures thereof; and at least one selected from the group including L-carnitine, coenzyme Q10, vitamin E and Se-L-methionine and pharmaceutically acceptable salts and derivatives thereof and mixtures thereof.

Excerpt(s): The present invention relates to a novel therapeutic use of L-acetylcarnitine, L-isovalerylcarnitine, L-propionylcarnitine or pharmacologically acceptable salts thereof for increasing the levels of IGF-1 (insulin-like growth factor 1) for the therapeutic treatment or prophylaxis of cytological disorders or diseases related to IGF-1. More particularly, the present invention relates to the use of L-acetylcarnitine, L-isovalerylcarnitine, L-propionylcarnitine or pharmacologically acceptable salts thereof for the therapeutic treatment or prophylaxis of individuals in whom IGF-1 contributes towards the pathogenesis of a particular disease or provokes cytological disorders. The present invention also relates to the use of any of L-acetylcarnitine, L-isovalerylcarnitine, L-propionylcarnitine or pharmacologically acceptable salts thereof in combination with any of L-carnitine, coenzyme Q10, vitamin E and/or Se-L-methionine and pharmaceutically acceptable salts and derivatives thereof in the treatment of hepatitis-C virus and/or for increasing the levels of IGF-1. Like other growth factors, IGF-1 promotes cell growth and differentiation. The administration of IGF-1 obtained as a protein purified by molecular biology methods has made it possible to confirm the effects observed in vitro with cells, on animal models and in man. Essentially, the action of IGF-1 is similar to that of insulin, that is to say an increase in the uptake of glucose, a reduction in ketones and fatty acids in the serum and an increase in protein synthesis. In accordance with these and other metabolic effects, clinical studies have been undertaken in order to evaluate the efficacy of IGF-1 in a range of diseases. IGF-1 has been administered to patients with type-II diabetes, to cachectic patients, to patients with ischemic damage at the neuronal, myocardial or renal level, and has been proposed for repairing and regenerating tissues (W. L. Lowe, Insulin-like growth factors, Scientific American Science and Medicine p. 62, March 1996). From the above, it is clear that the administration of IGF-1 may be therapeutically useful in various morbid conditions. Examples of diseases or disorders which may be prevented, cured or improved by the administration of IGF-1 include neuropathies of the optic nerve and of the olfactory nerve, neuralgia of the trigeminal nerve, Bell's paralysis, amyotrophic lateral sclerosis and other motor neuron diseases, degeneration of the retina, osteoporosis, arthropathy, arthritis, cervical spondylosis and hernia of the intervertebral discs, clinical syndromes of reduced height, **cachexia,** acute or chronic hepatic necrosis, Turner's syndrome, sarcopoenia, growth hormone insensitivity syndromes, diabetes, obesity, asthenia in general and in particular myasthenia and heart asthenia, immunodeficiencies and reperfusion injuries. IGF-1 moreover appears to be useful for the cicatrization of wounds, the healing of ulcers, the treatment of burns, tissue regeneration in general and in particular that of cutaneous, intestinal and hepatic tissue, and the formation of dentine.

Web site: http://www.delphion.com/details?pn=US06380252__

Patent Applications on Cachexia

As of December 2000, U.S. patent applications are open to public viewing.[9] Applications are patent requests which have yet to be granted. (The process to achieve a patent can take several years.) The following patent applications have been filed since December 2000 relating to cachexia:

- **Agent for preventing and/or treating multiple organ failure**

  Inventor(s): Arisawa, Hirohiko; (Kawachi-gun, JP), Higashio, Kanji; (Kawagoe-shi, JP), Masunaga, Hiroaki; (Shimotsuga-gun, JP), Ogawa, Hiromi; (Utsunomiya-shi, JP)

  Correspondence: Testa, Hurwitz & Thibeault, Llp; High Street Tower; 125 High Street; Boston; MA; 02110; US

  Patent Application Number: 20030153489

  Date filed: December 11, 2002

  Abstract: The present invention is to provide an agent for preventing and/or treating multiple organ failure comprising Tumor cytotoxic factor-II (TCF-II) or Hepatocyte growth factor (HGF) as an effective ingredient.The agent of the present invention will be useful for preventing and/or treating the development from burn, disseminated intravascular coagulation (DIC), circulatory failure, hemorrhagic shock, infectious disease, acute pancreatitis, ischemic disorder, hepatorenal syndrome, gastrointestinal hemorrhage, nutritional metabolic failure, terminal cancer, acquired immunodeficiency syndrome (AIDS), deterioration of systemic conditions due to radiation affection and **cachexia** etc. to multiple organ failure.

  Excerpt(s): The present invention relates to a novel agent for preventing and/or treating multiple organ failure. Development from burn, disseminated intravascular coagulation (DIC), circulatory failure, hemorrhagic shock, infectious disease, acute pancreatitis, ischemic disorder, hepatorenal syndrome, gastrointestinal hemorrhage, nutritional metabolic failure, terminal cancer, acquired immunodeficiency syndrome (AIDS), deterioration of systemic conditions due to radiation affection and **cachexia** etc. to multiple organ failure can be prevented or treated by the present invention. Onset or exacerbation of multiple organ failure can be classified into the following 3 categories with respect to mechanism: (1) Parallel induction of several organ disorders due to the same factor, (2) Induction of a specific organ dysfunction due to disorder of an organ; and (3) Participation of an iatrogenic factor. Excessive insults due to severe trauma or major surgeries, infectious diseases, shock etc. directly or through various kinds of mediator participate in the onset or deterioration of multiple organ failure by mechanism (1). In the case of multiple organ failure accompanied with organ disorder due to trauma or primary hepatic insufficiency, participation of mechanism (2) through organ correlation mechanism will largely contribute to the onset or deterioration thereof. By mechanism (3), medical care carried out during intensive care or care to correspond with an organ disorder may result in the other organ disorder. In patients, these 3 mechanisms participate to the development or deterioration of disorder in a complexed manner. The prognosis of patients of multiple organ failure is generally very poor and, in fact, the survival rate is low as 20-30% in spite of a wide variety of corresponding treatment.

  Web site: http://appft1.uspto.gov/netahtml/PTO/search-bool.html

---

[9] This has been a common practice outside the United States prior to December 2000.

- **Allenic aryl sulfonamide hydroxamic acids as matrix metalloproteinase and tace inhibitors**

  Inventor(s): Delos Santos, Efren Guillermo; (Nanuet, NY), Sandanayaka, Vincent Premaratna; (Northboro, MA)

  Correspondence: Daniel B. Moran; Five Giralda Farms; Madison; NJ; 07940; US

  Patent Application Number: 20030130238

  Date filed: November 1, 2002

  Abstract: Compounds of the formula 1are useful in treating disease conditions mediated by TNF-.alpha., such as rheumatoid arthritis, osteoarthritis, sepsis, AIDS, ulcerative colitis, multiple sclerosis, Crohn's disease, degenerative cartilage loss, graft rejection, **cachexia,** inflammation, fever, insulin resistance, septic shock, congestive heart failure, inflammatory disease of the central nervous system, inflammatory bowel disease and HIV.

  Excerpt(s): This invention relates to allenic aryl sulfonamide hydroxamic acids which act as inhibitors of TNF-.alpha. converting enzyme (TACE) and matrix metalloproteinase (MMP). The compounds of the present invention are useful in disease conditions mediated by MMP and TACE, such as rheumatoid arthritis, osteoarthritis, sepsis, AIDS, ulcerative colitis, multiple sclerosis, Crohn's disease, degenerative cartilage loss, graft rejection, **cachexia,** inflammation, fever, insulin resistance, septic shock, congestive heart failure, inflammatory disease of the central nervous system, inflammatory bowel disease and HIV. TNF-.alpha. converting enzyme (TACE) catalyzes the formation of TNF-.alpha. from membrane bound TNF-.alpha. precursor protein. TNF-.alpha. is a pro-inflammatory cytokine that is believed to have a role in rheumatoid arthritis [Shire, M. G.; Muller, G. W. Exp. Opin. Ther. Patents 1998, 8(5), 531; Grossman, J. M.; Brahn, E. J. Women's Health 1997, 6(6), 627; Isomaki, P.; Punnonen, J. Ann. Med. 1997, 29, 499; Camussi, G.; Lupia, E. Drugs, 1998, 55(5), 613.] septic shock [Mathison, et. al. J. Clin. Invest. 1988, 81, 1925; Miethke, et. al. J. Exp. Med. 1992, 175, 91.], graft rejection [Piguet, P. F.; Grau, G. E.; et. al. J. Exp. Med. 1987, 166, 1280.], **cachexia** [Beutler, B.; Cerami, A. Ann. Rev. Biochem. 1988, 57, 505.], anorexia, inflammation [Ksontini, R,; MacKay, S. L. D.; Moldawer, L. L. Arch. Surg. 1998, 133, 558.], congestive heart failure [Packer, M. Circulation, 1995, 92(6), 1379; Ferrari, R.; Bachetti, T.; et. al. Circulation, 1995, 92(6), 1479.], post-ischaemic reperfusion injury, inflammatory disease of the central nervous system, inflammatory bowel disease, insulin resistance [Hotamisligil, G. S.; Shargill, N. S.; Spiegelman, B. M.; et. al. Science, 1993, 259, 87.] and HIV infection [Peterson, P. K.; Gekker, G.; et. al. J. Clin. Invest. 1992, 89, 574; Pallares-Trujillo, J.; Lopez-Soriano, F. J. Argiles, J. M. Med. Res. Reviews, 1995, 15(6), 533.]], in addition to its well-documented antitumor properties [Old, L. Science, 1985, 230, 630.]. For example, research with anti-TNF-.alpha. antibodies and transgenic animals has demonstrated that blocking the formation of TNF-.alpha. inhibits the progression of arthritis [Rankin, E. C.; Choy, E. H.; Kassimos, D.; Kingsley, G. H.; Sopwith, A. M.; Isenberg, D. A.; Panayi, G. S. Br. J. Rheumatol. 1995, 34, 334; Pharmaprojects, 1996, Therapeutic Updates 17 (Oct.), au197-M2Z.]. This observation has recently been extended to humans as well as described in "TNF-.alpha. in Human Diseases", Current Pharmaceutical Design, 1996, 2, 662. Matrix metalloproteinases (MMPs) are a group of enzymes that have been implicated in the pathological destruction of connective tissue and basement membranes. These zinc containing endopeptidases consist of several subsets of enzymes including collagenases, stromelysins and gelatinases. Of these classes, the gelatinases have been shown to be the MMPs most intimately involved with the growth and spread of tumors. It is known that the level of expression of gelatinase is elevated in malignancies, and that gelatinase can degrade the basement membrane which leads to tumor metastasis. Angiogenesis, required for the growth of solid tumors, has also recently been shown to have a gelatinase component to its pathology. Furthermore, there is evidence to suggest that gelatinase is involved in plaque rupture associated with atherosclerosis. Other conditions mediated by MMPs are restenosis, MMP-mediated osteopenias, inflammatory diseases of the central nervous system, skin aging, tumor growth, osteoarthritis, rheumatoid arthritis, septic arthritis, corneal ulceration, abnormal wound healing, bone disease, proteinuria, aneurysmal aortic disease, degenerative cartilage loss following traumatic joint injury, demyelinating diseases of the nervous system, cirrhosis of the liver, glomerular disease of the kidney, premature rupture of fetal membranes, inflammatory bowel disease, periodontal disease, age related macular degeneration, diabetic retinopathy, proliferative vitreoretinopathy, retinopathy of prematurity, ocular inflammation, keratoconus, Sjogren's syndrome, myopia, ocular tumors, ocular angiogenesis/neo-vascularization and corneal graft rejection. For recent reviews, see: (1) Recent Advances in Matrix Metalloproteinase Inhibitor Research, R. P. Beckett, A. H. Davidson, A. H. Drummond, P. Huxley and M. Whittaker, Research Focus, Vol. 1,16-26, (1996), (2) Curr. Opin. Ther. Patents (1994) 4(1): 7-16, (3) Curr. Medicinal Chem. (1995) 2: 743-762, (4) Exp. Opin. Ther. Patents (1995) 5(2): 1087-110, (5) Exp. Opin. Ther. Patents (1995) 5(12): 1287-1196: (6) Exp. Opin. Ther. Patents (1998) 8(3): 281-259.

Web site: http://appft1.uspto.gov/netahtml/PTO/search-bool.html

- **GPCR-like retinoic acid-induced gene 1 protein and nucleic acid**

  Inventor(s): Lewin, David A.; (New Haven, CT), Stewart, Timothy A.; (San Francisco, CA)

  Correspondence: Sonnenschein Nath & Rosenthal; P.O. Box 061080; Wacker Drive Station; Chicago; IL; 60606-1080; US

  Patent Application Number: 20030207288

  Date filed: August 20, 2002

  Abstract: A novel G-protein coupled receptor-like retinoic acid induced molecule was identified as being differentially expressed (GPCR-like RAIG1) in an animal model of fasting and feeding. Compositions and methods pertaining to treatment and diagnosis of various metabolic disorders, such as **cachexia** and obesity.

  Excerpt(s): This application claims priority to No. 60/313,940 filed Aug. 20, 2001, the entirety of which is herein incorporated by reference. Millions of people throughout the world are affected daily by metabolic disorders such as obesity, anorexia, **cachexia,** and diabetes. Though the causes for these disorders are as varied as the disorders themselves, many candidate genes and gene products, such as insulin, leptin, and ghrelin, have been identified as potential drug targets for treatment of these disorders. Understanding metabolic disorders has been hampered by the absence of an animal model that immediately reflects the human situation. Human metabolic disorders do not generally follow a Mendelian inheritance pattern, wherein a single gene determines a metabolic disorder phenotype (physical manifestation of a gene's expression; Weigle and Kuijper, 1996), although there are several rodent models that do (Spiegelman and Flier, 1996; Weigle and Kuijper, 1996). Human metabolism is a quantitative trait with many genes, as well as environmental and behavioral aspects, responsible for metabolic activities and disorders (Clement et al., 1998; Montague et al., 1997; Comuzzie and Allison, 1998; Hill and Peters, 1998).

Web site: http://appft1.uspto.gov/netahtml/PTO/search-bool.html

- **Growth hormone secretagogues**

  Inventor(s): Carpino, Philip A.; (Groton, CT)

  Correspondence: Pfizer INC.; Patent Department, Ms8260-1611; Eastern Point Road; Groton; CT; 06340; US

  Patent Application Number: 20030130284

  Date filed: December 6, 2002

  Abstract: This invention is directed to compounds of the formula 1and the pharmaceutically-acceptable salts thereof, where the substituents are as defined in the specification, which are growth hormone secretogogues and which increase the level of endogenous growth hormone. The compounds of this invention are useful for the treatment and prevention of osteoporosis, congestive heart failure, frailty associated with aging, obesity; accelerating bone fracture repair, attenuating protein catabolic response after a major operation, reducing **cachexia** and protein loss due to chronic illness, accelerating wound healing, or accelerating the recovery of burn patients or patients having undergone major surgery; improving muscle strength, mobility, maintanence of skin thickness, metabolic homeostasis or renal homeostasis. The compounds of the present invention are also useful in treating osteoporosis when used in combination with: a bisphosphonate compound such as alendronate; estrogen, premarin, and optionally progesterone; a.beta.sub.3 adrenergic receptor agonist; an estrogen agonist or antagonist; or calcitonin, and pharmaceutical compositions useful therefor. Further, the present invention is directed to pharmaceutical compositions useful for increasing the endogenous production or release of growth hormone in a human or other animal which comprises an effective amount of a compound of the present invention and a growth hormone secretagogue selected from GHRP-6, Hexarelin, GHRP-1, growth hormone releasing factor (GRF), IGF-1, IGF-2 or B-HT920.

  Excerpt(s): This invention relates to dipeptide compounds, which are growth hormone secretagogues and are useful for the treatment and prevention of musculoskeletal frailty including osteoporosis. 3. Increased mobilization of free fatty acids and use of fatty acids for energy. Deficiency in growth hormone results in a variety of medical disorders. In children, it causes dwarfism. In adults, the consequences of acquired GH deficiency include profound reduction in lean body mass and concomitant increase in total body fat, particularly in the truncal region. Decreased skeletal and cardiac muscle mass and muscle strength lead to a significant reduction in exercise capacity. Bone density is also reduced. Administration of exogenous growth hormone has been shown to reverse many of the metabolic changes. Additional benefits of therapy have included reduction in LDL cholesterol and improved psychological well-being.

  Web site: http://appft1.uspto.gov/netahtml/PTO/search-bool.html

- **Method of screening agents for the treatment and prevention of cancer and cachexia and the new use of specific agents for the treatment and prevention of cancer and cachexia**

  Inventor(s): Ardies, C. Murray; (Chicago, IL)

  Correspondence: Cook, Alex, Mcfarron, Manzo, Cummings & Mehler Ltd; Suite 2850; 200 West Adams Street; Chicago; IL; 60606; US

  Patent Application Number: 20040115708

  Date filed: September 17, 2003

  Abstract: A method for screening agents to determine possible use as treatment and prevention drugs is provided. More specifically, cells, living organisms, mammals, or tissue are treated with the compound or agent of interest and then measured for transient activation of stress-response pathways. Activation of any of the genes or signaling molecules associated with a stress-response pathway is then determined. A transient activation of any of the genes within these pathways of transcription activation indicates the agent is a candidate for a drug, or a source of a drug for the treatment and prevention of **cachexia,** other wasting disorders, cancer, atherosclerosis, heart disease, autoimmune disease, chronic inflammatory disease, alcoholic hepatitis, non-alcoholic hepatitis, rheumatoid arthritis, osteoarthritis, type II diabetes, insulin insensitivity, Parkinson's disease, Alzheimer's disease, and any other condition caused or mediated by chronic oxygen radical damage or by chronic chemical toxicities. Methods of treatment and uses of specific agents are also provided.

  Excerpt(s): The present invention is directed to a method of screening chemical compounds, or agents, for potential use as drugs. More particularly, the present invention is directed to a method for screening of agents for potential use in the treatment and prevention of **cachexia** and other wasting disorders, cancer, atherosclerosis, heart disease, autoimmune disease, chronic inflammatory disease, alcoholic hepatitis, non-alcoholic hepatitis, rheumatoid arthritis, osteoarthritis, type II diabetes, insulin insensitivity, Parkinson's disease, Alzheimer's disease, and any other condition caused or mediated by chronic oxygen radical damage or by chronic chemical toxicities. The present invention also is directed to the new use of the following specific agents: diacylglycerol or any of its' derivatives or analogues; phospholipids, including but not limited to phosphatidylinositol or any of its' derivatives or analogues; hydrogen peroxide and any other lipid (including but not limited to short-, medium-, or long-chain fatty acid peroxides) or water soluble peroxide and peroxide derivative which retains any of the reactive properties of the original peroxide; oxygen radical generating system capable of generating superoxide anions, hydrogen peroxides, hydroxyl radicals or any other chemical oxidant; calcium; calcium ionophores such as A23187 or thapsigargin and their derivatives. The new use or uses of these specific agents is directed toward the treatment and prevention of **cachexia,** other wasting disorders, cancer, atherosclerosis, heart disease, acute or chronic autoimmune disease, chronic inflammatory disease, alcoholic hepatitis, non-alcoholic hepatitis, rheumatoid arthritis, osteoarthritis, type II diabetes, insulin insensitivity, Parkinson's disease, Alzheimer's disease, and any other condition caused or mediated by chronic oxygen radical damage or by chronic chemical toxicities. There is strong evidence that high endogenous expression and activity of the various protective antioxidant and phase H enzymes are important for protecting the body from disorders caused or mediated by chronic oxygen radical damage or chronic chemical toxicities, such as cancer, **cachexia** and other wasting disorders, atherosclerosis, heart disease, autoimmune disease, chronic inflammatory disease, alcoholic hepatitis, non-alcoholic hepatitis, rheumatoid arthritis, osteoarthritis, type II diabetes, insulin insensitivity, Parkinson's disease, and Alzheimer's disease. There also is strong evidence that enhancing activity or expression of any factor or factors related to the GLUT4 translocation or GLUT4 activation pathways will in turn enhance insulin sensitivity. There also is strong evidence that enhancing activation or expression of any factors related to or part of the growth hormone signal transduction pathway will enhance endogenous protein synthesis. It is desirable to use such knowledge to create drugs and agents for the treatment and prevention of such disorders.

Web site: http://appft1.uspto.gov/netahtml/PTO/search-bool.html

- **Method of treating anemia**

  Inventor(s): Creasy, Caretha; (Erdenheim, PA), Dillon, Susan B.; (Chester Springs, PA), Lord, Kenneth A.; (Collegeville, PA)

  Correspondence: Ratner & Prestia; P.O. Box 980; Valley Forge; PA; 19482-0980; US

  Patent Application Number: 20030176375

  Date filed: May 14, 2001

  Abstract: hYAK3-2 polypeptides and polynucleotides and methods for producing such polypeptides by recombinant techniques are disclosed. Also disclosed are methods for utilizing hYAK3-2 polypeptides and polynucleotides in the design of protocols for the treatment of bone loss including osteoporosis; inflammatory diseases such as Adult Respiratory Disease Syndrome (ARDS), Rheumatoid arthritis, Osteoarthritis, Inflammatory Bowel Disease (IBD), psoriasis, dermatitis, asthma, allergies; infections such as bacterial, fungal, protozoan and viral infections, particularly infections caused by HIV-1 or HIV-2; HIV-associated **cachexia** and other immunodeficiency disorders; septic shock; pain; injury; cancers including testicular cancer; anorexia; bulimia; neutropenia; cytopenia; anemias, including anemias due to renal insufficiency or to chronic disease, such as autoimmunity or cancer, and drug-induced anemias; polycythemia; myelosuppression; Parkinson's disease; cardiovascular disease including restenosis, atherosclerosis, acute heart failure, myocardial infarction; hypotension; hypertension; urinary retention; angina pectoris; ulcers; benign prostatic hypertrophy; and psychotic and neurological disorders, including anxiety, schizophrenia, manic depression, delirium, dementia, severe mental retardation and dyskinesias, such as Huntington's disease or Gilles dela Tourett's syndrome., among others, and diagnostic assays for such conditions.

  Excerpt(s): This application claims priority to U.S. Ser. No. 60/118,045 filed Feb. 1, 1999, which is incorporated by reference in its entirety. This invention relates to newly identified polynucleotides, polypeptides encoded by them and to the use of such polynucleotides and polypeptides, and to their production. More particularly, the polynucleotides and polypeptides of the present invention relate to a serine/threonine protein kinase, hereinafter referred to as hYAK3-2. The invention also relates to inhibiting or activating the action of such polynucleotides and polypeptides. A number of polypeptide growth factors and hormones mediate their cellular effects through a signal transduction pathway. Transduction of signals from the cell surface receptors for these ligands to intracellular effectors frequently involves phosphorylation or dephosphorylation of specific protein substrates by regulatory protein serine/threonine kinases (PSTK) and phosphatases. Serine/threonine phosphorylation is a major mediator of signal transduction in multicellular organisms. Receptor-bound, membrane-bound and intracellular PSTKs regulate cell proliferation, cell differentiation and signalling processes in many cell types.

Web site: http://appft1.uspto.gov/netahtml/PTO/search-bool.html

- **Methods and reagents for using mammalian melanocortin receptor antagonists to treat cachexia**

  Inventor(s): Cone, Roger D.; (Oregon City, OR), Marks, Daniel L.; (Portland, OR)

  Correspondence: Mcdonnell Boehnen Hulbert & Berghoff; 300 South Wacker Drive; Suite 3200; Chicago; IL; 60606; US

  Patent Application Number: 20030113263

  Date filed: February 13, 2002

  Abstract: The present invention provides recombinant expression constructs comprising nucleic acid encoding mammalian melanocortin receptors, in particular MC-4 melanocortin receptor, and mammalian cells into which said recombinant expression constructs have been introduced that express functional mammalian MC-4 melanocortin receptors. The invention particularly provides such genetically engineered cells expressing the human MC4-R melanocortin receptor for screening compounds for receptor agonist and antagonist activity. The invention also provides screening methods using genetically engineered cells expressing the human MC-4 melanocortin receptor to specifically detect and identify agonists and antagonists for this melanocortin receptor. Such screening methods are provided identifying compounds with MC-4 melanocortin receptor antagonist activity having the capacity to influence or modify metabolism and feeding behavior, particularly pathological feeding behavior such as illness-induced **cachexia.**

  Excerpt(s): This application claims priority to U.S. Serial No. 60/268,357, filed Feb. 13, 2001. The present invention relates to the cloning, expression and functional characterization of mammalian melanocortin MC4 receptor genes. The invention provides nucleic acid encoding mammalian, particularly human MC4 melanocortin receptors, recombinant expression constructs comprising said nucleic acids, and mammalian cells into which said recombinant expression constructs have been introduced, and that express functional mammalian MC4 melanocortin receptors. The invention also provides transgenic animals, most preferably transgenic mice wherein the endogenous murine MC4-R locus is either heterozygously or homozygously disrupted. The invention provides methods for using such genetically-engineered cells and animals to specifically detect and identify MC4-R receptor antagonists. Such screening methods provide a means for identifying compounds with MC4-R melanocortin receptor antagonist activity having the capacity to influence or modify physiological function and animal feeding behavior, particularly pathological feeding behavior such as illness-induced **cachexia.** Under normal circumstances, animals and humans respond to starvation with a complex neuroendocrine response that ultimately leads to an increase in appetite, a relative sparing of lean body mass and burning of fat stores, and an overall decrease in basal metabolic rate (Webber & Macdonald, 1994, Brit. J. Nutr. 71:437-447; Ahima et al., 1996, Nature 382:250-252). In contrast, in some diseases a devastating pathological state of malnutrition known as **cachexia** arises, brought about by a synergistic combination of a dramatic decrease in appetite and an increase in metabolic rate and metabolism of both fat and lean body mass, producing a relative wasting of lean body mass (Tisdale, 1997, J. Natl. Cancer Inst. 89: 1763-1773; Inui, 1999, Cancer Res. 59: 4493-4501; Fong et al., 1989, Amer. J. Phys. 256: R659-R665; Bruera, 1997, Brit. Med. J.

315: 1219-1222; Emery, 1999, Nutrition 15: 600-603). This combination is found in a number of disorders including cancer, cystic fibrosis, AIDS, rheumatoid arthritis, and renal failure (Tisdale, 1997, ibid.).

Web site: http://appft1.uspto.gov/netahtml/PTO/search-bool.html

- **Methods of treating cachexia with chimeric anti-TNF antibodies**

  Inventor(s): Daddona, Peter; (Menlo Park, CA), Ghrayeb, John; (Downingtown, PA), Knight, David; (Berwyn, PA), Le, Junming; (Jackson Heights, NY), Siegel, Scott; (Westborough, MA), Vilcek, Jan; (New York, NY)

  Correspondence: Hamilton, Brook, Smith & Reynolds, P.C.; 530 Virginia Road; P.O. Box 9133; Concord; MA; 01742-9133; US

  Patent Application Number: 20030054004

  Date filed: January 10, 2002

  Abstract: Anti-TNF antibodies, fragments and regions thereof which are specific for human tumor necrosis factor-.alpha.(TNF.alpha.) and are useful in vivo diagnosis and therapy of a number of TNF.alpha.-mediated pathologies and conditions, as well as polynucleotides coding for murine and chimeric antibodies, methods of producing the antibody, methods of use of the anti-TNF antibody, or fragment, region or derivative thereof, in immunoassays and immunotherapeutic approaches are provided.

  Excerpt(s): The present invention in the field of immunology and medicine relates to anti-tumor necrosis factor (TNF) antibodies, anti-TNF peptides and nucleic acids encoding therefor, and to pharmaceutical and diagnostic compositions and production, diagnostic and therapeutic methods thereof, and to methods for treating human TNF-mediated pathologies. Monocytes and macrophages secrete cytokines known as tumor necrosis factor-.alpha. (TNF.alpha.) and tumor necrosis factors-.beta. (TNF.beta.) in response to endotoxin or other stimuli. TNF.alpha. is a soluble homotrimer of 17 kD protein subunits (Smith, et al., J. Biol. Chem. 262:6951-6954 (1987)). A membrane-bound 26 kD precursor form of TNF also exists (Kriegler, et al., Cell 53:45-53 (1988)). For reviews of TNF, see Beutler, et al., Nature 320:584 (1986), Old, Science 230:630 (1986), and Le, et al., Lab. Invest. 56:234. Cells other than monocytes or macrophages also make TNF.alpha. For example, human non-monocytic tumor cell lines produce TNF (Rubin, et al., J. Exp. Med. 164:1350 (1986); Spriggs, et al., Proc. Natl. Acad. Sci. USA 84:6563 (1987)). CD4.sup.+ and CD8.sup.+ peripheral blood T lymphocytes and some cultured T and B cell lines (Cuturi, et al., J. Exp. Med. 165:1581 (1987); Sung, etal., J. Exp. Med. 168:1539 (1988)) also produce TNF.alpha.

  Web site: http://appft1.uspto.gov/netahtml/PTO/search-bool.html

- **Methods using TCF II**

  Inventor(s): Iemura, Akihiro; (Kurume-shi, JP), Kojiro, Masamichi; (Fukuoka, JP), Yano, Hirohisa; (Fukuoka, JP)

  Correspondence: Testa, Hurwitz & Thibeault, Llp; High Street Tower; 125 High Street; Boston; MA; 02110; US

  Patent Application Number: 20030082134

  Date filed: October 9, 2002

Abstract: The present invention provides an agent for preventing and/or treating **cachexia** comprising T-CF-II as an effective ingredient. An agent for preventing and treating **cachexia** caused by cancer, acquired immunodeficient syndrome (AIDS), cardiac diseases, infectious disease, shock, burn, endotoxinemia, organ inflammation, surgery, diabetes, collagen diseases, radiotherapy, chemotherapy is provided by the present invention.

Excerpt(s): The present invention relates to an agent for preventing and/or treating **cachexia** comprising Tumor Cytotoxic Factor-II (TCF-II) or hepatocyte growth factor (HGF) as an effective ingredient. In particular, the present invention relates to the use of TCF-II or HGF as agent for preventing and treating **cachexia** caused by one of the factors selected from the group consisting of cancer, acquired immunodeficient syndrome (AIDS), cardiac diseases, infectious disease, shock, burn, endotoxinemia, organ inflammation, surgery, diabetes, collagen diseases, radiotherapy, chemotherapy is provided by the present invention. Generally, a disease such as cancer, acquired immunodeficiency (AIDS), cardiac disease will accompany with anorexia, weight loss, physical exhaustion, marasmus, dermatrophia, xerosis, anemia, edema, abnormal blood coagulation-fibrinolysis and this pathology is defined as **cachexia.** After suffering from this systemic marasmus, a patient will eventually die (Tamaguma, M. et. al., Igakuno-ayumi, 149, 371-373 (1989)). Further, if radiotherapy and/or chemotherapy is carried out for a patient with progressive or terminal cancer for whom curative operation can not be expected, it may lead to extremely lowered biological body defensive function such as immunological function due to specific malnutrition, resulting in shortening life. Therefore, there are serious problems in practical treatment of **cachexia.** The cause of **cachexia** has been so far considered to be triggered by imbalance of nutritional equilibrium resulting from lowered nutrition intake combined with increased nutrition consumption, along with affection of humoric factors mobilized from the cancer or tile lesion oil systemic metabolism. In the above situations, positive alimentation is carried out using total parental nutrition in order to supplement extreme nutritional or energetic deficiency and enhance immunological function in the treatment of **cachexia.** However, in **cachexia,** intake of energy will be used not for saving patient's life but for proliferation of tumor cells, so that alimentation can not be sufficient for a cachexic patient. Recently, monokines or cytokines, such as Tumor Necrosis Factor (TNF) mobilized from macrophage, have been implicated in the pathogenesis of **cachexia.** TNF was found as a factor of affecting tumor cells and elucidated to be secreted by macrophages which is one of immunocytes and has a phagocytic action. Though it was originally studied as a potential anti-cancer drug because of its direct cytotoxic effect and strong anti-tumor activity, recently various kinds of action of TNF have been investigated since it was found that TNF may cause **cachexia** that is marasmus including weight loss of a patient with cancer, severe infectious disease, or a ringleader cytokine induced inflammation. The main actions of TNF are: (1) osteoclastic action, (2) induction of hyperlipidemia by inhibition of uptake of lipid into cell, (3) induction of production of interleukin 1 and colony stimulation factor, (4) impairment of angioendotherial cell, and (5) intervening reaction of exotoxin shock in grave infectious disease.

Web site: http://appft1.uspto.gov/netahtml/PTO/search-bool.html

- **Novel transcription factor regulating TNF-alpha**

  Inventor(s): Amar, Salomon; (Brookline, MA)

  Correspondence: Kevin M. Farrell; Pierce Atwood; Suite 350; One New Hampshire Avenue; Portsmouth; NH; 03801; US

  Patent Application Number: 20030166159

  Date filed: April 2, 2003

  Abstract: Disclosed herein is an isolated polypeptide which binds to the DNA binding domain located from -550 to -487 in the promoter of the human TNF-.alpha. gene. This isolated polypeptide is referred to herein as the LITAF protein. Polypeptides of human origin are specifically provided. Also disclosed is a nucleic acid sequence which encodes the LITAF protein. Such nucleic acids may be incorporated into an expression vector, which may be inserted into a cell. LITAF dependent induction of TNF-.alpha. gene expression in a cell can be inhibited by delivering an inhibitor of expression of the LITAF gene to the cell. Such an inhibitor is for example an antisense construct which encodes an antisense RNA molecule which is complementary to a portion of the LITAF mRNA which is greater than 200 nucleotides in length. Preferably, the antisense RNA molecule is complementary to the start site of translation, upstream adjacent 5' untranslated sequence, and downstream adjacent coding sequence of the LITAF mRNA. Optimal lengths and specific nucleotides for complementary are discussed. Inhibition of LITAF dependent induction of TNF-.alpha. gene expression in a cell can also be achieved by contacting an inhibitor of LITAF protein function to the LITAF protein within a cell. Such an inhibitor may be an antibody which binds the LITAF protein, or alternatively a small molecule which inhibits the function of the LITAF protein. One example of such an inhibitor is a recombinant mutant LITAF protein. Administration of a LITAF inhibitor can be performed as a therapeutic method for treating a patient with a disease associated with chronic inflammation. Such diseases include rheumatoid arthritis, gum disease Crohn's disease, and graft-versus-host disease. Therapeutic methods for treating a patient with a disease in which TNF-.alpha. plays a role in pathology are also provided. Examples of such diseases are diabetes mellitus, cancer, **cachexia,** breast cancer, HIV, sepsis, malaria, trypanomiasis and asthma. Other methods provided include a method for identifying genes which are regulated by the LITAF protein, a method for identifying a molecule which inhibits LITAF binding to the TNF-.alpha. promoter, and a method for identifying molecules which bind LITAF from a protein array.

  Excerpt(s): The innate host response to bacterial pathogens is characterized by an immediate release of biologically active compounds, including monokines and cytokines. These proinflammatory molecules, which are intended to enable the host to eliminate the pathogen, may also adversely affect the host. In acute situations, the pathogen is often eliminated, with resolution of inflammation and minimal tissue damage. However, failure to control the pathogen often leads to a state of metabolic anarchy in which the inflammatory response is not controlled and significant tissue damage results. Endotoxins, produced from the outer membrane of Gram-negative bacteria, and exotoxins, released from the cell wall of Gram-positive bacteria, are known to be potent inducers of the inflammatory response. Lipopolysaccharide (LPS), extracted from the outer membrane of Gram-negative bacteria, has been identified as a principal endotoxic component. Although the inflammatory response is mediated by a variety of secreted factors, the cytotoxic effects of LPS have been ascribed to TNF-.alpha. activity (Beutler et al., Science 229: 869-871 (1985); Tracey et al., Science 234: 470-474 (1986); Miethke et al., J. Exp. Med. 175: 91-98 (1992)). TNF-.alpha. is a pleiotropic cytokine which serves to either benefit the host or in some situations exert detrimental effects on the host (Beutler and Cerami, Nature 320: 584-588 (1986); Beutler et al., Science 232: 977-980 (1986); Beutler and Cerami, N. Engl. J. Med. 316: 379-385 (1987)). TNF-.alpha. benefits the host by helping to prevent cancer, protecting against infection, promoting tissue remodeling, and activating inflammatory responses. Conversely, in host responses which have gone awry, TNF-.alpha. mediates septic shock in chronic infections, is responsible for **cachexia** in cancer patients, causes inflammation in rheumatoid arthritis patients, and activates the human immunodeficiency virus. The pleiotropic effects of TNF-.alpha. are dose-dependent. Hence, the perceived need to control TNF-.alpha. production has raised interest into the understanding of the mechanisms that modulate TNF-.alpha. gene expression. It is well known that gene transcription is controlled by DNA-binding proteins. Recently, several groups have examined the transcriptional regulation of TNF-.alpha. by various inducers, such as virus, LPS, and PMA. The human TNF-.alpha. promoter contains motifs that resemble nuclear factor kappa B (NF-.kappa.B) binding sites; however, controversy exists as to the involvement of NF-.kappa.B in TNF-.alpha. gene regulation. The nature of the nuclear factor(s) involved in the regulation of LPS-induced TNF-.alpha. gene expression in humans remains unknown.

Web site: http://appft1.uspto.gov/netahtml/PTO/search-bool.html

- **Novel use for muscarinic receptor M5 in the diagnosis and treatment of metabolic disorders**

  Inventor(s): White, David W.; (Braintree, MA)

  Correspondence: Millennium Pharmaceuticals, INC.; 75 Sidney Street; Cambridge; MA; 02139; US

  Patent Application Number: 20030092041

  Date filed: August 22, 2002

  Abstract: The present invention relates to methods and compositions for the diagnosis and treatment of metabolic disorders, including, but not limited to, obesity, diabetes, overweight anorexia, or **cachexia.** The present invention describes methods for the diagnostic evaluation and prognosis of various metabolic disorders and obesity, for the identification of subjects exhibiting a predisposition to such conditions, as well as the diagnostic monitoring of patients undergoing clinical evaluation for the treatment of metabolic disease and obesity, and for monitoring the efficacy of compounds in clinical trials. The invention further provides methods for identifying a compound capable of modulating a metabolic activity as well as treating a metabolic disorder. In addition, the invention provides methods useful for modulating a metabolic activity as well as for treating a subject having a metabolic disorder characterized by either aberrant M5 polypeptide activity or aberrant M5 nucleic acid expression.

  Excerpt(s): Obesity represents the most prevalent of body weight disorders, affecting an estimated 30 to 50% of the middle-aged population in the western world. Other body weight disorders, such as anorexia nervosa and bulimia nervosa, which together affect approximately 0.2% of the female population of the western world, also pose serious health threats. Further, such disorders as anorexia and **cachexia** (wasting) are also prominent features of other diseases such as cancer, cystic fibrosis, and AIDS. Obesity, defined as a body mass index (BMI) of 30 kg/.sup.2m or more, contributes to diseases such as coronary artery disease, hypertension, stroke, diabetes, hyperlipidemia and some cancers. (See, e.g., Nishina, P. M. et al. (1994), Metab. 43:554-558; Grundy, S. M. &

Barnett, J. P. (1990), Dis. Mon. 36:641-731). Obesity is a complex multifactorial chronic disease that develops from an interaction of genotype and the environment and involves social, behavioral, cultural, physiological, metabolic and genetic factors. Diabetes mellitus is the most common metabolic disease worldwide. Daily 1700 new cases of diabetes are diagnosed in the United States, while at least one-third of the 16 million Americans with diabetes are unaware of it. Diabetes is the leading cause of blindness, renal failure, and lower limb amputations in adults and is a major risk factor for cardiovascular disease and stroke. Normal glucose homeostasis requires the finely tuned orchestration of insulin secretion by pancreatic beta cells in response to subtle changes in blood glucose levels, delicately balanced with secretion of counter-regulatory hormones such as glucagon. One of the fundamental actions of insulin is to stimulate uptake of glucose from the blood into tissues, especially muscle and fat. Type 1 diabetes results from autoimmune destruction of pancreatic beta cells causing insulin deficiency. Type 2 or non-insulin-dependent diabetes mellitus (NIDDM) accounts for >90% of cases and is characterized by a triad of (1) resistance to insulin action on glucose uptake in peripheral tissues, especially skeletal muscle and adipocytes, (2) impaired insulin action to inhibit hepatic glucose production, and (3) misregulated insulin secretion (DeFronzo, (1997) Diabetes Rev. 5:177-269). In most cases, type 2 diabetes is a polygenic disease with complex inheritance patterns (reviewed in Kahn et al., (1996) Annu. Rev. Med. 47:509-531).

Web site: http://appft1.uspto.gov/netahtml/PTO/search-bool.html

- **Nutritional compositions**

Inventor(s): Troup, John P.; (Commugny, CH), Wolfe, Robert R.; (League City, TX)

Correspondence: Thomas Hoxie; Novartis, Corporate Intellectual Property; One Health Plaza 430/2; East Hanover; NJ; 07936-1080; US

Patent Application Number: 20040087490

Date filed: September 15, 2003

Abstract: Compositions for the promotion of muscle protein synthesis and control of tumor-induced weight loss in patients that are, for example, suffering from cancer **cachexia,** and methods of administering such compositions.

Excerpt(s): This application claims the benefit of U.S. Provisional Application No. 60/412,370, filed Sep. 20, 2002; U.S. Provisional Application No. 60/417,203, filed Oct. 9, 2002; and U.S. Provisional Application No. 60/455,921 filed Mar. 19, 2003. Disclosed are methods and nutritional compositions for the promotion of muscle protein synthesis or the control of tumor-induced weight loss, such as cancer **cachexia.** Cachexia is a condition of severe malnutrition and negative nitrogen balance characterized by anorexia (i.e. a lack or severe loss of appetite), weight loss, and muscle atrophy. The physiological, metabolic, and behavioral changes in **cachexia** are associated with patient complaints of weakness, fatigue, gastrointestinal distress, sleep/wake disturbances, pain, listlessness, shortness of breath, lethargy, depression, malaise and the fear of being burdensome on family and friends. Although **cachexia** has been classically associated with chronic infections and malignant conditions, it has also been identified in patients after extensive traumatic injury and sepsis and in aging persons with failure to thrive syndrome.

Web site: http://appft1.uspto.gov/netahtml/PTO/search-bool.html

- **Plasmid mediated supplementation for treating chronically ill subjects**

  Inventor(s): Brenner, Malcolm K.; (Bellaire, TX), Carpenter, Robert H.; (Bastrop, TX), Draghia-Akli, Ruxandra; (Houston, TX), Hahn, Kevin; (Missouri City, TX), Kern, Douglas R.; (The Woodlands, TX), King, Glen; (Rosharon, TX), Schwartz, Robert J.; (Houston, TX)

  Correspondence: Jackson Walker Llp; 2435 North Central Expressway; Suite 600; Richardson; TX; 75080; US

  Patent Application Number: 20040057941

  Date filed: December 10, 2002

  Abstract: The present invention pertains to compositions and methods for plasmid-mediated supplementation. The compositions and method are useful for retarding the growth of the tumor, and retarding **cachexia,** wasting, anemia and other effects that are commonly associated in cancer bearing animals. Overall, the embodiments of the invention can be accomplished by delivering an effective amount of a nucleic acid expression construct that encodes a GHRH or functional biological equivalent thereof into a tissue of an animal and allowing expression of the encoded gene in the animal. For example, when such a nucleic acid sequence is delivered into the specific cells of the animal tissue specific constitutive expression is achieved. Furthermore, external regulation of the GHRH or functional biological equivalent thereof gene can be accomplished by utilizing inducible promoters that are regulated by molecular switch molecules, which are given to the animal. The preferred method to deliver the constitutive or inducible nucleic acid encoding sequences of GHRH or the functional biological equivalents thereof is directly into the cells of the animal by the process of in vivo electroporation. In addition, a treatment for retarding the growth of the tumor, and retarding **cachexia** or the wasting effects that are commonly associated with tumors is achieved by the delivery of recombinant GHRH or biological equivalent into the animal.

  Excerpt(s): This application claims priority to U.S. Provisional Patent Application Serial No. 60/339,610 entitled "Plasmid Mediated Treatment for Anemia, Wasting, Immune Dysfunction and Life Extension for the Chronically Ill," filed on Dec. 11, 2001, the entire content of which is hereby incorporated by reference. 10) extending life expectancy and increasing survival for the chronically ill subject. The present invention pertains to compositions and methods that are useful for retarding the growth rate of abnormal cells, tumor progression reduction, prevention of kidney failure, reduction of metastasis, and increased survival in cancer-bearing animals. Overall, the embodiments of the invention can be accomplished by delivering an effective amount of a nucleic acid expression construct that encodes a GHRH or functional biological equivalent thereof into a tissue of a subject and allowing expression of the encoded gene in the subject. For example, when such a nucleic acid sequence is delivered into the specific cells of the subject tissue specific constitutive expression is achieved. Furthermore, external regulation of the GHRH or functional biological equivalent thereof gene can be accomplished by utilizing inducible promoters that are regulated by molecular switch molecules, which are given to the subject. The preferred method to deliver the constitutive or inducible nucleic acid encoding sequences of GHRH or the functional biological equivalents thereof is directly into the cells of the subject by the process of in vivo electroporation. In addition, a treatment for retarding the growth of abnormal cells and tumor growth is achieved by the delivery of recombinant GHRH or biological equivalent into the subject. Anemia, wasting, tumor growth, immune dysfunction, kidney failure, cancer, decreased life expectancy, and other conditions also can be related to a specific cancer, tumor, disease or the effects of a disease treatment GHRH could be also delivered directly, as protein, by intravenous, subcutaneous or intranasal administration or through a slow release pump.

Web site: http://appft1.uspto.gov/netahtml/PTO/search-bool.html

- **Therapeutic agent for cachexia**

  Inventor(s): Ishii, Kimie; (Shizuoka, JP), Sato, Koh; (Shizuoka, JP), Tsunenari, Toshiaki; (Shizuoka, JP)

  Correspondence: Finnegan, Henderson, Farabow, Garrett &; Dunner Llp; 1300 I Street, NW; Washington; DC; 20006; US

  Patent Application Number: 20030138424

  Date filed: January 8, 2003

  Abstract: The invention relates to a therapeutic agent for **cachexia** comprising, as an active ingredient, a substance capab;le of inhibiting the binding between a parathyroid hormone related protein (PTHrP) and a receptor thereof.

  Excerpt(s): The present invention relates to a therapeutic agent for **cachexia** comprising a substance capable of inhibiting the binding between parathyroid hormone related protein (PTHrP) and a receptor thereof as an active ingredient. Cachexia found in terminal cancer patients is one of the common paraneoplastic syndromes of malignancy, and characterized by systemic disorders with anorexia, weight loss, anemia, electrolyte imbalance and compromised immune function as main symptoms. The development of **cachexia** in cancer patients leads to fatal and terminal symptoms; impairs the Quality-of-life (QOL) of the patients; and gives strong psychological, physical and social impacts on the patients and their families and surrounding people. Recently, it has been found that cachectin, which is believed to be a causative agent of cancer **cachexia,** is identical to tumor necrosis factor (TNF). Thereafter, it has also been found that cytokines (e.g., interleukin (IL)-1, IL-6, LIF, IFN) also have the same actions as cachectin and thus **cachexia** is induced by composite action of multiple factors.

  Web site: http://appft1.uspto.gov/netahtml/PTO/search-bool.html

- **Thiazole derivatives**

  Inventor(s): Cooper, Christopher B.; (Lawrenceville, NJ), Helal, Chris J.; (Mystic, CT), Sanner, Mark A.; (Old Saybrook, CT)

  Correspondence: Pfizer Inc; 150 East 42nd Street; 5th Floor - Stop 49; New York; NY; 10017-5612; US

  Patent Application Number: 20030078252

  Date filed: May 13, 2002

  Abstract: The invention provides compounds of formula 1 1wherein R.sup.1, R.sup.3, and R.sup.4 are as defined, and their pharmaceutically acceptable salts. Compounds of formula 1 are indicated to have activity inhibiting cdk5, cdk2, and GSK-3. Pharmaceutical compositions and methods comprising compounds of formula 1 for treating diseases and conditions comprising abnormal cell growth, such as cancer, and neurodegenerative diseases and conditions and those affected by dopamine neurotransmission are described. Also described are pharmaceutical compositions and methods comprising compounds of formula 1 for treating male fertility and sperm motility; diabetes mellitus; impaired glucose tolerance; metabolic syndrome or syndrome X; polycystic ovary syndrome; adipogenesis and obesity; myogenesis and frailty, for example age-related decline in physical performance; acute sarcopenia, for example muscle atrophy and/or **cachexia** associated with burns, bed rest, limb immobilization, or major thoracic, abdominal, and/or orthopedic surgery; sepsis; hair loss, hair thinning, and balding; and immunodeficiency.

Excerpt(s): This application claims priority under 35 U.S.C. 119(e) of U.S. application Ser. No. 60/290,466, filed May 11, 2001. The subject invention relates to thiazole derivatives, pharmaceutical compositions comprising such derivatives and methods of using such derivatives to treat abnormal cell growth and certain diseases and conditions of the central nervous system. The compounds of the present invention act as inhibitors of cyclin-dependent protein kinase enzymes cdk5 (cyclin-dependent protein kinase 5) and cdk2 (cyclin-dependent protein kinase 2). The compounds of the present invention also are inhibitors of the enzyme GSK-3 (glygogen synthase kinase-3) enzyme. The serine/threonine kinase cdk5 along with its cofactor p25 (or the longer cofactor, p35) has been linked to neurodegenerative disorders, and inhibitors of cdk5/p25 (or cdk5/p35) are therefore useful for the treatment of neurodegenerative disorders such as Alzheimer's disease, Parkinson's disease, stroke, or Huntington's disease. Treatment of such neurodegenerative disorders using cdk5 inhibitors is supported by the finding that cdk5 is involved in the phosphorylation of tau protein (J. Biochem, 117, 741-749 (1995)). cdk5 also phosphorylates Dopamine and Cyclic AMP-Regulated Phosphorprotein (DARPP-32) at threonine 75 and is thus indicated in having a role in dopaminergic neurotransmission (Nature, 402, 669-671 (1999)).

Web site: http://appft1.uspto.gov/netahtml/PTO/search-bool.html

- **Use for endothelin converting enzyme 2 (ECE-2) in the diagnosis and treatment of metabolic disorders**

  Inventor(s): White, David; (Braintree, MA)

  Correspondence: Kerri Pollard Schray; Millennium Pharmaceuticals, INC.; 75 Sidney Street; Cambridge; MA; 02139; US

  Patent Application Number: 20030232044

  Date filed: June 3, 2003

  Abstract: The invention relates to methods and compositions for the diagnosis and treatment of metabolic disorders including, but not limited to, obesity, diabetes, overweight, insulin resistance, anorexia, and **cachexia;** and disorders of appetite regulation, including hyperphagia. The invention further provides methods for identifying a compound capable of treating a metabolic disorder or a disorder of appetite regulation. The invention also provides methods for identifying a compound capable of modulating a metabolic activity or regulation of appetite. Yet further, the invention provides methods for modulating a metabolic activity and methods for modulating appetite regulation. In addition, the invention provides methods for treating a subject having a metabolic disorder or a disorder of appetite regulation characterized by aberrant ECE-2 polypeptide activity or aberrant ECE-2 nucleic acid expression.

  Excerpt(s): This application claims the benefit of U.S. Provisional Application No. 60/386,333, filed Jun. 5, 2002, the contents of which are incorporated herein by this reference. Obesity represents the most prevalent of body weight disorders, affecting an estimated 30 to 50% of the middle-aged population in the western world. Other body weight disorders, such as anorexia nervosa and bulimia nervosa, which together affect approximately 0.2% of the female population of the western world, also pose serious health threats. Further, such disorders as anorexia and **cachexia** (wasting) are also prominent features of other diseases such as cancer, cystic fibrosis, and AIDS. Obesity, defined as a body mass index (BMI) of 30 kg/M.sup.2 or more, contributes to diseases such as coronary artery disease, hypertension, stroke, diabetes, hyperlipidemia and some cancers. (See, e.g., Nishina, P. M. et al. (1994), Metab. 43:554-558; Grundy, S. M. & Barnett, J. P. (1990), Dis. Mon. 36:641-731). Obesity is a complex multifactorial chronic disease that develops from an interaction of genotype and the environment and involves social, behavioral, cultural, physiological, metabolic and genetic factors.

Web site: http://appft1.uspto.gov/netahtml/PTO/search-bool.html

- **Use of human not1and not1a orphan receptors**

  Inventor(s): Cairns, William John; (Essex, GB), Holder, Julie Caroline; (Hertfordshire, GB), Patel, Lisa; (Essex, GB)

  Correspondence: Smithkline Beecham Corporation; Corporate Intellectual Property-Us, Uw2220; P. O. Box 1539; King OF Prussia; PA; 19406-0939; US

  Patent Application Number: 20030153497

  Date filed: February 14, 2003

  Abstract: The use of NOT1 or NOT1 a polypeptides and polynucleotides in the design of protocols for the treatment of obesity, insulin resistance, type 2 diabetes, impaired glucose tolerance, **cachexia** or liposarcoma among others, and diagnostic assays for such conditions.

  Excerpt(s): This invention relates to new uses for polynucleotides and polypeptides encoded by them, to their use in therapy and in identifying compounds which may be agonists which are potentially useful in therapy. In one aspect, the invention relates to new uses of the orphan nuclear receptor, NOT1 or its splice variant NOT1a polynucleotides and polypeptides. Such uses include the treatment of obesity, insulin resistance, type 2 diabetes, impaired glucose tolerance, **cachexia** and liposarcoma, hereinafter referred to as "the Diseases", amongst others In another aspect the invention relates to methods for identifying compounds which activate NOT1 or NOT1a polypeptides, for example agonists, using NOT1 or NOT1a materials, and treating conditions associated with NOT1 or NOT1a imbalance with the identified agonist compounds. In a still further aspect, the invention relates to diagnostic assays for detecting diseases associated with inappropriateNOT1 or NOT1a activity or levels. (vi) liposarcoma.

  Web site: http://appft1.uspto.gov/netahtml/PTO/search-bool.html

Keeping Current

In order to stay informed about patents and patent applications dealing with cachexia, you can access the U.S. Patent Office archive via the Internet at the following Web address: **http://www.uspto.gov/patft/index.html**. You will see two broad options: (1) Issued Patent, and (2) Published Applications. To see a list of issued patents, perform the following steps: Under "Issued Patents," click "Quick Search." Then, type "cachexia" (or synonyms) into the

"Term 1" box. After clicking on the search button, scroll down to see the various patents which have been granted to date on cachexia.

You can also use this procedure to view pending patent applications concerning cachexia. Simply go back to **http://www.uspto.gov/patft/index.html**. Select "Quick Search" under "Published Applications." Then proceed with the steps listed above.

CHAPTER 5. BOOKS ON CACHEXIA

Overview

This chapter provides bibliographic book references relating to cachexia. In addition to online booksellers such as **www.amazon.com** and **www.bn.com**, excellent sources for book titles on cachexia include the Combined Health Information Database and the National Library of Medicine. Your local medical library also may have these titles available for loan.

Book Summaries: Online Booksellers

Commercial Internet-based booksellers, such as Amazon.com and Barnes&Noble.com, offer summaries which have been supplied by each title's publisher. Some summaries also include customer reviews. Your local bookseller may have access to in-house and commercial databases that index all published books (e.g. Books in Print®). **IMPORTANT NOTE:** Online booksellers typically produce search results for medical and non-medical books. When searching for "cachexia" at online booksellers' Web sites, you may discover non-medical books that use the generic term "cachexia" (or a synonym) in their titles. The following is indicative of the results you might find when searching for "cachexia" (sorted alphabetically by title; follow the hyperlink to view more details at Amazon.com):

- **Protein and Amino Acid Metabolism in Cancer Cachexia (Medical Intelligence Unit)** by Peter W. T. Pisters, Murray F. Brennan; ISBN: 0412100312; http://www.amazon.com/exec/obidos/ASIN/0412100312/icongroupinterna

CHAPTER 6. PERIODICALS AND NEWS ON CACHEXIA

Overview

In this chapter, we suggest a number of news sources and present various periodicals that cover cachexia.

News Services and Press Releases

One of the simplest ways of tracking press releases on cachexia is to search the news wires. In the following sample of sources, we will briefly describe how to access each service. These services only post recent news intended for public viewing.

PR Newswire

To access the PR Newswire archive, simply go to **http://www.prnewswire.com/**. Select your country. Type "cachexia" (or synonyms) into the search box. You will automatically receive information on relevant news releases posted within the last 30 days. The search results are shown by order of relevance.

Reuters Health

The Reuters' Medical News and Health eLine databases can be very useful in exploring news archives relating to cachexia. While some of the listed articles are free to view, others are available for purchase for a nominal fee. To access this archive, go to **http://www.reutershealth.com/en/index.html** and search by "cachexia" (or synonyms). The following was recently listed in this archive for cachexia:

- **NSAIDs reduce lung cancer growth, cachexia in mice**
  Source: Reuters Industry Breifing
  Date: June 09, 2004
- **Molecular mechanism behind skeletal muscle decay in cachexia elucidated**
  Source: Reuters Medical News
  Date: September 28, 2000

The NIH

Within MEDLINEplus, the NIH has made an agreement with the New York Times Syndicate, the AP News Service, and Reuters to deliver news that can be browsed by the public. Search news releases at **http://www.nlm.nih.gov/medlineplus/alphanews_a.html**. MEDLINEplus allows you to browse across an alphabetical index. Or you can search by date at the following Web page: **http://www.nlm.nih.gov/medlineplus/newsbydate.html**. Often, news items are indexed by MEDLINEplus within its search engine.

Business Wire

Business Wire is similar to PR Newswire. To access this archive, simply go to **http://www.businesswire.com/**. You can scan the news by industry category or company name.

Market Wire

Market Wire is more focused on technology than the other wires. To browse the latest press releases by topic, such as alternative medicine, biotechnology, fitness, healthcare, legal, nutrition, and pharmaceuticals, access Market Wire's Medical/Health channel at **http://www.marketwire.com/mw/release_index?channel=MedicalHealth**. Or simply go to Market Wire's home page at **http://www.marketwire.com/mw/home**, type "cachexia" (or synonyms) into the search box, and click on "Search News." As this service is technology oriented, you may wish to use it when searching for press releases covering diagnostic procedures or tests.

Search Engines

Medical news is also available in the news sections of commercial Internet search engines. See the health news page at Yahoo (**http://dir.yahoo.com/Health/News_and_Media/**), or you can use this Web site's general news search page at **http://news.yahoo.com/**. Type in "cachexia" (or synonyms). If you know the name of a company that is relevant to cachexia, you can go to any stock trading Web site (such as **http://www.etrade.com/**) and search for the company name there. News items across various news sources are reported on indicated hyperlinks. Google offers a similar service at **http://news.google.com/**.

BBC

Covering news from a more European perspective, the British Broadcasting Corporation (BBC) allows the public free access to their news archive located at **http://www.bbc.co.uk/**. Search by "cachexia" (or synonyms).

Academic Periodicals covering Cachexia

Numerous periodicals are currently indexed within the National Library of Medicine's PubMed database that are known to publish articles relating to cachexia. In addition to these sources, you can search for articles covering cachexia that have been published by any of the periodicals listed in previous chapters. To find the latest studies published, go to **http://www.ncbi.nlm.nih.gov/pubmed**, type the name of the periodical into the search box, and click "Go."

If you want complete details about the historical contents of a journal, you can also visit the following Web site: **http://www.ncbi.nlm.nih.gov/entrez/jrbrowser.cgi**. Here, type in the name of the journal or its abbreviation, and you will receive an index of published articles. At **http://locatorplus.gov/**, you can retrieve more indexing information on medical periodicals (e.g. the name of the publisher). Select the button "Search LOCATORplus." Then type in the name of the journal and select the advanced search option "Journal Title Search."

CHAPTER 7. RESEARCHING MEDICATIONS

Overview

While a number of hard copy or CD-ROM resources are available for researching medications, a more flexible method is to use Internet-based databases. Broadly speaking, there are two sources of information on approved medications: public sources and private sources. We will emphasize free-to-use public sources.

U.S. Pharmacopeia

Because of historical investments by various organizations and the emergence of the Internet, it has become rather simple to learn about the medications recommended for cachexia. One such source is the United States Pharmacopeia. In 1820, eleven physicians met in Washington, D.C. to establish the first compendium of standard drugs for the United States. They called this compendium the U.S. Pharmacopeia (USP). Today, the USP is a non-profit organization consisting of 800 volunteer scientists, eleven elected officials, and 400 representatives of state associations and colleges of medicine and pharmacy. The USP is located in Rockville, Maryland, and its home page is located at **http://www.usp.org/**. The USP currently provides standards for over 3,700 medications. The resulting USP DI® Advice for the Patient® can be accessed through the National Library of Medicine of the National Institutes of Health. The database is partially derived from lists of federally approved medications in the Food and Drug Administration's (FDA) Drug Approvals database, located at **http://www.fda.gov/cder/da/da.htm**.

While the FDA database is rather large and difficult to navigate, the Phamacopeia is both user-friendly and free to use. It covers more than 9,000 prescription and over-the-counter medications. To access this database, simply type the following hyperlink into your Web browser: **http://www.nlm.nih.gov/medlineplus/druginformation.html**. To view examples of a given medication (brand names, category, description, preparation, proper use, precautions, side effects, etc.), simply follow the hyperlinks indicated within the United States Pharmacopeia (USP).

Below, we have compiled a list of medications associated with cachexia. If you would like more information on a particular medication, the provided hyperlinks will direct you to ample documentation (e.g. typical dosage, side effects, drug-interaction risks, etc.). The following drugs have been mentioned in the Pharmacopeia and other sources as being potentially applicable to cachexia:

Progestins For Noncontraceptive Use

- **Systemic - U.S. Brands:** Amen; Aygestin; Crinone; Curretab; Cycrin; Depo-Provera; Gesterol 50; Gesterol LA 250; Hy/Gestrone; Hylutin; Megace; Prodrox; Prometrium; Pro-Span; Provera
  http://www.nlm.nih.gov/medlineplus/druginfo/uspdi/202758.html

Commercial Databases

In addition to the medications listed in the USP above, a number of commercial sites are available by subscription to physicians and their institutions. Or, you may be able to access these sources from your local medical library.

Mosby's Drug Consult™

Mosby's Drug Consult™ database (also available on CD-ROM and book format) covers 45,000 drug products including generics and international brands. It provides prescribing information, drug interactions, and patient information. Subscription information is available at the following hyperlink: **http://www.mosbysdrugconsult.com/**.

PDR*health*

The PDR*health* database is a free-to-use, drug information search engine that has been written for the public in layman's terms. It contains FDA-approved drug information adapted from the Physicians' Desk Reference (PDR) database. PDR*health* can be searched by brand name, generic name, or indication. It features multiple drug interactions reports. Search PDR*health* at **http://www.pdrhealth.com/drug_info/index.html**.

Other Web Sites

Drugs.com (**www.drugs.com**) reproduces the information in the Pharmacopeia as well as commercial information. You may also want to consider the Web site of the Medical Letter, Inc. (**http://www.medletter.com/**) which allows users to download articles on various drugs and therapeutics for a nominal fee.

Researching Orphan Drugs

Although the list of orphan drugs is revised on a daily basis, you can quickly research orphan drugs that might be applicable to cachexia by using the database managed by the National Organization for Rare Disorders, Inc. (NORD), at **http://www.rarediseases.org/**. Scroll down the page, and on the left toolbar, click on "Orphan Drug Designation Database." On this page (**http://www.rarediseases.org/search/noddsearch.html**), type "cachexia" (or synonyms) into the search box, and click "Submit Query." When you receive your results, note that not all of the drugs may be relevant, as some may have been withdrawn from orphan status. Write down or print out the name of each drug and the relevant contact information. From there, visit the Pharmacopeia Web site and type the name of each orphan drug into the search box at **http://www.nlm.nih.gov/medlineplus/druginformation.html**. You may need to contact the sponsor or NORD for further information.

NORD conducts "early access programs for investigational new drugs (IND) under the Food and Drug Administration's (FDA's) approval 'Treatment INDs' programs which allow for a limited number of individuals to receive investigational drugs before FDA marketing approval." If the orphan product about which you are seeking information is approved for marketing, information on side effects can be found on the product's label. If the product is not approved, you may need to contact the sponsor.

The following is a list of orphan drugs currently listed in the NORD Orphan Drug Designation Database for cachexia:

- **Megestrol acetate (trade name: Megace)**
  http://www.rarediseases.org/nord/search/nodd_full?code=208
- **Reduced L-glutathione (trade name: Cachexon)**
  http://www.rarediseases.org/nord/search/nodd_full?code=407

If you have any questions about a medical treatment, the FDA may have an office near you. Look for their number in the blue pages of the phone book. You can also contact the FDA through its toll-free number, 1-888-INFO-FDA (1-888-463-6332), or on the World Wide Web at **www.fda.gov**.

APPENDICES

Appendix A. Physician Resources

Overview

In this chapter, we focus on databases and Internet-based guidelines and information resources created or written for a professional audience.

NIH Guidelines

Commonly referred to as "clinical" or "professional" guidelines, the National Institutes of Health publish physician guidelines for the most common diseases. Publications are available at the following by relevant Institute[10]:

- Office of the Director (OD); guidelines consolidated across agencies available at **http://www.nih.gov/health/consumer/conkey.htm**
- National Institute of General Medical Sciences (NIGMS); fact sheets available at **http://www.nigms.nih.gov/news/facts/**
- National Library of Medicine (NLM); extensive encyclopedia (A.D.A.M., Inc.) with guidelines: **http://www.nlm.nih.gov/medlineplus/healthtopics.html**
- National Cancer Institute (NCI); guidelines available at **http://www.cancer.gov/cancerinfo/list.aspx?viewid=5f35036e-5497-4d86-8c2c-714a9f7c8d25**
- National Eye Institute (NEI); guidelines available at **http://www.nei.nih.gov/order/index.htm**
- National Heart, Lung, and Blood Institute (NHLBI); guidelines available at **http://www.nhlbi.nih.gov/guidelines/index.htm**
- National Human Genome Research Institute (NHGRI); research available at **http://www.genome.gov/page.cfm?pageID=10000375**
- National Institute on Aging (NIA); guidelines available at **http://www.nia.nih.gov/health/**

---

[10] These publications are typically written by one or more of the various NIH Institutes.

- National Institute on Alcohol Abuse and Alcoholism (NIAAA); guidelines available at **http://www.niaaa.nih.gov/publications/publications.htm**
- National Institute of Allergy and Infectious Diseases (NIAID); guidelines available at **http://www.niaid.nih.gov/publications/**
- National Institute of Arthritis and Musculoskeletal and Skin Diseases (NIAMS); fact sheets and guidelines available at **http://www.niams.nih.gov/hi/index.htm**
- National Institute of Child Health and Human Development (NICHD); guidelines available at **http://www.nichd.nih.gov/publications/pubskey.cfm**
- National Institute on Deafness and Other Communication Disorders (NIDCD); fact sheets and guidelines at **http://www.nidcd.nih.gov/health/**
- National Institute of Dental and Craniofacial Research (NIDCR); guidelines available at **http://www.nidr.nih.gov/health/**
- National Institute of Diabetes and Digestive and Kidney Diseases (NIDDK); guidelines available at **http://www.niddk.nih.gov/health/health.htm**
- National Institute on Drug Abuse (NIDA); guidelines available at **http://www.nida.nih.gov/DrugAbuse.html**
- National Institute of Environmental Health Sciences (NIEHS); environmental health information available at **http://www.niehs.nih.gov/external/facts.htm**
- National Institute of Mental Health (NIMH); guidelines available at **http://www.nimh.nih.gov/practitioners/index.cfm**
- National Institute of Neurological Disorders and Stroke (NINDS); neurological disorder information pages available at **http://www.ninds.nih.gov/health_and_medical/disorder_index.htm**
- National Institute of Nursing Research (NINR); publications on selected illnesses at **http://www.nih.gov/ninr/news-info/publications.html**
- National Institute of Biomedical Imaging and Bioengineering; general information at **http://grants.nih.gov/grants/becon/becon_info.htm**
- Center for Information Technology (CIT); referrals to other agencies based on keyword searches available at **http://kb.nih.gov/www_query_main.asp**
- National Center for Complementary and Alternative Medicine (NCCAM); health information available at **http://nccam.nih.gov/health/**
- National Center for Research Resources (NCRR); various information directories available at **http://www.ncrr.nih.gov/publications.asp**
- Office of Rare Diseases; various fact sheets available at **http://rarediseases.info.nih.gov/html/resources/rep_pubs.html**
- Centers for Disease Control and Prevention; various fact sheets on infectious diseases available at **http://www.cdc.gov/publications.htm**

NIH Databases

In addition to the various Institutes of Health that publish professional guidelines, the NIH has designed a number of databases for professionals.[11] Physician-oriented resources provide a wide variety of information related to the biomedical and health sciences, both past and present. The format of these resources varies. Searchable databases, bibliographic citations, full-text articles (when available), archival collections, and images are all available. The following are referenced by the National Library of Medicine:[12]

- **Bioethics:** Access to published literature on the ethical, legal, and public policy issues surrounding healthcare and biomedical research. This information is provided in conjunction with the Kennedy Institute of Ethics located at Georgetown University, Washington, D.C.: **http://www.nlm.nih.gov/databases/databases_bioethics.html**
- **HIV/AIDS Resources:** Describes various links and databases dedicated to HIV/AIDS research: **http://www.nlm.nih.gov/pubs/factsheets/aidsinfs.html**
- **NLM Online Exhibitions:** Describes "Exhibitions in the History of Medicine": **http://www.nlm.nih.gov/exhibition/exhibition.html**. Additional resources for historical scholarship in medicine: **http://www.nlm.nih.gov/hmd/hmd.html**
- **Biotechnology Information:** Access to public databases. The National Center for Biotechnology Information conducts research in computational biology, develops software tools for analyzing genome data, and disseminates biomedical information for the better understanding of molecular processes affecting human health and disease: **http://www.ncbi.nlm.nih.gov/**
- **Population Information:** The National Library of Medicine provides access to worldwide coverage of population, family planning, and related health issues, including family planning technology and programs, fertility, and population law and policy: **http://www.nlm.nih.gov/databases/databases_population.html**
- **Cancer Information:** Access to cancer-oriented databases: **http://www.nlm.nih.gov/databases/databases_cancer.html**
- **Profiles in Science:** Offering the archival collections of prominent twentieth-century biomedical scientists to the public through modern digital technology: **http://www.profiles.nlm.nih.gov/**
- **Chemical Information:** Provides links to various chemical databases and references: **http://sis.nlm.nih.gov/Chem/ChemMain.html**
- **Clinical Alerts:** Reports the release of findings from the NIH-funded clinical trials where such release could significantly affect morbidity and mortality: **http://www.nlm.nih.gov/databases/alerts/clinical_alerts.html**
- **Space Life Sciences:** Provides links and information to space-based research (including NASA): **http://www.nlm.nih.gov/databases/databases_space.html**
- **MEDLINE:** Bibliographic database covering the fields of medicine, nursing, dentistry, veterinary medicine, the healthcare system, and the pre-clinical sciences: **http://www.nlm.nih.gov/databases/databases_medline.html**

---

[11] Remember, for the general public, the National Library of Medicine recommends the databases referenced in MEDLINE*plus* (**http://medlineplus.gov/** or **http://www.nlm.nih.gov/medlineplus/databases.html**).

[12] See **http://www.nlm.nih.gov/databases/databases.html.**

- **Toxicology and Environmental Health Information (TOXNET):** Databases covering toxicology and environmental health: **http://sis.nlm.nih.gov/Tox/ToxMain.html**
- **Visible Human Interface:** Anatomically detailed, three-dimensional representations of normal male and female human bodies: **http://www.nlm.nih.gov/research/visible/visible_human.html**

The NLM Gateway[13]

The NLM (National Library of Medicine) Gateway is a Web-based system that lets users search simultaneously in multiple retrieval systems at the U.S. National Library of Medicine (NLM). It allows users of NLM services to initiate searches from one Web interface, providing one-stop searching for many of NLM's information resources or databases.[14] To use the NLM Gateway, simply go to the search site at **http://gateway.nlm.nih.gov/gw/Cmd**. Type "cachexia" (or synonyms) into the search box and click "Search." The results will be presented in a tabular form, indicating the number of references in each database category.

Results Summary

Category	Items Found
Journal Articles	3868
Books / Periodicals / Audio Visual	54
Consumer Health	712
Meeting Abstracts	99
Other Collections	60
Total	4793

HSTAT[15]

HSTAT is a free, Web-based resource that provides access to full-text documents used in healthcare decision-making.[16] These documents include clinical practice guidelines, quick-reference guides for clinicians, consumer health brochures, evidence reports and technology assessments from the Agency for Healthcare Research and Quality (AHRQ), as well as AHRQ's Put Prevention Into Practice.[17] Simply search by "cachexia" (or synonyms) at the following Web site: **http://text.nlm.nih.gov**.

---

13 Adapted from NLM: **http://gateway.nlm.nih.gov/gw/Cmd?Overview.x.**

14 The NLM Gateway is currently being developed by the Lister Hill National Center for Biomedical Communications (LHNCBC) at the National Library of Medicine (NLM) of the National Institutes of Health (NIH).

15 Adapted from HSTAT: **http://www.nlm.nih.gov/pubs/factsheets/hstat.html.**

16 The HSTAT URL is **http://hstat.nlm.nih.gov/.**

17 Other important documents in HSTAT include: the National Institutes of Health (NIH) Consensus Conference Reports and Technology Assessment Reports; the HIV/AIDS Treatment Information Service (ATIS) resource documents; the Substance Abuse and Mental Health Services Administration's Center for Substance Abuse Treatment (SAMHSA/CSAT) Treatment Improvement Protocols (TIP) and Center for Substance Abuse Prevention (SAMHSA/CSAP) Prevention Enhancement Protocols System (PEPS); the Public Health Service (PHS) Preventive Services Task Force's *Guide to Clinical Preventive Services*; the independent, nonfederal Task Force on Community Services' *Guide to Community Preventive Services*; and the Health Technology Advisory Committee (HTAC) of the Minnesota Health Care Commission (MHCC) health technology evaluations.

Coffee Break: Tutorials for Biologists[18]

Coffee Break is a general healthcare site that takes a scientific view of the news and covers recent breakthroughs in biology that may one day assist physicians in developing treatments. Here you will find a collection of short reports on recent biological discoveries. Each report incorporates interactive tutorials that demonstrate how bioinformatics tools are used as a part of the research process. Currently, all Coffee Breaks are written by NCBI staff.[19] Each report is about 400 words and is usually based on a discovery reported in one or more articles from recently published, peer-reviewed literature.[20] This site has new articles every few weeks, so it can be considered an online magazine of sorts. It is intended for general background information. You can access the Coffee Break Web site at the following hyperlink: **http://www.ncbi.nlm.nih.gov/Coffeebreak/**.

Other Commercial Databases

In addition to resources maintained by official agencies, other databases exist that are commercial ventures addressing medical professionals. Here are some examples that may interest you:

- **CliniWeb International:** Index and table of contents to selected clinical information on the Internet; see **http://www.ohsu.edu/cliniweb/**.
- **Medical World Search:** Searches full text from thousands of selected medical sites on the Internet; see **http://www.mwsearch.com/**.

---

[18] Adapted from **http://www.ncbi.nlm.nih.gov/Coffeebreak/Archive/FAQ.html**.

[19] The figure that accompanies each article is frequently supplied by an expert external to NCBI, in which case the source of the figure is cited. The result is an interactive tutorial that tells a biological story.

[20] After a brief introduction that sets the work described into a broader context, the report focuses on how a molecular understanding can provide explanations of observed biology and lead to therapies for diseases. Each vignette is accompanied by a figure and hypertext links that lead to a series of pages that interactively show how NCBI tools and resources are used in the research process.

APPENDIX B. PATIENT RESOURCES

Overview

Official agencies, as well as federally funded institutions supported by national grants, frequently publish a variety of guidelines written with the patient in mind. These are typically called "Fact Sheets" or "Guidelines." They can take the form of a brochure, information kit, pamphlet, or flyer. Often they are only a few pages in length. Since new guidelines on cachexia can appear at any moment and be published by a number of sources, the best approach to finding guidelines is to systematically scan the Internet-based services that post them.

Patient Guideline Sources

The remainder of this chapter directs you to sources which either publish or can help you find additional guidelines on topics related to cachexia. Due to space limitations, these sources are listed in a concise manner. Do not hesitate to consult the following sources by either using the Internet hyperlink provided, or, in cases where the contact information is provided, contacting the publisher or author directly.

The National Institutes of Health

The NIH gateway to patients is located at **http://health.nih.gov/**. From this site, you can search across various sources and institutes, a number of which are summarized below.

Topic Pages: MEDLINEplus

The National Library of Medicine has created a vast and patient-oriented healthcare information portal called MEDLINEplus. Within this Internet-based system are "health topic pages" which list links to available materials relevant to cachexia. To access this system, log on to **http://www.nlm.nih.gov/medlineplus/healthtopics.html**. From there you can either search using the alphabetical index or browse by broad topic areas. Recently, MEDLINEplus listed the following when searched for "cachexia":

Cancer
http://www.nlm.nih.gov/medlineplus/cancer.html

Cancer Alternative Therapy
http://www.nlm.nih.gov/medlineplus/canceralternativetherapy.html

Eating Disorders
http://www.nlm.nih.gov/medlineplus/eatingdisorders.html

Nutritional Support
http://www.nlm.nih.gov/medlineplus/nutritionalsupport.html

You may also choose to use the search utility provided by MEDLINEplus at the following Web address: **http://www.nlm.nih.gov/medlineplus/**. Simply type a keyword into the search box and click "Search." This utility is similar to the NIH search utility, with the exception that it only includes materials that are linked within the MEDLINEplus system (mostly patient-oriented information). It also has the disadvantage of generating unstructured results. We recommend, therefore, that you use this method only if you have a very targeted search.

The Combined Health Information Database (CHID)

CHID Online is a reference tool that maintains a database directory of thousands of journal articles and patient education guidelines on cachexia. CHID offers summaries that describe the guidelines available, including contact information and pricing. CHID's general Web site is **http://chid.nih.gov/**. To search this database, go to **http://chid.nih.gov/detail/detail.html**. In particular, you can use the advanced search options to look up pamphlets, reports, brochures, and information kits. The following was recently posted in this archive:

- **National Cancer Institute Studies of Hydrazine Sulfate**

  Source: Bethesda, MD: National Cancer Institute. 2001. 4 p.

  Contact: Available from National Center for Complementary and Alternative Medicine Clearinghouse. P.O. Box 7923, Gaithersburg, MD 20898. (888) 644-6226; INTERNATIONAL PHONE: (301) 519-3153; TTY: (866) 464-3615; FAX: (866) 464-3616; E-MAIL: info@nccam.nih.gov. PRICE: Free. Publication Number: D170.

  Summary: This Cancer Facts fact sheet discusses National Cancer Institute (NCI)-sponsored studies of hydrazine sulfate, a compound used to treat cancer and help reverse cancer **cachexia.** It provides information about the development of hydrazine sulfate and the history of its use, as well as NCI clinical trials testing the compound. A list of sources of NCI information is given.

- **Marijuana Use in Supportive Care for Cancer Patients**

  Source: Bethesda, MD: National Cancer Institute. 2000. 3 p.

  Contact: Available from National Cancer Institute. Publications Ordering Service, P.O. Box 24128, Baltimore, MD 21227. (800) 4-CANCER or (800) 422-6237; TTY: (800) 332-8615; FAX: (301) 330-7968. PRICE: Free.

  Summary: This fact sheet, developed by the National Cancer Institute (NCI), discusses the use of marijuana for chemotherapy-induced nausea and vomiting, anorexia, and **cachexia.** It specifies the forms of marijuana that have been used to treat these conditions, and provides examples of other therapies, drugs, or combinations of drugs that can be used in place of marijuana. The fact sheet also briefly reviews the findings of a National Institutes of Health (NIH) meeting convened in February 1997 to explore the potential medical uses of marijuana. 1 reference.

Healthfinder™

Healthfinder™ is sponsored by the U.S. Department of Health and Human Services and offers links to hundreds of other sites that contain healthcare information. This Web site is located at **http://www.healthfinder.gov**. Again, keyword searches can be used to find guidelines. The following was recently found in this database:

- **Marijuana Use in Supportive Care for Cancer Patients**

  Summary: A fact sheet about marijuana use to treat chemotherapy-induced nausea, vomiting, anorexia and cachexia in cancer patients

  Source: Cancer Information Service, National Cancer Institute

  http://www.healthfinder.gov/scripts/recordpass.asp?RecordType=0&RecordID=7054

The NIH Search Utility

The NIH search utility allows you to search for documents on over 100 selected Web sites that comprise the NIH-WEB-SPACE. Each of these servers is "crawled" and indexed on an ongoing basis. Your search will produce a list of various documents, all of which will relate in some way to cachexia. The drawbacks of this approach are that the information is not organized by theme and that the references are often a mix of information for professionals and patients. Nevertheless, a large number of the listed Web sites provide useful background information. We can only recommend this route, therefore, for relatively rare or specific disorders, or when using highly targeted searches. To use the NIH search utility, visit the following Web page: **http://search.nih.gov/index.html**.

Additional Web Sources

A number of Web sites are available to the public that often link to government sites. These can also point you in the direction of essential information. The following is a representative sample:

- AOL: **http://search.aol.com/cat.adp?id=168&layer=&from=subcats**
- Family Village: **http://www.familyvillage.wisc.edu/specific.htm**
- Google: **http://directory.google.com/Top/Health/Conditions_and_Diseases/**
- Med Help International: **http://www.medhelp.org/HealthTopics/A.html**
- Open Directory Project: **http://dmoz.org/Health/Conditions_and_Diseases/**
- Yahoo.com: **http://dir.yahoo.com/Health/Diseases_and_Conditions/**
- WebMD®Health: **http://my.webmd.com/health_topics**

Finding Associations

There are several Internet directories that provide lists of medical associations with information on or resources relating to cachexia. By consulting all of associations listed in this chapter, you will have nearly exhausted all sources for patient associations concerned with cachexia.

The National Health Information Center (NHIC)

The National Health Information Center (NHIC) offers a free referral service to help people find organizations that provide information about cachexia. For more information, see the NHIC's Web site at **http://www.health.gov/NHIC/** or contact an information specialist by calling 1-800-336-4797.

Directory of Health Organizations

The Directory of Health Organizations, provided by the National Library of Medicine Specialized Information Services, is a comprehensive source of information on associations. The Directory of Health Organizations database can be accessed via the Internet at **http://www.sis.nlm.nih.gov/Dir/DirMain.html**. It is composed of two parts: DIRLINE and Health Hotlines.

The DIRLINE database comprises some 10,000 records of organizations, research centers, and government institutes and associations that primarily focus on health and biomedicine. To access DIRLINE directly, go to the following Web site: **http://dirline.nlm.nih.gov/**. Simply type in "cachexia" (or a synonym), and you will receive information on all relevant organizations listed in the database.

Health Hotlines directs you to toll-free numbers to over 300 organizations. You can access this database directly at **http://www.sis.nlm.nih.gov/hotlines/**. On this page, you are given the option to search by keyword or by browsing the subject list. When you have received your search results, click on the name of the organization for its description and contact information.

The Combined Health Information Database

Another comprehensive source of information on healthcare associations is the Combined Health Information Database. Using the "Detailed Search" option, you will need to limit your search to "Organizations" and "cachexia". Type the following hyperlink into your Web browser: **http://chid.nih.gov/detail/detail.html**. To find associations, use the drop boxes at the bottom of the search page where "You may refine your search by." For publication date, select "All Years." Then, select your preferred language and the format option "Organization Resource Sheet." Type "cachexia" (or synonyms) into the "For these words:" box. You should check back periodically with this database since it is updated every three months.

The National Organization for Rare Disorders, Inc.

The National Organization for Rare Disorders, Inc. has prepared a Web site that provides, at no charge, lists of associations organized by health topic. You can access this database at the following Web site: **http://www.rarediseases.org/search/orgsearch.html**. Type "cachexia" (or a synonym) into the search box, and click "Submit Query."

APPENDIX C. FINDING MEDICAL LIBRARIES

Overview

In this Appendix, we show you how to quickly find a medical library in your area.

Preparation

Your local public library and medical libraries have interlibrary loan programs with the National Library of Medicine (NLM), one of the largest medical collections in the world. According to the NLM, most of the literature in the general and historical collections of the National Library of Medicine is available on interlibrary loan to any library. If you would like to access NLM medical literature, then visit a library in your area that can request the publications for you.[21]

Finding a Local Medical Library

The quickest method to locate medical libraries is to use the Internet-based directory published by the National Network of Libraries of Medicine (NN/LM). This network includes 4626 members and affiliates that provide many services to librarians, health professionals, and the public. To find a library in your area, simply visit **http://nnlm.gov/members/adv.html** or call 1-800-338-7657.

Medical Libraries in the U.S. and Canada

In addition to the NN/LM, the National Library of Medicine (NLM) lists a number of libraries with reference facilities that are open to the public. The following is the NLM's list and includes hyperlinks to each library's Web site. These Web pages can provide information on hours of operation and other restrictions. The list below is a small sample of

---

[21] Adapted from the NLM: **http://www.nlm.nih.gov/psd/cas/interlibrary.html.**

libraries recommended by the National Library of Medicine (sorted alphabetically by name of the U.S. state or Canadian province where the library is located)[22]:

- **Alabama:** Health InfoNet of Jefferson County (Jefferson County Library Cooperative, Lister Hill Library of the Health Sciences), **http://www.uab.edu/infonet/**
- **Alabama:** Richard M. Scrushy Library (American Sports Medicine Institute)
- **Arizona:** Samaritan Regional Medical Center: The Learning Center (Samaritan Health System, Phoenix, Arizona), **http://www.samaritan.edu/library/bannerlibs.htm**
- **California:** Kris Kelly Health Information Center (St. Joseph Health System, Humboldt), **http://www.humboldt1.com/~kkhic/index.html**
- **California:** Community Health Library of Los Gatos, **http://www.healthlib.org/orgresources.html**
- **California:** Consumer Health Program and Services (CHIPS) (County of Los Angeles Public Library, Los Angeles County Harbor-UCLA Medical Center Library) - Carson, CA, **http://www.colapublib.org/services/chips.html**
- **California:** Gateway Health Library (Sutter Gould Medical Foundation)
- **California:** Health Library (Stanford University Medical Center), **http://www-med.stanford.edu/healthlibrary/**
- **California:** Patient Education Resource Center - Health Information and Resources (University of California, San Francisco), **http://sfghdean.ucsf.edu/barnett/PERC/default.asp**
- **California:** Redwood Health Library (Petaluma Health Care District), **http://www.phcd.org/rdwdlib.html**
- **California:** Los Gatos PlaneTree Health Library, **http://planetreesanjose.org/**
- **California:** Sutter Resource Library (Sutter Hospitals Foundation, Sacramento), **http://suttermedicalcenter.org/library/**
- **California:** Health Sciences Libraries (University of California, Davis), **http://www.lib.ucdavis.edu/healthsci/**
- **California:** ValleyCare Health Library & Ryan Comer Cancer Resource Center (ValleyCare Health System, Pleasanton), **http://gaelnet.stmarys-ca.edu/other.libs/gbal/east/vchl.html**
- **California:** Washington Community Health Resource Library (Fremont), **http://www.healthlibrary.org/**
- **Colorado:** William V. Gervasini Memorial Library (Exempla Healthcare), **http://www.saintjosephdenver.org/yourhealth/libraries/**
- **Connecticut:** Hartford Hospital Health Science Libraries (Hartford Hospital), **http://www.harthosp.org/library/**
- **Connecticut:** Healthnet: Connecticut Consumer Health Information Center (University of Connecticut Health Center, Lyman Maynard Stowe Library), **http://library.uchc.edu/departm/hnet/**

---

[22] Abstracted from **http://www.nlm.nih.gov/medlineplus/libraries.html.**

- **Connecticut:** Waterbury Hospital Health Center Library (Waterbury Hospital, Waterbury), **http://www.waterburyhospital.com/library/consumer.shtml**
- **Delaware:** Consumer Health Library (Christiana Care Health System, Eugene du Pont Preventive Medicine & Rehabilitation Institute, Wilmington), **http://www.christianacare.org/health_guide/health_guide_pmri_health_info.cfm**
- **Delaware:** Lewis B. Flinn Library (Delaware Academy of Medicine, Wilmington), **http://www.delamed.org/chls.html**
- **Georgia:** Family Resource Library (Medical College of Georgia, Augusta), **http://cmc.mcg.edu/kids_families/fam_resources/fam_res_lib/frl.htm**
- **Georgia:** Health Resource Center (Medical Center of Central Georgia, Macon), **http://www.mccg.org/hrc/hrchome.asp**
- **Hawaii:** Hawaii Medical Library: Consumer Health Information Service (Hawaii Medical Library, Honolulu), **http://hml.org/CHIS/**
- **Idaho:** DeArmond Consumer Health Library (Kootenai Medical Center, Coeur d'Alene), **http://www.nicon.org/DeArmond/index.htm**
- **Illinois:** Health Learning Center of Northwestern Memorial Hospital (Chicago), **http://www.nmh.org/health_info/hlc.html**
- **Illinois:** Medical Library (OSF Saint Francis Medical Center, Peoria), **http://www.osfsaintfrancis.org/general/library/**
- **Kentucky:** Medical Library - Services for Patients, Families, Students & the Public (Central Baptist Hospital, Lexington), **http://www.centralbap.com/education/community/library.cfm**
- **Kentucky:** University of Kentucky - Health Information Library (Chandler Medical Center, Lexington), **http://www.mc.uky.edu/PatientEd/**
- **Louisiana:** Alton Ochsner Medical Foundation Library (Alton Ochsner Medical Foundation, New Orleans), **http://www.ochsner.org/library/**
- **Louisiana:** Louisiana State University Health Sciences Center Medical Library-Shreveport, **http://lib-sh.lsuhsc.edu/**
- **Maine:** Franklin Memorial Hospital Medical Library (Franklin Memorial Hospital, Farmington), **http://www.fchn.org/fmh/lib.htm**
- **Maine:** Gerrish-True Health Sciences Library (Central Maine Medical Center, Lewiston), **http://www.cmmc.org/library/library.html**
- **Maine:** Hadley Parrot Health Science Library (Eastern Maine Healthcare, Bangor), **http://www.emh.org/hll/hpl/guide.htm**
- **Maine:** Maine Medical Center Library (Maine Medical Center, Portland), **http://www.mmc.org/library/**
- **Maine:** Parkview Hospital (Brunswick), **http://www.parkviewhospital.org/**
- **Maine:** Southern Maine Medical Center Health Sciences Library (Southern Maine Medical Center, Biddeford), **http://www.smmc.org/services/service.php3?choice=10**
- **Maine:** Stephens Memorial Hospital's Health Information Library (Western Maine Health, Norway), **http://www.wmhcc.org/Library/**

- **Manitoba, Canada:** Consumer & Patient Health Information Service (University of Manitoba Libraries), **http://www.umanitoba.ca/libraries/units/health/reference/chis.html**
- **Manitoba, Canada:** J.W. Crane Memorial Library (Deer Lodge Centre, Winnipeg), **http://www.deerlodge.mb.ca/crane_library/about.asp**
- **Maryland:** Health Information Center at the Wheaton Regional Library (Montgomery County, Dept. of Public Libraries, Wheaton Regional Library), **http://www.mont.lib.md.us/healthinfo/hic.asp**
- **Massachusetts:** Baystate Medical Center Library (Baystate Health System), **http://www.baystatehealth.com/1024/**
- **Massachusetts:** Boston University Medical Center Alumni Medical Library (Boston University Medical Center), **http://med-libwww.bu.edu/library/lib.html**
- **Massachusetts:** Lowell General Hospital Health Sciences Library (Lowell General Hospital, Lowell), **http://www.lowellgeneral.org/library/HomePageLinks/WWW.htm**
- **Massachusetts:** Paul E. Woodard Health Sciences Library (New England Baptist Hospital, Boston), **http://www.nebh.org/health_lib.asp**
- **Massachusetts:** St. Luke's Hospital Health Sciences Library (St. Luke's Hospital, Southcoast Health System, New Bedford), **http://www.southcoast.org/library/**
- **Massachusetts:** Treadwell Library Consumer Health Reference Center (Massachusetts General Hospital), **http://www.mgh.harvard.edu/library/chrcindex.html**
- **Massachusetts:** UMass HealthNet (University of Massachusetts Medical School, Worchester), **http://healthnet.umassmed.edu/**
- **Michigan:** Botsford General Hospital Library - Consumer Health (Botsford General Hospital, Library & Internet Services), **http://www.botsfordlibrary.org/consumer.htm**
- **Michigan:** Helen DeRoy Medical Library (Providence Hospital and Medical Centers), **http://www.providence-hospital.org/library/**
- **Michigan:** Marquette General Hospital - Consumer Health Library (Marquette General Hospital, Health Information Center), **http://www.mgh.org/center.html**
- **Michigan:** Patient Education Resouce Center - University of Michigan Cancer Center (University of Michigan Comprehensive Cancer Center, Ann Arbor), **http://www.cancer.med.umich.edu/learn/leares.htm**
- **Michigan:** Sladen Library & Center for Health Information Resources - Consumer Health Information (Detroit), **http://www.henryford.com/body.cfm?id=39330**
- **Montana:** Center for Health Information (St. Patrick Hospital and Health Sciences Center, Missoula)
- **National:** Consumer Health Library Directory (Medical Library Association, Consumer and Patient Health Information Section), **http://caphis.mlanet.org/directory/index.html**
- **National:** National Network of Libraries of Medicine (National Library of Medicine) - provides library services for health professionals in the United States who do not have access to a medical library, **http://nnlm.gov/**
- **National:** NN/LM List of Libraries Serving the Public (National Network of Libraries of Medicine), **http://nnlm.gov/members/**

- **Nevada:** Health Science Library, West Charleston Library (Las Vegas-Clark County Library District, Las Vegas), **http://www.lvccld.org/special_collections/medical/index.htm**
- **New Hampshire:** Dartmouth Biomedical Libraries (Dartmouth College Library, Hanover), **http://www.dartmouth.edu/~biomed/resources.htmld/conshealth.htmld/**
- **New Jersey:** Consumer Health Library (Rahway Hospital, Rahway), **http://www.rahwayhospital.com/library.htm**
- **New Jersey:** Dr. Walter Phillips Health Sciences Library (Englewood Hospital and Medical Center, Englewood), **http://www.englewoodhospital.com/links/index.htm**
- **New Jersey:** Meland Foundation (Englewood Hospital and Medical Center, Englewood), **http://www.geocities.com/ResearchTriangle/9360/**
- **New York:** Choices in Health Information (New York Public Library) - NLM Consumer Pilot Project participant, **http://www.nypl.org/branch/health/links.html**
- **New York:** Health Information Center (Upstate Medical University, State University of New York, Syracuse), **http://www.upstate.edu/library/hic/**
- **New York:** Health Sciences Library (Long Island Jewish Medical Center, New Hyde Park), **http://www.lij.edu/library/library.html**
- **New York:** ViaHealth Medical Library (Rochester General Hospital), **http://www.nyam.org/library/**
- **Ohio:** Consumer Health Library (Akron General Medical Center, Medical & Consumer Health Library), **http://www.akrongeneral.org/hwlibrary.htm**
- **Oklahoma:** The Health Information Center at Saint Francis Hospital (Saint Francis Health System, Tulsa), **http://www.sfh-tulsa.com/services/healthinfo.asp**
- **Oregon:** Planetree Health Resource Center (Mid-Columbia Medical Center, The Dalles), **http://www.mcmc.net/phrc/**
- **Pennsylvania:** Community Health Information Library (Milton S. Hershey Medical Center, Hershey), **http://www.hmc.psu.edu/commhealth/**
- **Pennsylvania:** Community Health Resource Library (Geisinger Medical Center, Danville), **http://www.geisinger.edu/education/commlib.shtml**
- **Pennsylvania:** HealthInfo Library (Moses Taylor Hospital, Scranton), **http://www.mth.org/healthwellness.html**
- **Pennsylvania:** Hopwood Library (University of Pittsburgh, Health Sciences Library System, Pittsburgh), **http://www.hsls.pitt.edu/guides/chi/hopwood/index_html**
- **Pennsylvania:** Koop Community Health Information Center (College of Physicians of Philadelphia), **http://www.collphyphil.org/kooppg1.shtml**
- **Pennsylvania:** Learning Resources Center - Medical Library (Susquehanna Health System, Williamsport), **http://www.shscares.org/services/lrc/index.asp**
- **Pennsylvania:** Medical Library (UPMC Health System, Pittsburgh), **http://www.upmc.edu/passavant/library.htm**
- **Quebec, Canada:** Medical Library (Montreal General Hospital), **http://www.mghlib.mcgill.ca/**

- **South Dakota:** Rapid City Regional Hospital Medical Library (Rapid City Regional Hospital), **http://www.rcrh.org/Services/Library/Default.asp**
- **Texas:** Houston HealthWays (Houston Academy of Medicine-Texas Medical Center Library), **http://hhw.library.tmc.edu/**
- **Washington:** Community Health Library (Kittitas Valley Community Hospital), **http://www.kvch.com/**
- **Washington:** Southwest Washington Medical Center Library (Southwest Washington Medical Center, Vancouver), **http://www.swmedicalcenter.com/body.cfm?id=72**

ONLINE GLOSSARIES

The Internet provides access to a number of free-to-use medical dictionaries. The National Library of Medicine has compiled the following list of online dictionaries:

- ADAM Medical Encyclopedia (A.D.A.M., Inc.), comprehensive medical reference: **http://www.nlm.nih.gov/medlineplus/encyclopedia.html**
- MedicineNet.com Medical Dictionary (MedicineNet, Inc.): **http://www.medterms.com/Script/Main/hp.asp**
- Merriam-Webster Medical Dictionary (Inteli-Health, Inc.): **http://www.intelihealth.com/IH/**
- Multilingual Glossary of Technical and Popular Medical Terms in Eight European Languages (European Commission) - Danish, Dutch, English, French, German, Italian, Portuguese, and Spanish: **http://allserv.rug.ac.be/~rvdstich/eugloss/welcome.html**
- On-line Medical Dictionary (CancerWEB): **http://cancerweb.ncl.ac.uk/omd/**
- Rare Diseases Terms (Office of Rare Diseases): **http://ord.aspensys.com/asp/diseases/diseases.asp**
- Technology Glossary (National Library of Medicine) - Health Care Technology: **http://www.nlm.nih.gov/nichsr/ta101/ta10108.htm**

Beyond these, MEDLINEplus contains a very patient-friendly encyclopedia covering every aspect of medicine (licensed from A.D.A.M., Inc.). The ADAM Medical Encyclopedia can be accessed at **http://www.nlm.nih.gov/medlineplus/encyclopedia.html**. ADAM is also available on commercial Web sites such as drkoop.com (**http://www.drkoop.com/**) and Web MD (**http://my.webmd.com/adam/asset/adam_disease_articles/a_to_z/a**).

Online Dictionary Directories

The following are additional online directories compiled by the National Library of Medicine, including a number of specialized medical dictionaries:

- Medical Dictionaries: Medical & Biological (World Health Organization): **http://www.who.int/hlt/virtuallibrary/English/diction.htm#Medical**
- MEL-Michigan Electronic Library List of Online Health and Medical Dictionaries (Michigan Electronic Library): **http://mel.lib.mi.us/health/health-dictionaries.html**
- Patient Education: Glossaries (DMOZ Open Directory Project): **http://dmoz.org/Health/Education/Patient_Education/Glossaries/**
- Web of Online Dictionaries (Bucknell University): **http://www.yourdictionary.com/diction5.html#medicine**

CACHEXIA DICTIONARY

The definitions below are derived from official public sources, including the National Institutes of Health [NIH] and the European Union [EU].

5-Hydroxytryptophan: Precursor of serotonin used as antiepileptic and antidepressant. [NIH]

Abdomen: That portion of the body that lies between the thorax and the pelvis. [NIH]

Abdominal: Having to do with the abdomen, which is the part of the body between the chest and the hips that contains the pancreas, stomach, intestines, liver, gallbladder, and other organs. [NIH]

Abdominal fat: Fat (adipose tissue) that is centrally distributed between the thorax and pelvis and that induces greater health risk. [NIH]

Abdominal Pain: Sensation of discomfort, distress, or agony in the abdominal region. [NIH]

Aberrant: Wandering or deviating from the usual or normal course. [EU]

Ablation: The removal of an organ by surgery. [NIH]

Acceptor: A substance which, while normally not oxidized by oxygen or reduced by hydrogen, can be oxidized or reduced in presence of a substance which is itself undergoing oxidation or reduction. [NIH]

Accommodation: Adjustment, especially that of the eye for various distances. [EU]

Acetylcarnitine: An acetic acid ester of carnitine that facilitates movement of acetyl CoA into the matrices of mammalian mitochondria during the oxidation of fatty acids. [NIH]

Acetylcholine: A neurotransmitter. Acetylcholine in vertebrates is the major transmitter at neuromuscular junctions, autonomic ganglia, parasympathetic effector junctions, a subset of sympathetic effector junctions, and at many sites in the central nervous system. It is generally not used as an administered drug because it is broken down very rapidly by cholinesterases, but it is useful in some ophthalmological applications. [NIH]

Acetylcysteine: The N-acetyl derivative of cysteine. It is used as a mucolytic agent to reduce the viscosity of mucous secretions. It has also been shown to have antiviral effects in patients with HIV due to inhibition of viral stimulation by reactive oxygen intermediates. [NIH]

Acquired Immunodeficiency Syndrome: An acquired defect of cellular immunity associated with infection by the human immunodeficiency virus (HIV), a CD4-positive T-lymphocyte count under 200 cells/microliter or less than 14% of total lymphocytes, and increased susceptibility to opportunistic infections and malignant neoplasms. Clinical manifestations also include emaciation (wasting) and dementia. These elements reflect criteria for AIDS as defined by the CDC in 1993. [NIH]

Actin: Essential component of the cell skeleton. [NIH]

Activities of Daily Living: The performance of the basic activities of self care, such as dressing, ambulation, eating, etc., in rehabilitation. [NIH]

Acute renal: A condition in which the kidneys suddenly stop working. In most cases, kidneys can recover from almost complete loss of function. [NIH]

Acute tubular: A severe form of acute renal failure that develops in people with severe illnesses like infections or with low blood pressure. Patients may need dialysis. Kidney function often improves if the underlying disease is successfully treated. [NIH]

Adaptability: Ability to develop some form of tolerance to conditions extremely different from those under which a living organism evolved. [NIH]

Adaptation: 1. The adjustment of an organism to its environment, or the process by which it enhances such fitness. 2. The normal ability of the eye to adjust itself to variations in the intensity of light; the adjustment to such variations. 3. The decline in the frequency of firing of a neuron, particularly of a receptor, under conditions of constant stimulation. 4. In dentistry, (a) the proper fitting of a denture, (b) the degree of proximity and interlocking of restorative material to a tooth preparation, (c) the exact adjustment of bands to teeth. 5. In microbiology, the adjustment of bacterial physiology to a new environment. [EU]

Adenocarcinoma: A malignant epithelial tumor with a glandular organization. [NIH]

Adenosine: A nucleoside that is composed of adenine and d-ribose. Adenosine or adenosine derivatives play many important biological roles in addition to being components of DNA and RNA. Adenosine itself is a neurotransmitter. [NIH]

Adipocytes: Fat-storing cells found mostly in the abdominal cavity and subcutaneous tissue. Fat is usually stored in the form of tryglycerides. [NIH]

Adipose Tissue: Connective tissue composed of fat cells lodged in the meshes of areolar tissue. [NIH]

Adjustment: The dynamic process wherein the thoughts, feelings, behavior, and biophysiological mechanisms of the individual continually change to adjust to the environment. [NIH]

Adjuvant: A substance which aids another, such as an auxiliary remedy; in immunology, nonspecific stimulator (e.g., BCG vaccine) of the immune response. [EU]

Adrenal Cortex: The outer layer of the adrenal gland. It secretes mineralocorticoids, androgens, and glucocorticoids. [NIH]

Adrenal Glands: Paired glands situated in the retroperitoneal tissues at the superior pole of each kidney. [NIH]

Adrenal insufficiency: The reduced secretion of adrenal glands. [NIH]

Adrenaline: A hormone. Also called epinephrine. [NIH]

Adrenergic: Activated by, characteristic of, or secreting epinephrine or substances with similar activity; the term is applied to those nerve fibres that liberate norepinephrine at a synapse when a nerve impulse passes, i.e., the sympathetic fibres. [EU]

Adverse Effect: An unwanted side effect of treatment. [NIH]

Aerobic: In biochemistry, reactions that need oxygen to happen or happen when oxygen is present. [NIH]

Aerobic Metabolism: A chemical process in which oxygen is used to make energy from carbohydrates (sugars). Also known as aerobic respiration, oxidative metabolism, or cell respiration. [NIH]

Aerobic Respiration: A chemical process in which oxygen is used to make energy from carbohydrates (sugars). Also known as oxidative metabolism, cell respiration, or aerobic metabolism. [NIH]

Aerosols: Colloids with a gaseous dispersing phase and either liquid (fog) or solid (smoke) dispersed phase; used in fumigation or in inhalation therapy; may contain propellent agents. [NIH]

Afferent: Concerned with the transmission of neural impulse toward the central part of the nervous system. [NIH]

Affinity: 1. Inherent likeness or relationship. 2. A special attraction for a specific element, organ, or structure. 3. Chemical affinity; the force that binds atoms in molecules; the tendency of substances to combine by chemical reaction. 4. The strength of noncovalent chemical binding between two substances as measured by the dissociation constant of the complex. 5. In immunology, a thermodynamic expression of the strength of interaction between a single antigen-binding site and a single antigenic determinant (and thus of the stereochemical compatibility between them), most accurately applied to interactions among simple, uniform antigenic determinants such as haptens. Expressed as the association constant (K litres mole -1), which, owing to the heterogeneity of affinities in a population of antibody molecules of a given specificity, actually represents an average value (mean intrinsic association constant). 6. The reciprocal of the dissociation constant. [EU]

Agar: A complex sulfated polymer of galactose units, extracted from Gelidium cartilagineum, Gracilaria confervoides, and related red algae. It is used as a gel in the preparation of solid culture media for microorganisms, as a bulk laxative, in making emulsions, and as a supporting medium for immunodiffusion and immunoelectrophoresis. [NIH]

Age of Onset: The age or period of life at which a disease or the initial symptoms or manifestations of a disease appear in an individual. [NIH]

Agonist: In anatomy, a prime mover. In pharmacology, a drug that has affinity for and stimulates physiologic activity at cell receptors normally stimulated by naturally occurring substances. [EU]

Albumin: 1. Any protein that is soluble in water and moderately concentrated salt solutions and is coagulable by heat. 2. Serum albumin; the major plasma protein (approximately 60 per cent of the total), which is responsible for much of the plasma colloidal osmotic pressure and serves as a transport protein carrying large organic anions, such as fatty acids, bilirubin, and many drugs, and also carrying certain hormones, such as cortisol and thyroxine, when their specific binding globulins are saturated. Albumin is synthesized in the liver. Low serum levels occur in protein malnutrition, active inflammation and serious hepatic and renal disease. [EU]

Alendronate: A nonhormonal medication for the treatment of postmenopausal osteoporosis in women. This drug builds healthy bone, restoring some of the bone loss as a result of osteoporosis. [NIH]

Algorithms: A procedure consisting of a sequence of algebraic formulas and/or logical steps to calculate or determine a given task. [NIH]

Alimentary: Pertaining to food or nutritive material, or to the organs of digestion. [EU]

Alkaline: Having the reactions of an alkali. [EU]

Alkylating Agents: Highly reactive chemicals that introduce alkyl radicals into biologically active molecules and thereby prevent their proper functioning. Many are used as antineoplastic agents, but most are very toxic, with carcinogenic, mutagenic, teratogenic, and immunosuppressant actions. They have also been used as components in poison gases. [NIH]

Allantois: An embryonic diverticulum of the hindgut of reptiles, birds, and mammals; in man its blood vessels give rise to those of the umbilical cord. [NIH]

Allogeneic: Taken from different individuals of the same species. [NIH]

Allograft: An organ or tissue transplant between two humans. [NIH]

Allylamine: Possesses an unusual and selective cytotoxicity for vascular smooth muscle cells in dogs and rats. Useful for experiments dealing with arterial injury, myocardial fibrosis or cardiac decompensation. [NIH]

Alopecia: Absence of hair from areas where it is normally present. [NIH]

Alpha Particles: Positively charged particles composed of two protons and two neutrons, i.e., helium nuclei, emitted during disintegration of very heavy isotopes; a beam of alpha particles or an alpha ray has very strong ionizing power, but weak penetrability. [NIH]

Alpha-1: A protein with the property of inactivating proteolytic enzymes such as leucocyte collagenase and elastase. [NIH]

Alpha-Linolenic Acid: A fatty acid that is found in plants and involved in the formation of prostaglandins. [NIH]

Alternative medicine: Practices not generally recognized by the medical community as standard or conventional medical approaches and used instead of standard treatments. Alternative medicine includes the taking of dietary supplements, megadose vitamins, and herbal preparations; the drinking of special teas; and practices such as massage therapy, magnet therapy, spiritual healing, and meditation. [NIH]

Ameliorating: A changeable condition which prevents the consequence of a failure or accident from becoming as bad as it otherwise would. [NIH]

Amenorrhea: Absence of menstruation. [NIH]

Amine: An organic compound containing nitrogen; any member of a group of chemical compounds formed from ammonia by replacement of one or more of the hydrogen atoms by organic (hydrocarbon) radicals. The amines are distinguished as primary, secondary, and tertiary, according to whether one, two, or three hydrogen atoms are replaced. The amines include allylamine, amylamine, ethylamine, methylamine, phenylamine, propylamine, and many other compounds. [EU]

Amino Acid Sequence: The order of amino acids as they occur in a polypeptide chain. This is referred to as the primary structure of proteins. It is of fundamental importance in determining protein conformation. [NIH]

Amino Acids: Organic compounds that generally contain an amino (-NH2) and a carboxyl (-COOH) group. Twenty alpha-amino acids are the subunits which are polymerized to form proteins. [NIH]

Amino Acids: Organic compounds that generally contain an amino (-NH2) and a carboxyl (-COOH) group. Twenty alpha-amino acids are the subunits which are polymerized to form proteins. [NIH]

Amitriptyline: Tricyclic antidepressant with anticholinergic and sedative properties. It appears to prevent the re-uptake of norepinephrine and serotonin at nerve terminals, thus potentiating the action of these neurotransmitters. Amitriptyline also appears to antaganize cholinergic and alpha-1 adrenergic responses to bioactive amines. [NIH]

Ammonia: A colorless alkaline gas. It is formed in the body during decomposition of organic materials during a large number of metabolically important reactions. [NIH]

Amnion: The extraembryonic membrane which contains the embryo and amniotic fluid. [NIH]

Amplification: The production of additional copies of a chromosomal DNA sequence, found as either intrachromosomal or extrachromosomal DNA. [NIH]

Amyotrophy: A type of diabetic neuropathy that causes muscle weakness and wasting. [NIH]

Anabolic: Relating to, characterized by, or promoting anabolism. [EU]

Anaesthesia: Loss of feeling or sensation. Although the term is used for loss of tactile sensibility, or of any of the other senses, it is applied especially to loss of the sensation of pain, as it is induced to permit performance of surgery or other painful procedures. [EU]

Analgesic: An agent that alleviates pain without causing loss of consciousness. [EU]

Analog: In chemistry, a substance that is similar, but not identical, to another. [NIH]

Analogous: Resembling or similar in some respects, as in function or appearance, but not in origin or development;. [EU]

Anaplastic: A term used to describe cancer cells that divide rapidly and bear little or no resemblance to normal cells. [NIH]

Anatomical: Pertaining to anatomy, or to the structure of the organism. [EU]

Androgens: A class of sex hormones associated with the development and maintenance of the secondary male sex characteristics, sperm induction, and sexual differentiation. In addition to increasing virility and libido, they also increase nitrogen and water retention and stimulate skeletal growth. [NIH]

Anemia: A reduction in the number of circulating erythrocytes or in the quantity of hemoglobin. [NIH]

Anergy: Absence of immune response to particular substances. [NIH]

Anesthesia: A state characterized by loss of feeling or sensation. This depression of nerve function is usually the result of pharmacologic action and is induced to allow performance of surgery or other painful procedures. [NIH]

Angina: Chest pain that originates in the heart. [NIH]

Angina Pectoris: The symptom of paroxysmal pain consequent to myocardial ischemia usually of distinctive character, location and radiation, and provoked by a transient stressful situation during which the oxygen requirements of the myocardium exceed the capacity of the coronary circulation to supply it. [NIH]

Animal model: An animal with a disease either the same as or like a disease in humans. Animal models are used to study the development and progression of diseases and to test new treatments before they are given to humans. Animals with transplanted human cancers or other tissues are called xenograft models. [NIH]

Anions: Negatively charged atoms, radicals or groups of atoms which travel to the anode or positive pole during electrolysis. [NIH]

Anode: Electrode held at a positive potential with respect to a cathode. [NIH]

Anorexia: Lack or loss of appetite for food. Appetite is psychologic, dependent on memory and associations. Anorexia can be brought about by unattractive food, surroundings, or company. [NIH]

Anorexia Nervosa: The chief symptoms are inability to eat, weight loss, and amenorrhea. [NIH]

Anosmia: Absence of the sense of smell; called also anosphrasia and olfactory anaesthesia. [EU]

Anovulation: Suspension or cessation of ovulation in animals and humans. [NIH]

Antagonism: Interference with, or inhibition of, the growth of a living organism by another living organism, due either to creation of unfavorable conditions (e. g. exhaustion of food supplies) or to production of a specific antibiotic substance (e. g. penicillin). [NIH]

Anthropometry: The technique that deals with the measurement of the size, weight, and proportions of the human or other primate body. [NIH]

Antiallergic: Counteracting allergy or allergic conditions. [EU]

Antibiotic: A drug used to treat infections caused by bacteria and other microorganisms. [NIH]

Antibodies: Immunoglobulin molecules having a specific amino acid sequence by virtue of which they interact only with the antigen that induced their synthesis in cells of the lymphoid series (especially plasma cells), or with an antigen closely related to it. [NIH]

Antibody: A type of protein made by certain white blood cells in response to a foreign substance (antigen). Each antibody can bind to only a specific antigen. The purpose of this binding is to help destroy the antigen. Antibodies can work in several ways, depending on the nature of the antigen. Some antibodies destroy antigens directly. Others make it easier for white blood cells to destroy the antigen. [NIH]

Anticholinergic: An agent that blocks the parasympathetic nerves. Called also parasympatholytic. [EU]

Anticoagulant: A drug that helps prevent blood clots from forming. Also called a blood thinner. [NIH]

Antidepressant: A drug used to treat depression. [NIH]

Antiepileptic: An agent that combats epilepsy. [EU]

Antigen: Any substance which is capable, under appropriate conditions, of inducing a specific immune response and of reacting with the products of that response, that is, with specific antibody or specifically sensitized T-lymphocytes, or both. Antigens may be soluble substances, such as toxins and foreign proteins, or particulate, such as bacteria and tissue cells; however, only the portion of the protein or polysaccharide molecule known as the antigenic determinant (q.v.) combines with antibody or a specific receptor on a lymphocyte. Abbreviated Ag. [EU]

Anti-infective: An agent that so acts. [EU]

Anti-inflammatory: Having to do with reducing inflammation. [NIH]

Anti-Inflammatory Agents: Substances that reduce or suppress inflammation. [NIH]

Antimetabolite: A chemical that is very similar to one required in a normal biochemical reaction in cells. Antimetabolites can stop or slow down the reaction. [NIH]

Antineoplastic: Inhibiting or preventing the development of neoplasms, checking the maturation and proliferation of malignant cells. [EU]

Antioxidant: A substance that prevents damage caused by free radicals. Free radicals are highly reactive chemicals that often contain oxygen. They are produced when molecules are split to give products that have unpaired electrons. This process is called oxidation. [NIH]

Antipruritic: Relieving or preventing itching. [EU]

Antipyretic: An agent that relieves or reduces fever. Called also antifebrile, antithermic and febrifuge. [EU]

Antiviral: Destroying viruses or suppressing their replication. [EU]

Anuria: Inability to form or excrete urine. [NIH]

Anus: The opening of the rectum to the outside of the body. [NIH]

Anxiety: Persistent feeling of dread, apprehension, and impending disaster. [NIH]

Apnoea: Cessation of breathing. [EU]

Apolipoproteins: The protein components of lipoproteins which remain after the lipids to which the proteins are bound have been removed. They play an important role in lipid transport and metabolism. [NIH]

Apoptosis: One of the two mechanisms by which cell death occurs (the other being the pathological process of necrosis). Apoptosis is the mechanism responsible for the physiological deletion of cells and appears to be intrinsically programmed. It is characterized by distinctive morphologic changes in the nucleus and cytoplasm, chromatin cleavage at regularly spaced sites, and the endonucleolytic cleavage of genomic DNA (DNA fragmentation) at internucleosomal sites. This mode of cell death serves as a balance to mitosis in regulating the size of animal tissues and in mediating pathologic processes associated with tumor growth. [NIH]

Aqueous: Having to do with water. [NIH]

Arachidonic Acid: An unsaturated, essential fatty acid. It is found in animal and human fat as well as in the liver, brain, and glandular organs, and is a constituent of animal phosphatides. It is formed by the synthesis from dietary linoleic acid and is a precursor in the biosynthesis of prostaglandins, thromboxanes, and leukotrienes. [NIH]

Arcuate Nucleus: A nucleus located in the middle hypothalamus in the most ventral part of the third ventricle near the entrance of the infundibular recess. Its small cells are in close contact with the ependyma. [NIH]

Arginine: An essential amino acid that is physiologically active in the L-form. [NIH]

Argon: A noble gas with the atomic symbol Ar, atomic number 18, and atomic weight 39.948. It is used in fluorescent tubes and wherever an inert atmosphere is desired and nitrogen cannot be used. [NIH]

Arterial: Pertaining to an artery or to the arteries. [EU]

Arteries: The vessels carrying blood away from the heart. [NIH]

Arterioles: The smallest divisions of the arteries located between the muscular arteries and the capillaries. [NIH]

Arteriovenous: Both arterial and venous; pertaining to or affecting an artery and a vein. [EU]

Artery: Vessel-carrying blood from the heart to various parts of the body. [NIH]

Arthropathy: Any joint disease. [EU]

Articular: Of or pertaining to a joint. [EU]

Asbestos: Fibrous incombustible mineral composed of magnesium and calcium silicates with or without other elements. It is relatively inert chemically and used in thermal insulation and fireproofing. Inhalation of dust causes asbestosis and later lung and gastrointestinal neoplasms. [NIH]

Ascites: Accumulation or retention of free fluid within the peritoneal cavity. [NIH]

Assay: Determination of the amount of a particular constituent of a mixture, or of the biological or pharmacological potency of a drug. [EU]

Asthenia: Clinical sign or symptom manifested as debility, or lack or loss of strength and energy. [NIH]

Astrocytes: The largest and most numerous neuroglial cells in the brain and spinal cord. Astrocytes (from "star" cells) are irregularly shaped with many long processes, including those with "end feet" which form the glial (limiting) membrane and directly and indirectly contribute to the blood brain barrier. They regulate the extracellular ionic and chemical environment, and "reactive astrocytes" (along with microglia) respond to injury. Astrocytes have high- affinity transmitter uptake systems, voltage-dependent and transmitter-gated ion channels, and can release transmitter, but their role in signaling (as in many other functions) is not well understood. [NIH]

Asymptomatic: Having no signs or symptoms of disease. [NIH]

Atrophy: Decrease in the size of a cell, tissue, organ, or multiple organs, associated with a variety of pathological conditions such as abnormal cellular changes, ischemia, malnutrition, or hormonal changes. [NIH]

Attenuated: Strain with weakened or reduced virulence. [NIH]

Attenuation: Reduction of transmitted sound energy or its electrical equivalent. [NIH]

Autodigestion: Autolysis; a condition found in disease of the stomach: the stomach wall is digested by the gastric juice. [NIH]

Autoimmune disease: A condition in which the body recognizes its own tissues as foreign and directs an immune response against them. [NIH]

Autoimmunity: Process whereby the immune system reacts against the body's own tissues. Autoimmunity may produce or be caused by autoimmune diseases. [NIH]

Autonomic Nervous System: The enteric, parasympathetic, and sympathetic nervous systems taken together. Generally speaking, the autonomic nervous system regulates the internal environment during both peaceful activity and physical or emotional stress. Autonomic activity is controlled and integrated by the central nervous system, especially the hypothalamus and the solitary nucleus, which receive information relayed from visceral afferents; these and related central and sensory structures are sometimes (but not here) considered to be part of the autonomic nervous system itself. [NIH]

Autopsy: Postmortem examination of the body. [NIH]

Autosuggestion: Suggestion coming from the subject himself. [NIH]

Axons: Nerve fibers that are capable of rapidly conducting impulses away from the neuron cell body. [NIH]

Bacteria: Unicellular prokaryotic microorganisms which generally possess rigid cell walls, multiply by cell division, and exhibit three principal forms: round or coccal, rodlike or bacillary, and spiral or spirochetal. [NIH]

Bacterial Infections: Infections by bacteria, general or unspecified. [NIH]

Bacterial Physiology: Physiological processes and activities of bacteria. [NIH]

Bacterium: Microscopic organism which may have a spherical, rod-like, or spiral unicellular or non-cellular body. Bacteria usually reproduce through asexual processes. [NIH]

Barbiturate: A drug with sedative and hypnotic effects. Barbiturates have been used as sedatives and anesthetics, and they have been used to treat the convulsions associated with epilepsy. [NIH]

Basal cells: Small, round cells found in the lower part (or base) of the epidermis, the outer layer of the skin. [NIH]

Basal Ganglia: Large subcortical nuclear masses derived from the telencephalon and located in the basal regions of the cerebral hemispheres. [NIH]

Basal Ganglia Diseases: Diseases of the basal ganglia including the putamen; globus pallidus; claustrum; amygdala; and caudate nucleus. Dyskinesias (most notably involuntary movements and alterations of the rate of movement) represent the primary clinical manifestations of these disorders. Common etiologies include cerebrovascular disease; neurodegenerative diseases; and craniocerebral trauma. [NIH]

Basal metabolic rate: Represents the minimum energy expenditure required for the maintenance of vital functions; normally the amount of energy expended, measured in calories, per unit of time at rest; measured after 14-18 hours of rest. [NIH]

Base: In chemistry, the nonacid part of a salt; a substance that combines with acids to form salts; a substance that dissociates to give hydroxide ions in aqueous solutions; a substance whose molecule or ion can combine with a proton (hydrogen ion); a substance capable of donating a pair of electrons (to an acid) for the formation of a coordinate covalent bond. [EU]

Basement Membrane: Ubiquitous supportive tissue adjacent to epithelium and around smooth and striated muscle cells. This tissue contains intrinsic macromolecular components such as collagen, laminin, and sulfated proteoglycans. As seen by light microscopy one of its subdivisions is the basal (basement) lamina. [NIH]

Basophil: A type of white blood cell. Basophils are granulocytes. [NIH]

Bed Rest: Confinement of an individual to bed for therapeutic or experimental reasons. [NIH]

Benign: Not cancerous; does not invade nearby tissue or spread to other parts of the body. [NIH]

Beta-Thromboglobulin: A platelet-specific protein which is released when platelets aggregate. Elevated plasma levels have been reported after deep venous thrombosis, pre-eclampsia, myocardial infarction with mural thrombosis, and myeloproliferative disorders. Measurement of beta-thromboglobulin in biological fluids by radioimmunoassay is used for the diagnosis and assessment of progress of thromboembolic disorders. [NIH]

Bewilderment: Impairment or loss of will power. [NIH]

Bilateral: Affecting both the right and left side of body. [NIH]

Bile: An emulsifying agent produced in the liver and secreted into the duodenum. Its composition includes bile acids and salts, cholesterol, and electrolytes. It aids digestion of fats in the duodenum. [NIH]

Bile Acids: Acids made by the liver that work with bile to break down fats. [NIH]

Biliary: Having to do with the liver, bile ducts, and/or gallbladder. [NIH]

Biliary Tract: The gallbladder and its ducts. [NIH]

Bilirubin: A bile pigment that is a degradation product of heme. [NIH]

Binding Sites: The reactive parts of a macromolecule that directly participate in its specific combination with another molecule. [NIH]

Bioassays: Determination of the relative effective strength of a substance (as a vitamin, hormone, or drug) by comparing its effect on a test organism with that of a standard preparation. [NIH]

Bioavailability: The degree to which a drug or other substance becomes available to the target tissue after administration. [EU]

Biochemical: Relating to biochemistry; characterized by, produced by, or involving chemical reactions in living organisms. [EU]

Biogenesis: The origin of life. It includes studies of the potential basis for life in organic compounds but excludes studies of the development of altered forms of life through mutation and natural selection, which is evolution. [NIH]

Biological response modifier: BRM. A substance that stimulates the body's response to infection and disease. [NIH]

Biological therapy: Treatment to stimulate or restore the ability of the immune system to fight infection and disease. Also used to lessen side effects that may be caused by some cancer treatments. Also known as immunotherapy, biotherapy, or biological response modifier (BRM) therapy. [NIH]

Biomarkers: Substances sometimes found in an increased amount in the blood, other body fluids, or tissues and that may suggest the presence of some types of cancer. Biomarkers include CA 125 (ovarian cancer), CA 15-3 (breast cancer), CEA (ovarian, lung, breast, pancreas, and GI tract cancers), and PSA (prostate cancer). Also called tumor markers. [NIH]

Biopsy: Removal and pathologic examination of specimens in the form of small pieces of tissue from the living body. [NIH]

Biopterin: A natural product that has been considered as a growth factor for some insects. [NIH]

Biosynthesis: The building up of a chemical compound in the physiologic processes of a living organism. [EU]

Biotechnology: Body of knowledge related to the use of organisms, cells or cell-derived constituents for the purpose of developing products which are technically, scientifically and clinically useful. Alteration of biologic function at the molecular level (i.e., genetic engineering) is a central focus; laboratory methods used include transfection and cloning technologies, sequence and structure analysis algorithms, computer databases, and gene and protein structure function analysis and prediction. [NIH]

Bladder: The organ that stores urine. [NIH]

Blood Coagulation: The process of the interaction of blood coagulation factors that results in an insoluble fibrin clot. [NIH]

Blood Coagulation Factors: Endogenous substances, usually proteins, that are involved in the blood coagulation process. [NIH]

Blood Glucose: Glucose in blood. [NIH]

Blood Platelets: Non-nucleated disk-shaped cells formed in the megakaryocyte and found in the blood of all mammals. They are mainly involved in blood coagulation. [NIH]

Blood pressure: The pressure of blood against the walls of a blood vessel or heart chamber. Unless there is reference to another location, such as the pulmonary artery or one of the heart chambers, it refers to the pressure in the systemic arteries, as measured, for example, in the forearm. [NIH]

Blood vessel: A tube in the body through which blood circulates. Blood vessels include a network of arteries, arterioles, capillaries, venules, and veins. [NIH]

Blot: To transfer DNA, RNA, or proteins to an immobilizing matrix such as nitrocellulose. [NIH]

Body Composition: The relative amounts of various components in the body, such as percent body fat. [NIH]

Body Fluids: Liquid components of living organisms. [NIH]

Body Mass Index: One of the anthropometric measures of body mass; it has the highest correlation with skinfold thickness or body density. [NIH]

Bone Marrow: The soft tissue filling the cavities of bones. Bone marrow exists in two types, yellow and red. Yellow marrow is found in the large cavities of large bones and consists mostly of fat cells and a few primitive blood cells. Red marrow is a hematopoietic tissue and is the site of production of erythrocytes and granular leukocytes. Bone marrow is made up of a framework of connective tissue containing branching fibers with the frame being filled with marrow cells. [NIH]

Bone Marrow Transplantation: The transference of bone marrow from one human or animal to another. [NIH]

Bowel: The long tube-shaped organ in the abdomen that completes the process of digestion. There is both a small and a large bowel. Also called the intestine. [NIH]

Bowel Movement: Body wastes passed through the rectum and anus. [NIH]

Brachytherapy: A collective term for interstitial, intracavity, and surface radiotherapy. It uses small sealed or partly-sealed sources that may be placed on or near the body surface or within a natural body cavity or implanted directly into the tissues. [NIH]

Bradykinin: A nonapeptide messenger that is enzymatically produced from kallidin in the blood where it is a potent but short-lived agent of arteriolar dilation and increased capillary permeability. Bradykinin is also released from mast cells during asthma attacks, from gut walls as a gastrointestinal vasodilator, from damaged tissues as a pain signal, and may be a neurotransmitter. [NIH]

Brain Stem: The part of the brain that connects the cerebral hemispheres with the spinal cord. It consists of the mesencephalon, pons, and medulla oblongata. [NIH]

Breast Neoplasms: Tumors or cancer of the breast. [NIH]

Bronchial: Pertaining to one or more bronchi. [EU]

Bronchitis: Inflammation (swelling and reddening) of the bronchi. [NIH]

Bronchodilator: A drug that relaxes the smooth muscles in the constricted airway. [NIH]

Buccal: Pertaining to or directed toward the cheek. In dental anatomy, used to refer to the buccal surface of a tooth. [EU]

Bulimia: Episodic binge eating. The episodes may be associated with the fear of not being able to stop eating, depressed mood, or self-deprecating thoughts (binge-eating disorder) and may frequently be terminated by self-induced vomiting (bulimia nervosa). [NIH]

Calcitonin: A peptide hormone that lowers calcium concentration in the blood. In humans, it is released by thyroid cells and acts to decrease the formation and absorptive activity of osteoclasts. Its role in regulating plasma calcium is much greater in children and in certain diseases than in normal adults. [NIH]

Calcium: A basic element found in nearly all organized tissues. It is a member of the alkaline earth family of metals with the atomic symbol Ca, atomic number 20, and atomic weight 40. Calcium is the most abundant mineral in the body and combines with phosphorus to form calcium phosphate in the bones and teeth. It is essential for the normal functioning of nerves and muscles and plays a role in blood coagulation (as factor IV) and in many enzymatic processes. [NIH]

Caloric intake: Refers to the number of calories (energy content) consumed. [NIH]

Calpain: Cysteine proteinase found in many tissues. Hydrolyzes a variety of endogenous proteins including neuropeptides, cytoskeletal proteins, proteins from smooth muscle, cardiac muscle, liver, platelets and erythrocytes. Two subclasses having high and low calcium sensitivity are known. Removes Z-discs and M-lines from myofibrils. Activates phosphorylase kinase and cyclic nucleotide-independent protein kinase. [NIH]

Cannabidiol: Compound isolated from Cannabis sativa extract. [NIH]

Cannabinoids: Compounds extracted from Cannabis sativa L. and metabolites having the cannabinoid structure. The most active constituents are tetrahydrocannabinol, cannabinol, and cannabidiol. [NIH]

Cannabinol: A physiologically inactive constituent of Cannabis sativa L. [NIH]

Capillary: Any one of the minute vessels that connect the arterioles and venules, forming a network in nearly all parts of the body. Their walls act as semipermeable membranes for the interchange of various substances, including fluids, between the blood and tissue fluid; called also vas capillare. [EU]

Capsules: Hard or soft soluble containers used for the oral administration of medicine. [NIH]

Carbohydrate: An aldehyde or ketone derivative of a polyhydric alcohol, particularly of the pentahydric and hexahydric alcohols. They are so named because the hydrogen and oxygen are usually in the proportion to form water, $(CH2O)n$. The most important carbohydrates are the starches, sugars, celluloses, and gums. They are classified into mono-, di-, tri-, poly- and heterosaccharides. [EU]

Carbon Dioxide: A colorless, odorless gas that can be formed by the body and is necessary for the respiration cycle of plants and animals. [NIH]

Carcinogenic: Producing carcinoma. [EU]

Carcinoma: Cancer that begins in the skin or in tissues that line or cover internal organs. [NIH]

Cardiac: Having to do with the heart. [NIH]

Cardiovascular: Having to do with the heart and blood vessels. [NIH]

Cardiovascular disease: Any abnormal condition characterized by dysfunction of the heart and blood vessels. CVD includes atherosclerosis (especially coronary heart disease, which can lead to heart attacks), cerebrovascular disease (e.g., stroke), and hypertension (high blood pressure). [NIH]

Carmustine: An anticancer drug that belongs to the family of drugs called alkylating agents. [NIH]

Carnitine: Constituent of striated muscle and liver. It is used therapeutically to stimulate gastric and pancreatic secretions and in the treatment of hyperlipoproteinemias. [NIH]

Carotene: The general name for a group of pigments found in green, yellow, and leafy vegetables, and yellow fruits. The pigments are fat-soluble, unsaturated aliphatic hydrocarbons functioning as provitamins and are converted to vitamin A through enzymatic processes in the intestinal wall. [NIH]

Case report: A detailed report of the diagnosis, treatment, and follow-up of an individual patient. Case reports also contain some demographic information about the patient (for example, age, gender, ethnic origin). [NIH]

Case series: A group or series of case reports involving patients who were given similar treatment. Reports of case series usually contain detailed information about the individual patients. This includes demographic information (for example, age, gender, ethnic origin) and information on diagnosis, treatment, response to treatment, and follow-up after treatment. [NIH]

Caspase: Enzyme released by the cell at a crucial stage in apoptosis in order to shred all cellular proteins. [NIH]

Catabolism: Any destructive metabolic process by which organisms convert substances into excreted compounds. [EU]

Cataract: An opacity, partial or complete, of one or both eyes, on or in the lens or capsule, especially an opacity impairing vision or causing blindness. The many kinds of cataract are classified by their morphology (size, shape, location) or etiology (cause and time of occurrence). [EU]

Catecholamine: A group of chemical substances manufactured by the adrenal medulla and secreted during physiological stress. [NIH]

Caudal: Denoting a position more toward the cauda, or tail, than some specified point of reference; same as inferior, in human anatomy. [EU]

Causal: Pertaining to a cause; directed against a cause. [EU]

Cause of Death: Factors which produce cessation of all vital bodily functions. They can be analyzed from an epidemiologic viewpoint. [NIH]

Cell: The individual unit that makes up all of the tissues of the body. All living things are made up of one or more cells. [NIH]

Cell Cycle: The complex series of phenomena, occurring between the end of one cell division and the end of the next, by which cellular material is divided between daughter cells. [NIH]

Cell Death: The termination of the cell's ability to carry out vital functions such as metabolism, growth, reproduction, responsiveness, and adaptability. [NIH]

Cell Differentiation: Progressive restriction of the developmental potential and increasing specialization of function which takes place during the development of the embryo and leads to the formation of specialized cells, tissues, and organs. [NIH]

Cell Division: The fission of a cell. [NIH]

Cell Fusion: Fusion of somatic cells in vitro or in vivo, which results in somatic cell hybridization. [NIH]

Cell membrane: Cell membrane = plasma membrane. The structure enveloping a cell, enclosing the cytoplasm, and forming a selective permeability barrier; it consists of lipids, proteins, and some carbohydrates, the lipids thought to form a bilayer in which integral proteins are embedded to varying degrees. [EU]

Cell motility: The ability of a cell to move. [NIH]

Cell proliferation: An increase in the number of cells as a result of cell growth and cell division. [NIH]

Cell Respiration: The metabolic process of all living cells (animal and plant) in which oxygen is used to provide a source of energy for the cell. [NIH]

Cell Survival: The span of viability of a cell characterized by the capacity to perform certain functions such as metabolism, growth, reproduction, some form of responsiveness, and adaptability. [NIH]

Central Nervous System: The main information-processing organs of the nervous system, consisting of the brain, spinal cord, and meninges. [NIH]

Ceramide: A type of fat produced in the body. It may cause some types of cells to die, and is being studied in cancer treatment. [NIH]

Cerebral: Of or pertaining of the cerebrum or the brain. [EU]

Cerebrovascular: Pertaining to the blood vessels of the cerebrum, or brain. [EU]

Cerebrum: The largest part of the brain. It is divided into two hemispheres, or halves, called the cerebral hemispheres. The cerebrum controls muscle functions of the body and also controls speech, emotions, reading, writing, and learning. [NIH]

Cervical: Relating to the neck, or to the neck of any organ or structure. Cervical lymph nodes are located in the neck; cervical cancer refers to cancer of the uterine cervix, which is the lower, narrow end (the "neck") of the uterus. [NIH]

Cervix: The lower, narrow end of the uterus that forms a canal between the uterus and vagina. [NIH]

Character: In current usage, approximately equivalent to personality. The sum of the relatively fixed personality traits and habitual modes of response of an individual. [NIH]

Chemoprevention: The use of drugs, vitamins, or other agents to try to reduce the risk of, or delay the development or recurrence of, cancer. [NIH]

Chemotherapeutic agent: A drug used to treat cancer. [NIH]

Chemotherapy: Treatment with anticancer drugs. [NIH]

Chin: The anatomical frontal portion of the mandible, also known as the mentum, that contains the line of fusion of the two separate halves of the mandible (symphysis menti). This line of fusion divides inferiorly to enclose a triangular area called the mental protuberance. On each side, inferior to the second premolar tooth, is the mental foramen for the passage of blood vessels and a nerve. [NIH]

Chlorambucil: An anticancer drug that belongs to the family of drugs called alkylating agents. [NIH]

Chlorpromazine: The prototypical phenothiazine antipsychotic drug. Like the other drugs in this class chlorpromazine's antipsychotic actions are thought to be due to long-term adaptation by the brain to blocking dopamine receptors. Chlorpromazine has several other actions and therapeutic uses, including as an antiemetic and in the treatment of intractable hiccup. [NIH]

Cholesterol: The principal sterol of all higher animals, distributed in body tissues, especially the brain and spinal cord, and in animal fats and oils. [NIH]

Cholesterol Esters: Fatty acid esters of cholesterol which constitute about two-thirds of the cholesterol in the plasma. The accumulation of cholesterol esters in the arterial intima is a characteristic feature of atherosclerosis. [NIH]

Choline: A basic constituent of lecithin that is found in many plants and animal organs. It is important as a precursor of acetylcholine, as a methyl donor in various metabolic processes, and in lipid metabolism. [NIH]

Choline Kinase: An enzyme that is active in the first step of choline phosphoglyceride (lecithin) biosynthesis by catalyzing the phosphorylation of choline to phosphorylcholine in the presence of ATP. Ethanolamine and its methyl and ethyl derivatives can also act as acceptors. EC 2.7.1.32. [NIH]

Cholinergic: Resembling acetylcholine in pharmacological action; stimulated by or releasing acetylcholine or a related compound. [EU]

Chondrocytes: Polymorphic cells that form cartilage. [NIH]

Chorda Tympani Nerve: A branch of the facial (7th cranial) nerve which passes through the middle ear and continues through the petrotympanic fissure. The chorda tympani nerve carries taste sensation from the anterior two-thirds of the tongue and conveys parasympathetic efferents to the salivary glands. [NIH]

Chorion: The outermost extraembryonic membrane. [NIH]

Choroid: The thin, highly vascular membrane covering most of the posterior of the eye between the retina and sclera. [NIH]

Chromatin: The material of chromosomes. It is a complex of DNA, histones, and nonhistone proteins (chromosomal proteins, non-histone) found within the nucleus of a cell. [NIH]

Chromosomal: Pertaining to chromosomes. [EU]

Chromosome: Part of a cell that contains genetic information. Except for sperm and eggs, all human cells contain 46 chromosomes. [NIH]

Chronic: A disease or condition that persists or progresses over a long period of time. [NIH]

Chronic Disease: Disease or ailment of long duration. [NIH]

Chronic Obstructive Pulmonary Disease: Collective term for chronic bronchitis and emphysema. [NIH]

Chronic renal: Slow and progressive loss of kidney function over several years, often resulting in end-stage renal disease. People with end-stage renal disease need dialysis or transplantation to replace the work of the kidneys. [NIH]

Chylomicrons: A class of lipoproteins that carry dietary cholesterol and triglycerides from the small intestines to the tissues. [NIH]

Cicatrix: The formation of new tissue in the process of wound healing. [NIH]

Cicatrization: The formation of a cicatrix or scar. [EU]

Circadian: Repeated more or less daily, i. e. on a 23- to 25-hour cycle. [NIH]

Circadian Rhythm: The regular recurrence, in cycles of about 24 hours, of biological processes or activities, such as sensitivity to drugs and stimuli, hormone secretion, sleeping, feeding, etc. This rhythm seems to be set by a 'biological clock' which seems to be set by recurring daylight and darkness. [NIH]

Cirrhosis: A type of chronic, progressive liver disease. [NIH]

CIS: Cancer Information Service. The CIS is the National Cancer Institute's link to the public, interpreting and explaining research findings in a clear and understandable manner, and providing personalized responses to specific questions about cancer. Access the CIS by calling 1-800-4-CANCER, or by using the Web site at http://cis.nci.nih.gov. [NIH]

Cisplatin: An inorganic and water-soluble platinum complex. After undergoing hydrolysis, it reacts with DNA to produce both intra and interstrand crosslinks. These crosslinks appear to impair replication and transcription of DNA. The cytotoxicity of cisplatin correlates with cellular arrest in the G2 phase of the cell cycle. [NIH]

Clamp: A u-shaped steel rod used with a pin or wire for skeletal traction in the treatment of certain fractures. [NIH]

Clear cell carcinoma: A rare type of tumor of the female genital tract in which the inside of the cells looks clear when viewed under a microscope. [NIH]

Clenbuterol: A substituted phenylaminoethanol that has beta-2 adrenomimetic properties at very low doses. It is used as a bronchodilator in asthma. [NIH]

Clinical Medicine: The study and practice of medicine by direct examination of the patient. [NIH]

Clinical study: A research study in which patients receive treatment in a clinic or other medical facility. Reports of clinical studies can contain results for single patients (case reports) or many patients (case series or clinical trials). [NIH]

Clinical trial: A research study that tests how well new medical treatments or other interventions work in people. Each study is designed to test new methods of screening, prevention, diagnosis, or treatment of a disease. [NIH]

Cloning: The production of a number of genetically identical individuals; in genetic engineering, a process for the efficient replication of a great number of identical DNA molecules. [NIH]

Coagulation: 1. The process of clot formation. 2. In colloid chemistry, the solidification of a sol into a gelatinous mass; an alteration of a disperse phase or of a dissolved solid which causes the separation of the system into a liquid phase and an insoluble mass called the clot or curd. Coagulation is usually irreversible. 3. In surgery, the disruption of tissue by physical means to form an amorphous residuum, as in electrocoagulation and photocoagulation. [EU]

Coenzyme: An organic nonprotein molecule, frequently a phosphorylated derivative of a water-soluble vitamin, that binds with the protein molecule (apoenzyme) to form the active enzyme (holoenzyme). [EU]

Cofactor: A substance, microorganism or environmental factor that activates or enhances the action of another entity such as a disease-causing agent. [NIH]

Colitis: Inflammation of the colon. [NIH]

Collagen: A polypeptide substance comprising about one third of the total protein in mammalian organisms. It is the main constituent of skin, connective tissue, and the organic substance of bones and teeth. Different forms of collagen are produced in the body but all consist of three alpha-polypeptide chains arranged in a triple helix. Collagen is differentiated from other fibrous proteins, such as elastin, by the content of proline, hydroxyproline, and hydroxylysine; by the absence of tryptophan; and particularly by the high content of polar groups which are responsible for its swelling properties. [NIH]

Collagen disease: A term previously used to describe chronic diseases of the connective tissue (e.g., rheumatoid arthritis, systemic lupus erythematosus, and systemic sclerosis), but now is thought to be more appropriate for diseases associated with defects in collagen, which is a component of the connective tissue. [NIH]

Collagenases: Enzymes that catalyze the degradation of collagen by acting on the peptide bonds. EC 3.4.24.-. [NIH]

Colloidal: Of the nature of a colloid. [EU]

Colon: The long, coiled, tubelike organ that removes water from digested food. The remaining material, solid waste called stool, moves through the colon to the rectum and leaves the body through the anus. [NIH]

Combination Therapy: Association of 3 drugs to treat AIDS (AZT + DDC or DDI + protease inhibitor). [NIH]

Complement: A term originally used to refer to the heat-labile factor in serum that causes immune cytolysis, the lysis of antibody-coated cells, and now referring to the entire functionally related system comprising at least 20 distinct serum proteins that is the effector not only of immune cytolysis but also of other biologic functions. Complement activation occurs by two different sequences, the classic and alternative pathways. The proteins of the classic pathway are termed 'components of complement' and are designated by the symbols C1 through C9. C1 is a calcium-dependent complex of three distinct proteins C1q, C1r and C1s. The proteins of the alternative pathway (collectively referred to as the properdin system) and complement regulatory proteins are known by semisystematic or trivial names. Fragments resulting from proteolytic cleavage of complement proteins are designated with lower-case letter suffixes, e.g., C3a. Inactivated fragments may be designated with the suffix 'i', e.g. C3bi. Activated components or complexes with biological activity are designated by a bar over the symbol e.g. C1 or C4b,2a. The classic pathway is activated by the binding of C1 to classic pathway activators, primarily antigen-antibody complexes containing IgM, IgG1, IgG3; C1q binds to a single IgM molecule or two adjacent IgG molecules. The alternative pathway can be activated by IgA immune complexes and also by nonimmunologic materials including bacterial endotoxins, microbial polysaccharides, and cell walls. Activation of the classic pathway triggers an enzymatic cascade involving C1, C4, C2 and C3; activation of the alternative pathway triggers a cascade involving C3 and factors B, D and P. Both result in the cleavage of C5 and the formation of the membrane attack complex. Complement activation also results in the formation of many biologically active complement fragments that act as anaphylatoxins, opsonins, or chemotactic factors. [EU]

Complementary and alternative medicine: CAM. Forms of treatment that are used in addition to (complementary) or instead of (alternative) standard treatments. These practices are not considered standard medical approaches. CAM includes dietary supplements, megadose vitamins, herbal preparations, special teas, massage therapy, magnet therapy, spiritual healing, and meditation. [NIH]

Complementary medicine: Practices not generally recognized by the medical community as standard or conventional medical approaches and used to enhance or complement the standard treatments. Complementary medicine includes the taking of dietary supplements, megadose vitamins, and herbal preparations; the drinking of special teas; and practices such as massage therapy, magnet therapy, spiritual healing, and meditation. [NIH]

Compliance: Distensibility measure of a chamber such as the lungs (lung compliance) or bladder. Compliance is expressed as a change in volume per unit change in pressure. [NIH]

Computational Biology: A field of biology concerned with the development of techniques for the collection and manipulation of biological data, and the use of such data to make biological discoveries or predictions. This field encompasses all computational methods and theories applicable to molecular biology and areas of computer-based techniques for solving biological problems including manipulation of models and datasets. [NIH]

Concomitant: Accompanying; accessory; joined with another. [EU]

Confusion: A mental state characterized by bewilderment, emotional disturbance, lack of clear thinking, and perceptual disorientation. [NIH]

Congestive heart failure: Weakness of the heart muscle that leads to a buildup of fluid in body tissues. [NIH]

Conjugated: Acting or operating as if joined; simultaneous. [EU]

Conjugation: 1. The act of joining together or the state of being conjugated. 2. A sexual process seen in bacteria, ciliate protozoa, and certain fungi in which nuclear material is exchanged during the temporary fusion of two cells (conjugants). In bacterial genetics a form of sexual reproduction in which a donor bacterium (male) contributes some, or all, of its DNA (in the form of a replicated set) to a recipient (female) which then incorporates differing genetic information into its own chromosome by recombination and passes the recombined set on to its progeny by replication. In ciliate protozoa, two conjugants of separate mating types exchange micronuclear material and then separate, each now being a fertilized cell. In certain fungi, the process involves fusion of two gametes, resulting in union of their nuclei and formation of a zygote. 3. In chemistry, the joining together of two compounds to produce another compound, such as the combination of a toxic product with some substance in the body to form a detoxified product, which is then eliminated. [EU]

Conjunctiva: The mucous membrane that lines the inner surface of the eyelids and the anterior part of the sclera. [NIH]

Connective Tissue: Tissue that supports and binds other tissues. It consists of connective tissue cells embedded in a large amount of extracellular matrix. [NIH]

Connective Tissue: Tissue that supports and binds other tissues. It consists of connective tissue cells embedded in a large amount of extracellular matrix. [NIH]

Connective Tissue Cells: A group of cells that includes fibroblasts, cartilage cells, adipocytes, smooth muscle cells, and bone cells. [NIH]

Consciousness: Sense of awareness of self and of the environment. [NIH]

Constitutional: 1. Affecting the whole constitution of the body; not local. 2. Pertaining to the constitution. [EU]

Contraceptive: An agent that diminishes the likelihood of or prevents conception. [EU]

Contraindications: Any factor or sign that it is unwise to pursue a certain kind of action or treatment, e. g. giving a general anesthetic to a person with pneumonia. [NIH]

Contralateral: Having to do with the opposite side of the body. [NIH]

Control group: In a clinical trial, the group that does not receive the new treatment being studied. This group is compared to the group that receives the new treatment, to see if the new treatment works. [NIH]

Controlled study: An experiment or clinical trial that includes a comparison (control) group. [NIH]

Coordination: Muscular or motor regulation or the harmonious cooperation of muscles or groups of muscles, in a complex action or series of actions. [NIH]

Cornea: The transparent part of the eye that covers the iris and the pupil and allows light to enter the inside. [NIH]

Corneal Ulcer: Loss of epithelial tissue from the surface of the cornea due to progressive erosion and necrosis of the tissue; usually caused by bacterial, fungal, or viral infection. [NIH]

Coronary: Encircling in the manner of a crown; a term applied to vessels; nerves, ligaments, etc. The term usually denotes the arteries that supply the heart muscle and, by extension, a pathologic involvement of them. [EU]

Coronary Circulation: The circulation of blood through the coronary vessels of the heart. [NIH]

Coronary heart disease: A type of heart disease caused by narrowing of the coronary arteries that feed the heart, which needs a constant supply of oxygen and nutrients carried by the blood in the coronary arteries. When the coronary arteries become narrowed or clogged by fat and cholesterol deposits and cannot supply enough blood to the heart, CHD results. [NIH]

Coronary Thrombosis: Presence of a thrombus in a coronary artery, often causing a myocardial infarction. [NIH]

Corpus: The body of the uterus. [NIH]

Corpus Luteum: The yellow glandular mass formed in the ovary by an ovarian follicle that has ruptured and discharged its ovum. [NIH]

Cortex: The outer layer of an organ or other body structure, as distinguished from the internal substance. [EU]

Cortical: Pertaining to or of the nature of a cortex or bark. [EU]

Corticosteroids: Hormones that have antitumor activity in lymphomas and lymphoid leukemias; in addition, corticosteroids (steroids) may be used for hormone replacement and for the management of some of the complications of cancer and its treatment. [NIH]

Cortisol: A steroid hormone secreted by the adrenal cortex as part of the body's response to stress. [NIH]

Cortisone: A natural steroid hormone produced in the adrenal gland. It can also be made in the laboratory. Cortisone reduces swelling and can suppress immune responses. [NIH]

Cranial: Pertaining to the cranium, or to the anterior (in animals) or superior (in humans) end of the body. [EU]

Croton Oil: Viscous, nauseating oil obtained from the shrub Croton tiglium (Euphorbaceae). It is a vesicant and skin irritant used as pharmacologic standard for skin inflammation and allergy and causes skin cancer. It was formerly used as an emetic and cathartic with frequent mortality. [NIH]

Curative: Tending to overcome disease and promote recovery. [EU]

Cutaneous: Having to do with the skin. [NIH]

Cyclic: Pertaining to or occurring in a cycle or cycles; the term is applied to chemical compounds that contain a ring of atoms in the nucleus. [EU]

Cyclin: Molecule that regulates the cell cycle. [NIH]

Cyclophosphamide: Precursor of an alkylating nitrogen mustard antineoplastic and immunosuppressive agent that must be activated in the liver to form the active aldophosphamide. It is used in the treatment of lymphomas, leukemias, etc. Its side effect, alopecia, has been made use of in defleecing sheep. Cyclophosphamide may also cause sterility, birth defects, mutations, and cancer. [NIH]

Cyproheptadine: A serotonin antagonist and a histamine H1 blocker used as antipruritic, appetite stimulant, antiallergic, and for the post-gastrectomy dumping syndrome, etc. [NIH]

Cysteine: A thiol-containing non-essential amino acid that is oxidized to form cystine. [NIH]

Cystine: A covalently linked dimeric nonessential amino acid formed by the oxidation of cysteine. Two molecules of cysteine are joined together by a disulfide bridge to form cystine. [NIH]

Cytochrome: Any electron transfer hemoprotein having a mode of action in which the transfer of a single electron is effected by a reversible valence change of the central iron atom of the heme prosthetic group between the +2 and +3 oxidation states; classified as cytochromes a in which the heme contains a formyl side chain, cytochromes b, which contain protoheme or a closely similar heme that is not covalently bound to the protein, cytochromes c in which protoheme or other heme is covalently bound to the protein, and cytochromes d in which the iron-tetrapyrrole has fewer conjugated double bonds than the hemes have. Well-known cytochromes have been numbered consecutively within groups and are designated by subscripts (beginning with no subscript), e.g. cytochromes c, c1, C2, . New cytochromes are named according to the wavelength in nanometres of the absorption maximum of the a-band of the iron (II) form in pyridine, e.g., c-555. [EU]

Cytogenetics: A branch of genetics which deals with the cytological and molecular behavior of genes and chromosomes during cell division. [NIH]

Cytokine: Small but highly potent protein that modulates the activity of many cell types, including T and B cells. [NIH]

Cytopenia: A reduction in the number of blood cells. [NIH]

Cytoplasm: The protoplasm of a cell exclusive of that of the nucleus; it consists of a continuous aqueous solution (cytosol) and the organelles and inclusions suspended in it (phaneroplasm), and is the site of most of the chemical activities of the cell. [EU]

Cytoskeletal Proteins: Major constituent of the cytoskeleton found in the cytoplasm of eukaryotic cells. They form a flexible framework for the cell, provide attachment points for organelles and formed bodies, and make communication between parts of the cell possible. [NIH]

Cytotoxic: Cell-killing. [NIH]

Cytotoxic chemotherapy: Anticancer drugs that kill cells, especially cancer cells. [NIH]

Cytotoxicity: Quality of being capable of producing a specific toxic action upon cells of special organs. [NIH]

Dactinomycin: An anticancer drug that belongs to the family of drugs called antitumor antibiotics. [NIH]

Dantrolene: Skeletal muscle relaxant that acts by interfering with excitation-contraction coupling in the muscle fiber. It is used in spasticity and other neuromuscular abnormalities. Although the mechanism of action is probably not central, dantrolene is usually grouped with the central muscle relaxants. [NIH]

Daunorubicin: Very toxic anthracycline aminoglycoside antibiotic isolated from Streptomyces peucetius and others, used in treatment of leukemias and other neoplasms. [NIH]

Deamination: The removal of an amino group (NH2) from a chemical compound. [NIH]

Decarboxylation: The removal of a carboxyl group, usually in the form of carbon dioxide, from a chemical compound. [NIH]

Decidua: The epithelial lining of the endometrium that is formed before the fertilized ovum reaches the uterus. The fertilized ovum embeds in the decidua. If the ovum is not fertilized, the decidua is shed during menstruation. [NIH]

Degenerative: Undergoing degeneration : tending to degenerate; having the character of or involving degeneration; causing or tending to cause degeneration. [EU]

Dehydration: The condition that results from excessive loss of body water. [NIH]

Dehydroepiandrosterone: DHEA. A substance that is being studied as a cancer prevention drug. It belongs to the family of drugs called steroids. [NIH]

Deletion: A genetic rearrangement through loss of segments of DNA (chromosomes), bringing sequences, which are normally separated, into close proximity. [NIH]

Delirium: (DSM III-R) an acute, reversible organic mental disorder characterized by reduced ability to maintain attention to external stimuli and disorganized thinking as manifested by rambling, irrelevant, or incoherent speech; there are also a reduced level of consciousness, sensory misperceptions, disturbance of the sleep-wakefulness cycle and level of psychomotor activity, disorientation to time, place, or person, and memory impairment. Delirium may be caused by a large number of conditions resulting in derangement of cerebral metabolism, including systemic infection, poisoning, drug intoxication or withdrawal, seizures or head trauma, and metabolic disturbances such as hypoxia, hypoglycaemia, fluid, electrolyte, or acid-base imbalances, or hepatic or renal failure. Called also acute confusional state and acute brain syndrome. [EU]

Delivery of Health Care: The concept concerned with all aspects of providing and distributing health services to a patient population. [NIH]

Dementia: An acquired organic mental disorder with loss of intellectual abilities of sufficient severity to interfere with social or occupational functioning. The dysfunction is multifaceted and involves memory, behavior, personality, judgment, attention, spatial relations, language, abstract thought, and other executive functions. The intellectual decline is usually progressive, and initially spares the level of consciousness. [NIH]

Demyelinating Diseases: Diseases characterized by loss or dysfunction of myelin in the central or peripheral nervous system. [NIH]

Dendrites: Extensions of the nerve cell body. They are short and branched and receive stimuli from other neurons. [NIH]

Depolarization: The process or act of neutralizing polarity. In neurophysiology, the reversal of the resting potential in excitable cell membranes when stimulated, i.e., the tendency of the cell membrane potential to become positive with respect to the potential outside the cell. [EU]

Deprivation: Loss or absence of parts, organs, powers, or things that are needed. [EU]

Dermatitis: Any inflammation of the skin. [NIH]

DES: Diethylstilbestrol. A synthetic hormone that was prescribed from the early 1940s until 1971 to help women with complications of pregnancy. DES has been linked to an increased risk of clear cell carcinoma of the vagina in daughters of women who used DES. DES may also increase the risk of breast cancer in women who used DES. [NIH]

Desensitization: The prevention or reduction of immediate hypersensitivity reactions by administration of graded doses of allergen; called also hyposensitization and immunotherapy. [EU]

Deuterium: Deuterium. The stable isotope of hydrogen. It has one neutron and one proton in the nucleus. [NIH]

Dexamethasone: (11 beta,16 alpha)-9-Fluoro-11,17,21-trihydroxy-16-methylpregna-1,4-

diene-3,20-dione. An anti-inflammatory glucocorticoid used either in the free alcohol or esterified form in treatment of conditions that respond generally to cortisone. [NIH]

Diabetes Mellitus: A heterogeneous group of disorders that share glucose intolerance in common. [NIH]

Diabetic Retinopathy: Retinopathy associated with diabetes mellitus, which may be of the background type, progressively characterized by microaneurysms, interretinal punctuate macular edema, or of the proliferative type, characterized by neovascularization of the retina and optic disk, which may project into the vitreous, proliferation of fibrous tissue, vitreous hemorrhage, and retinal detachment. [NIH]

Diagnostic procedure: A method used to identify a disease. [NIH]

Dialyzer: A part of the hemodialysis machine. (See hemodialysis under dialysis.) The dialyzer has two sections separated by a membrane. One section holds dialysate. The other holds the patient's blood. [NIH]

Diarrhea: Passage of excessively liquid or excessively frequent stools. [NIH]

Diastolic: Of or pertaining to the diastole. [EU]

Dietary Fats: Fats present in food, especially in animal products such as meat, meat products, butter, ghee. They are present in lower amounts in nuts, seeds, and avocados. [NIH]

Digestion: The process of breakdown of food for metabolism and use by the body. [NIH]

Digestive system: The organs that take in food and turn it into products that the body can use to stay healthy. Waste products the body cannot use leave the body through bowel movements. The digestive system includes the salivary glands, mouth, esophagus, stomach, liver, pancreas, gallbladder, small and large intestines, and rectum. [NIH]

Digestive tract: The organs through which food passes when food is eaten. These organs are the mouth, esophagus, stomach, small and large intestines, and rectum. [NIH]

Dihydrotestosterone: Anabolic agent. [NIH]

Diltiazem: A benzothiazepine derivative with vasodilating action due to its antagonism of the actions of the calcium ion in membrane functions. It is also teratogenic. [NIH]

Direct: 1. Straight; in a straight line. 2. Performed immediately and without the intervention of subsidiary means. [EU]

Discrete: Made up of separate parts or characterized by lesions which do not become blended; not running together; separate. [NIH]

Disease Progression: The worsening of a disease over time. This concept is most often used for chronic and incurable diseases where the stage of the disease is an important determinant of therapy and prognosis. [NIH]

Disorientation: The loss of proper bearings, or a state of mental confusion as to time, place, or identity. [EU]

Dissection: Cutting up of an organism for study. [NIH]

Dissociation: 1. The act of separating or state of being separated. 2. The separation of a molecule into two or more fragments (atoms, molecules, ions, or free radicals) produced by the absorption of light or thermal energy or by solvation. 3. In psychology, a defense mechanism in which a group of mental processes are segregated from the rest of a person's mental activity in order to avoid emotional distress, as in the dissociative disorders (q.v.), or in which an idea or object is segregated from its emotional significance; in the first sense it is roughly equivalent to splitting, in the second, to isolation. 4. A defect of mental integration in which one or more groups of mental processes become separated off from normal consciousness and, thus separated, function as a unitary whole. [EU]

Distal: Remote; farther from any point of reference; opposed to proximal. In dentistry, used to designate a position on the dental arch farther from the median line of the jaw. [EU]

Diuretic: A drug that increases the production of urine. [NIH]

Diverticulum: A pathological condition manifested as a pouch or sac opening from a tubular or sacular organ. [NIH]

Dopamine: An endogenous catecholamine and prominent neurotransmitter in several systems of the brain. In the synthesis of catecholamines from tyrosine, it is the immediate precursor to norepinephrine and epinephrine. Dopamine is a major transmitter in the extrapyramidal system of the brain, and important in regulating movement. A family of dopaminergic receptor subtypes mediate its action. Dopamine is used pharmacologically for its direct (beta adrenergic agonist) and indirect (adrenergic releasing) sympathomimetic effects including its actions as an inotropic agent and as a renal vasodilator. [NIH]

Dose-dependent: Refers to the effects of treatment with a drug. If the effects change when the dose of the drug is changed, the effects are said to be dose dependent. [NIH]

Double-blind: Pertaining to a clinical trial or other experiment in which neither the subject nor the person administering treatment knows which treatment any particular subject is receiving. [EU]

Doxorubicin: Antineoplastic antibiotic obtained from Streptomyces peucetics. It is a hydroxy derivative of daunorubicin and is used in treatment of both leukemia and solid tumors. [NIH]

Drinking Behavior: Behaviors associated with the ingesting of water and other liquids; includes rhythmic patterns of drinking (time intervals - onset and duration), frequency and satiety. [NIH]

Drive: A state of internal activity of an organism that is a necessary condition before a given stimulus will elicit a class of responses; e.g., a certain level of hunger (drive) must be present before food will elicit an eating response. [NIH]

Dronabinol: A synthetic pill form of delta-9-tetrahydrocannabinol (THC), an active ingredient in marijuana that is used to treat nausea and vomiting associated with cancer chemotherapy. [NIH]

Drug Interactions: The action of a drug that may affect the activity, metabolism, or toxicity of another drug. [NIH]

Dumping Syndrome: Gastrointestinal symptoms resulting from an absent or nonfunctioning pylorus. [NIH]

Duodenum: The first part of the small intestine. [NIH]

Dura mater: The outermost, toughest, and most fibrous of the three membranes (meninges) covering the brain and spinal cord; called also pachymeninx. [EU]

Dwarfism: The condition of being undersized as a result of premature arrest of skeletal growth. It may be caused by insufficient secretion of growth hormone (pituitary dwarfism). [NIH]

Dysgeusia: A condition characterized by alterations of the sense of taste which may range from mild to severe, including gross distortions of taste quality. [NIH]

Dyskinesia: Impairment of the power of voluntary movement, resulting in fragmentary or incomplete movements. [EU]

Dysmenorrhea: Painful menstruation. [NIH]

Dyspepsia: Impaired digestion, especially after eating. [NIH]

Dysphagia: Difficulty in swallowing. [EU]

Dyspnea: Difficult or labored breathing. [NIH]

Dystrophin: A muscle protein localized in surface membranes which is the product of the Duchenne/Becker muscular dystrophy gene. Individuals with Duchenne muscular dystrophy usually lack dystrophin completely while those with Becker muscular dystrophy have dystrophin of an altered size. It shares features with other cytoskeletal proteins such as spectrin and alpha-actinin but the precise function of dystrophin is not clear. One possible role might be to preserve the integrity and alignment of the plasma membrane to the myofibrils during muscle contraction and relaxation. MW 400 kDa. [NIH]

Dystrophy: Any disorder arising from defective or faulty nutrition, especially the muscular dystrophies. [EU]

Eating Disorders: A group of disorders characterized by physiological and psychological disturbances in appetite or food intake. [NIH]

Edema: Excessive amount of watery fluid accumulated in the intercellular spaces, most commonly present in subcutaneous tissue. [NIH]

Effector: It is often an enzyme that converts an inactive precursor molecule into an active second messenger. [NIH]

Efficacy: The extent to which a specific intervention, procedure, regimen, or service produces a beneficial result under ideal conditions. Ideally, the determination of efficacy is based on the results of a randomized control trial. [NIH]

Eicosanoids: A class of oxygenated, endogenous, unsaturated fatty acids derived from arachidonic acid. They include prostaglandins, leukotrienes, thromboxanes, and hydroxyeicosatetraenoic acid compounds (HETE). They are hormone-like substances that act near the site of synthesis without altering functions throughout the body. [NIH]

Elasticity: Resistance and recovery from distortion of shape. [NIH]

Elastin: The protein that gives flexibility to tissues. [NIH]

Elective: Subject to the choice or decision of the patient or physician; applied to procedures that are advantageous to the patient but not urgent. [EU]

Electrocoagulation: Electrosurgical procedures used to treat hemorrhage (e.g., bleeding ulcers) and to ablate tumors, mucosal lesions, and refractory arrhythmias. [NIH]

Electrolysis: Destruction by passage of a galvanic electric current, as in disintegration of a chemical compound in solution. [NIH]

Electrolyte: A substance that dissociates into ions when fused or in solution, and thus becomes capable of conducting electricity; an ionic solute. [EU]

Electrons: Stable elementary particles having the smallest known negative charge, present in all elements; also called negatrons. Positively charged electrons are called positrons. The numbers, energies and arrangement of electrons around atomic nuclei determine the chemical identities of elements. Beams of electrons are called cathode rays or beta rays, the latter being a high-energy biproduct of nuclear decay. [NIH]

Electrophoresis: An electrochemical process in which macromolecules or colloidal particles with a net electric charge migrate in a solution under the influence of an electric current. [NIH]

Electroporation: A technique in which electric pulses of intensity in kilovolts per centimeter and of microsecond-to-millisecond duration cause a temporary loss of the semipermeability of cell membranes, thus leading to ion leakage, escape of metabolites, and increased uptake by cells of drugs, molecular probes, and DNA. Some applications of electroporation include introduction of plasmids or foreign DNA into living cells for transfection, fusion of cells to prepare hybridomas, and insertion of proteins into cell membranes. [NIH]

Emaciation: Clinical manifestation of excessive leanness usually caused by disease or a lack of nutrition. [NIH]

Embryo: The prenatal stage of mammalian development characterized by rapid morphological changes and the differentiation of basic structures. [NIH]

Emesis: Vomiting; an act of vomiting. Also used as a word termination, as in haematemesis. [EU]

Emetic: An agent that causes vomiting. [EU]

Emollient: Softening or soothing; called also malactic. [EU]

Emphysema: A pathological accumulation of air in tissues or organs. [NIH]

Emulsion: A preparation of one liquid distributed in small globules throughout the body of a second liquid. The dispersed liquid is the discontinuous phase, and the dispersion medium is the continuous phase. When oil is the dispersed liquid and an aqueous solution is the continuous phase, it is known as an oil-in-water emulsion, whereas when water or aqueous solution is the dispersed phase and oil or oleaginous substance is the continuous phase, it is known as a water-in-oil emulsion. Pharmaceutical emulsions for which official standards have been promulgated include cod liver oil emulsion, cod liver oil emulsion with malt, liquid petrolatum emulsion, and phenolphthalein in liquid petrolatum emulsion. [EU]

Enalapril: An angiotensin-converting enzyme inhibitor that is used to treat hypertension. [NIH]

Endemic: Present or usually prevalent in a population or geographical area at all times; said of a disease or agent. Called also endemial. [EU]

Endocrine System: The system of glands that release their secretions (hormones) directly into the circulatory system. In addition to the endocrine glands, included are the chromaffin system and the neurosecretory systems. [NIH]

Endogenous: Produced inside an organism or cell. The opposite is external (exogenous) production. [NIH]

Endorphins: One of the three major groups of endogenous opioid peptides. They are large peptides derived from the pro-opiomelanocortin precursor. The known members of this group are alpha-, beta-, and gamma-endorphin. The term endorphin is also sometimes used to refer to all opioid peptides, but the narrower sense is used here; opioid peptides is used for the broader group. [NIH]

Endothelial cell: The main type of cell found in the inside lining of blood vessels, lymph vessels, and the heart. [NIH]

Endothelium: A layer of epithelium that lines the heart, blood vessels (endothelium, vascular), lymph vessels (endothelium, lymphatic), and the serous cavities of the body. [NIH]

Endothelium-derived: Small molecule that diffuses to the adjacent muscle layer and relaxes it. [NIH]

Endotoxemia: A condition characterized by the presence of endotoxins in the blood. If endotoxemia is the result of gram-negative rod-shaped bacteria, shock may occur. [NIH]

Endotoxic: Of, relating to, or acting as an endotoxin (= a heat-stable toxin, associated with the outer membranes of certain gram-negative bacteria. Endotoxins are not secreted and are released only when the cells are disrupted). [EU]

Endotoxin: Toxin from cell walls of bacteria. [NIH]

End-stage renal: Total chronic kidney failure. When the kidneys fail, the body retains fluid and harmful wastes build up. A person with ESRD needs treatment to replace the work of the failed kidneys. [NIH]

Energetic: Exhibiting energy : strenuous; operating with force, vigour, or effect. [EU]

Energy balance: Energy is the capacity of a body or a physical system for doing work. Energy balance is the state in which the total energy intake equals total energy needs. [NIH]

Enhancer: Transcriptional element in the virus genome. [NIH]

Enkephalins: One of the three major families of endogenous opioid peptides. The enkephalins are pentapeptides that are widespread in the central and peripheral nervous systems and in the adrenal medulla. [NIH]

Environmental Exposure: The exposure to potentially harmful chemical, physical, or biological agents in the environment or to environmental factors that may include ionizing radiation, pathogenic organisms, or toxic chemicals. [NIH]

Environmental Health: The science of controlling or modifying those conditions, influences, or forces surrounding man which relate to promoting, establishing, and maintaining health. [NIH]

Enzymatic: Phase where enzyme cuts the precursor protein. [NIH]

Enzyme: A protein that speeds up chemical reactions in the body. [NIH]

Ependyma: A thin membrane that lines the ventricles of the brain and the central canal of the spinal cord. [NIH]

Epidermal: Pertaining to or resembling epidermis. Called also epidermic or epidermoid. [EU]

Epidermal Growth Factor: A 6 kD polypeptide growth factor initially discovered in mouse submaxillary glands. Human epidermal growth factor was originally isolated from urine based on its ability to inhibit gastric secretion and called urogastrone. epidermal growth factor exerts a wide variety of biological effects including the promotion of proliferation and differentiation of mesenchymal and epithelial cells. [NIH]

Epidermis: Nonvascular layer of the skin. It is made up, from within outward, of five layers: 1) basal layer (stratum basale epidermidis); 2) spinous layer (stratum spinosum epidermidis); 3) granular layer (stratum granulosum epidermidis); 4) clear layer (stratum lucidum epidermidis); and 5) horny layer (stratum corneum epidermidis). [NIH]

Epidermoid carcinoma: A type of cancer in which the cells are flat and look like fish scales. Also called squamous cell carcinoma. [NIH]

Epigastric: Having to do with the upper middle area of the abdomen. [NIH]

Epinephrine: The active sympathomimetic hormone from the adrenal medulla in most species. It stimulates both the alpha- and beta- adrenergic systems, causes systemic vasoconstriction and gastrointestinal relaxation, stimulates the heart, and dilates bronchi and cerebral vessels. It is used in asthma and cardiac failure and to delay absorption of local anesthetics. [NIH]

Epithelial: Refers to the cells that line the internal and external surfaces of the body. [NIH]

Epithelial Cells: Cells that line the inner and outer surfaces of the body. [NIH]

Epithelium: One or more layers of epithelial cells, supported by the basal lamina, which covers the inner or outer surfaces of the body. [NIH]

Erythrocytes: Red blood cells. Mature erythrocytes are non-nucleated, biconcave disks containing hemoglobin whose function is to transport oxygen. [NIH]

Erythroid Progenitor Cells: Committed, erythroid stem cells derived from myeloid stem cells. The progenitor cells develop in two phases: erythroid burst-forming units (BFU-E) followed by erythroid colony-forming units (CFU-E). BFU-E differentiate into CFU-E on stimulation by erythropoietin, and then further differentiate into erythroblasts when stimulated by other factors. [NIH]

Esophageal: Having to do with the esophagus, the muscular tube through which food passes from the throat to the stomach. [NIH]

Esophagitis: Inflammation, acute or chronic, of the esophagus caused by bacteria, chemicals, or trauma. [NIH]

Esophagus: The muscular tube through which food passes from the throat to the stomach. [NIH]

Estrogen: One of the two female sex hormones. [NIH]

Etoposide: A semisynthetic derivative of podophyllotoxin that exhibits antitumor activity. Etoposide inhibits DNA synthesis by forming a complex with topoisomerase II and DNA. This complex induces breaks in double stranded DNA and prevents repair by topoisomerase II binding. Accumulated breaks in DNA prevent entry into the mitotic phase of cell division, and lead to cell death. Etoposide acts primarily in the G2 and S phases of the cell cycle. [NIH]

Eukaryotic Cells: Cells of the higher organisms, containing a true nucleus bounded by a nuclear membrane. [NIH]

Evoke: The electric response recorded from the cerebral cortex after stimulation of a peripheral sense organ. [NIH]

Excipients: Usually inert substances added to a prescription in order to provide suitable consistency to the dosage form; a binder, matrix, base or diluent in pills, tablets, creams, salves, etc. [NIH]

Excitation: An act of irritation or stimulation or of responding to a stimulus; the addition of energy, as the excitation of a molecule by absorption of photons. [EU]

Excitatory: When cortical neurons are excited, their output increases and each new input they receive while they are still excited raises their output markedly. [NIH]

Excrete: To get rid of waste from the body. [NIH]

Exhaustion: The feeling of weariness of mind and body. [NIH]

Exocrine: Secreting outwardly, via a duct. [EU]

Exocytosis: Cellular release of material within membrane-limited vesicles by fusion of the vesicles with the cell membrane. [NIH]

Exogenous: Developed or originating outside the organism, as exogenous disease. [EU]

Exotoxin: Toxic substance excreted by living bacterial cells. [NIH]

Expiration: The act of breathing out, or expelling air from the lungs. [EU]

Extensor: A muscle whose contraction tends to straighten a limb; the antagonist of a flexor. [NIH]

External-beam radiation: Radiation therapy that uses a machine to aim high-energy rays at the cancer. Also called external radiation. [NIH]

Extracellular: Outside a cell or cells. [EU]

Extracellular Matrix: A meshwork-like substance found within the extracellular space and in association with the basement membrane of the cell surface. It promotes cellular proliferation and provides a supporting structure to which cells or cell lysates in culture dishes adhere. [NIH]

Extracellular Matrix Proteins: Macromolecular organic compounds that contain carbon, hydrogen, oxygen, nitrogen, and usually, sulfur. These macromolecules (proteins) form an intricate meshwork in which cells are embedded to construct tissues. Variations in the relative types of macromolecules and their organization determine the type of extracellular matrix, each adapted to the functional requirements of the tissue. The two main classes of macromolecules that form the extracellular matrix are: glycosaminoglycans, usually linked to proteins (proteoglycans), and fibrous proteins (e.g., collagen, elastin, fibronectins and laminin). [NIH]

Extracellular Space: Interstitial space between cells, occupied by fluid as well as amorphous and fibrous substances. [NIH]

Extraction: The process or act of pulling or drawing out. [EU]

Extrapyramidal: Outside of the pyramidal tracts. [EU]

Extremity: A limb; an arm or leg (membrum); sometimes applied specifically to a hand or foot. [EU]

Facial: Of or pertaining to the face. [EU]

Facial Nerve: The 7th cranial nerve. The facial nerve has two parts, the larger motor root which may be called the facial nerve proper, and the smaller intermediate or sensory root. Together they provide efferent innervation to the muscles of facial expression and to the lacrimal and salivary glands, and convey afferent information for taste from the anterior two-thirds of the tongue and for touch from the external ear. [NIH]

Failure to Thrive: A condition in which an infant or child's weight gain and growth are far below usual levels for age. [NIH]

Family Planning: Programs or services designed to assist the family in controlling reproduction by either improving or diminishing fertility. [NIH]

Fat: Total lipids including phospholipids. [NIH]

Fatigue: The state of weariness following a period of exertion, mental or physical, characterized by a decreased capacity for work and reduced efficiency to respond to stimuli. [NIH]

Fatty acids: A major component of fats that are used by the body for energy and tissue development. [NIH]

Feces: The excrement discharged from the intestines, consisting of bacteria, cells exfoliated from the intestines, secretions, chiefly of the liver, and a small amount of food residue. [EU]

Feeding Behavior: Behavioral responses or sequences associated with eating including modes of feeding, rhythmic patterns of eating, and time intervals. [NIH]

Fetal Membranes: Thin layers of tissue which surround the embryo or fetus and provide for its nutrition, respiration, excretion and protection; they are the yolk sac, allantois, amnion, and chorion. [NIH]

Fetus: The developing offspring from 7 to 8 weeks after conception until birth. [NIH]

Fibrin: A protein derived from fibrinogen in the presence of thrombin, which forms part of the blood clot. [NIH]

Fibrinogen: Plasma glycoprotein clotted by thrombin, composed of a dimer of three non-identical pairs of polypeptide chains (alpha, beta, gamma) held together by disulfide bonds. Fibrinogen clotting is a sol-gel change involving complex molecular arrangements: whereas fibrinogen is cleaved by thrombin to form polypeptides A and B, the proteolytic action of other enzymes yields different fibrinogen degradation products. [NIH]

Fibrinolysis: The natural enzymatic dissolution of fibrin. [NIH]

Fibroblast Growth Factor: Peptide isolated from the pituitary gland and from the brain. It is a potent mitogen which stimulates growth of a variety of mesodermal cells including chondrocytes, granulosa, and endothelial cells. The peptide may be active in wound healing and animal limb regeneration. [NIH]

Fibroblasts: Connective tissue cells which secrete an extracellular matrix rich in collagen and other macromolecules. [NIH]

Fibronectins: Glycoproteins found on the surfaces of cells, particularly in fibrillar structures. The proteins are lost or reduced when these cells undergo viral or chemical transformation. They are highly susceptible to proteolysis and are substrates for activated blood coagulation factor VIII. The forms present in plasma are called cold-insoluble globulins. [NIH]

Fibrosarcoma: A type of soft tissue sarcoma that begins in fibrous tissue, which holds bones, muscles, and other organs in place. [NIH]

Fibrosis: Any pathological condition where fibrous connective tissue invades any organ, usually as a consequence of inflammation or other injury. [NIH]

Fluid Therapy: Therapy whose basic objective is to restore the volume and composition of the body fluids to normal with respect to water-electrolyte balance. Fluids may be administered intravenously, orally, by intermittent gavage, or by hypodermoclysis. [NIH]

Fluorouracil: A pyrimidine analog that acts as an antineoplastic antimetabolite and also has immunosuppressant. It interferes with DNA synthesis by blocking the thymidylate synthetase conversion of deoxyuridylic acid to thymidylic acid. [NIH]

Fluoxymesterone: An anabolic steroid that has been used in the treatment of male hypogonadism, delayed puberty in males, and in the treatment of breast neoplasms in women. [NIH]

Fluphenazine: A phenothiazine used in the treatment of psychoses. Its properties and uses are generally similar to those of chlorpromazine. [NIH]

Folate: A B-complex vitamin that is being studied as a cancer prevention agent. Also called folic acid. [NIH]

Folic Acid: N-(4-(((2-Amino-1,4-dihydro-4-oxo-6-pteridinyl)methyl)amino)benzoyl)-L-glutamic acid. A member of the vitamin B family that stimulates the hematopoietic system. It is present in the liver and kidney and is found in mushrooms, spinach, yeast, green leaves, and grasses. Folic acid is used in the treatment and prevention of folate deficiencies and megaloblastic anemia. [NIH]

Follicles: Shafts through which hair grows. [NIH]

Forearm: The part between the elbow and the wrist. [NIH]

Free Radicals: Highly reactive molecules with an unsatisfied electron valence pair. Free radicals are produced in both normal and pathological processes. They are proven or suspected agents of tissue damage in a wide variety of circumstances including radiation, damage from environment chemicals, and aging. Natural and pharmacological prevention of free radical damage is being actively investigated. [NIH]

Fumigation: The application of smoke, vapor, or gas for the purpose of disinfecting or destroying pests or microorganisms. [NIH]

Gallbladder: The pear-shaped organ that sits below the liver. Bile is concentrated and stored in the gallbladder. [NIH]

Gamma Rays: Very powerful and penetrating, high-energy electromagnetic radiation of shorter wavelength than that of x-rays. They are emitted by a decaying nucleus, usually between 0.01 and 10 MeV. They are also called nuclear x-rays. [NIH]

Gamma-interferon: Interferon produced by T-lymphocytes in response to various mitogens and antigens. Gamma interferon appears to have potent antineoplastic, immunoregulatory and antiviral activity. [NIH]

Ganglia: Clusters of multipolar neurons surrounded by a capsule of loosely organized connective tissue located outside the central nervous system. [NIH]

Ganglion: 1. A knot, or knotlike mass. 2. A general term for a group of nerve cell bodies located outside the central nervous system; occasionally applied to certain nuclear groups within the brain or spinal cord, e.g. basal ganglia. 3. A benign cystic tumour occurring on a aponeurosis or tendon, as in the wrist or dorsum of the foot; it consists of a thin fibrous capsule enclosing a clear mucinous fluid. [EU]

Gas: Air that comes from normal breakdown of food. The gases are passed out of the body through the rectum (flatus) or the mouth (burp). [NIH]

Gastrectomy: An operation to remove all or part of the stomach. [NIH]

Gastric: Having to do with the stomach. [NIH]

Gastrin: A hormone released after eating. Gastrin causes the stomach to produce more acid. [NIH]

Gastroesophageal Reflux: Reflux of gastric juice and/or duodenal contents (bile acids, pancreatic juice) into the distal esophagus, commonly due to incompetence of the lower esophageal sphincter. Gastric regurgitation is an extension of this process with entry of fluid into the pharynx or mouth. [NIH]

Gastrointestinal: Refers to the stomach and intestines. [NIH]

Gastrointestinal Hemorrhage: Bleeding in the gastrointestinal tract. [NIH]

Gastrointestinal tract: The stomach and intestines. [NIH]

Gelatinases: A class of enzymes that catalyzes the degradation of gelatin by acting on the peptide bonds. EC 3.4.24.-. [NIH]

Gemcitabine: An anticancer drug that belongs to the family of drugs called antimetabolites. [NIH]

Gene: The functional and physical unit of heredity passed from parent to offspring. Genes are pieces of DNA, and most genes contain the information for making a specific protein. [NIH]

Gene Expression: The phenotypic manifestation of a gene or genes by the processes of gene action. [NIH]

Gene Targeting: The integration of exogenous DNA into the genome of an organism at sites where its expression can be suitably controlled. This integration occurs as a result of homologous recombination. [NIH]

Gene Therapy: The introduction of new genes into cells for the purpose of treating disease by restoring or adding gene expression. Techniques include insertion of retroviral vectors, transfection, homologous recombination, and injection of new genes into the nuclei of single cell embryos. The entire gene therapy process may consist of multiple steps. The new genes may be introduced into proliferating cells in vivo (e.g., bone marrow) or in vitro (e.g., fibroblast cultures) and the modified cells transferred to the site where the gene expression is required. Gene therapy may be particularly useful for treating enzyme deficiency diseases, hemoglobinopathies, and leukemias and may also prove useful in restoring drug sensitivity, particularly for leukemia. [NIH]

Genetic Code: The specifications for how information, stored in nucleic acid sequence (base sequence), is translated into protein sequence (amino acid sequence). The start, stop, and order of amino acids of a protein is specified by consecutive triplets of nucleotides called codons (codon). [NIH]

Genetic Engineering: Directed modification of the gene complement of a living organism by such techniques as altering the DNA, substituting genetic material by means of a virus, transplanting whole nuclei, transplanting cell hybrids, etc. [NIH]

Genetics: The biological science that deals with the phenomena and mechanisms of heredity. [NIH]

Genotype: The genetic constitution of the individual; the characterization of the genes. [NIH]

Geriatric: Pertaining to the treatment of the aged. [EU]

Germ Cells: The reproductive cells in multicellular organisms. [NIH]

Germline mutation: A gene change in the body's reproductive cells (egg or sperm) that becomes incorporated into the DNA of every cell in the body of offspring; germline mutations are passed on from parents to offspring. Also called hereditary mutation. [NIH]

Ginseng: An araliaceous genus of plants that contains a number of pharmacologically active agents used as stimulants, sedatives, and tonics, especially in traditional medicine. [NIH]

Gland: An organ that produces and releases one or more substances for use in the body. Some glands produce fluids that affect tissues or organs. Others produce hormones or participate in blood production. [NIH]

Glomerular: Pertaining to or of the nature of a glomerulus, especially a renal glomerulus. [EU]

Glomerular Filtration Rate: The volume of water filtered out of plasma through glomerular capillary walls into Bowman's capsules per unit of time. It is considered to be equivalent to inulin clearance. [NIH]

Glomerulus: A tiny set of looping blood vessels in the nephron where blood is filtered in the kidney. [NIH]

Glossopharyngeal Nerve: The 9th cranial nerve. The glossopharyngeal nerve is a mixed motor and sensory nerve; it conveys somatic and autonomic efferents as well as general, special, and visceral afferents. Among the connections are motor fibers to the stylopharyngeus muscle, parasympathetic fibers to the parotid glands, general and taste afferents from the posterior third of the tongue, the nasopharynx, and the palate, and afferents from baroreceptors and chemoreceptors of the carotid sinus. [NIH]

Glucocorticoid: A compound that belongs to the family of compounds called corticosteroids (steroids). Glucocorticoids affect metabolism and have anti-inflammatory and immunosuppressive effects. They may be naturally produced (hormones) or synthetic (drugs). [NIH]

Gluconeogenesis: The process by which glucose is formed from a non-carbohydrate source. [NIH]

Glucose: D-Glucose. A primary source of energy for living organisms. It is naturally occurring and is found in fruits and other parts of plants in its free state. It is used therapeutically in fluid and nutrient replacement. [NIH]

Glucose Intolerance: A pathological state in which the fasting plasma glucose level is less than 140 mg per deciliter and the 30-, 60-, or 90-minute plasma glucose concentration following a glucose tolerance test exceeds 200 mg per deciliter. This condition is seen frequently in diabetes mellitus but also occurs with other diseases. [NIH]

Glucose tolerance: The power of the normal liver to absorb and store large quantities of glucose and the effectiveness of intestinal absorption of glucose. The glucose tolerance test is a metabolic test of carbohydrate tolerance that measures active insulin, a hepatic function based on the ability of the liver to absorb glucose. The test consists of ingesting 100 grams of glucose into a fasting stomach; blood sugar should return to normal in 2 to 21 hours after ingestion. [NIH]

Glucose Tolerance Test: Determination of whole blood or plasma sugar in a fasting state before and at prescribed intervals (usually 1/2 hr, 1 hr, 3 hr, 4 hr) after taking a specified amount (usually 100 gm orally) of glucose. [NIH]

Glucuronic Acid: Derivatives of uronic acid found throughout the plant and animal kingdoms. They detoxify drugs and toxins by conjugating with them to form glucuronides in the liver which are more water-soluble metabolites that can be easily eliminated from the body. [NIH]

Glutamate: Excitatory neurotransmitter of the brain. [NIH]

Glutamic Acid: A non-essential amino acid naturally occurring in the L-form. Glutamic acid (glutamate) is the most common excitatory neurotransmitter in the central nervous system. [NIH]

Glutamine: A non-essential amino acid present abundantly throught the body and is involved in many metabolic processes. It is synthesized from glutamic acid and ammonia. It is the principal carrier of nitrogen in the body and is an important energy source for many cells. [NIH]

Glutathione Peroxidase: An enzyme catalyzing the oxidation of 2 moles of glutathione in the presence of hydrogen peroxide to yield oxidized glutathione and water. EC 1.11.1.9. [NIH]

Glycerol: A trihydroxy sugar alcohol that is an intermediate in carbohydrate and lipid metabolism. It is used as a solvent, emollient, pharmaceutical agent, and sweetening agent. [NIH]

Glycerophospholipids: Derivatives of phosphatidic acid in which the hydrophobic regions are composed of two fatty acids and a polar alcohol is joined to the C-3 position of glycerol through a phosphodiester bond. They are named according to their polar head groups, such as phosphatidylcholine and phosphatidylethanolamine. [NIH]

Glycine: A non-essential amino acid. It is found primarily in gelatin and silk fibroin and used therapeutically as a nutrient. It is also a fast inhibitory neurotransmitter. [NIH]

Glycogen: A sugar stored in the liver and muscles. It releases glucose into the blood when cells need it for energy. Glycogen is the chief source of stored fuel in the body. [NIH]

Glycols: A generic grouping for dihydric alcohols with the hydroxy groups (-OH) located on different carbon atoms. They are viscous liquids with high boiling points for their molecular weights. [NIH]

Glycoprotein: A protein that has sugar molecules attached to it. [NIH]

Glycosaminoglycans: Heteropolysaccharides which contain an N-acetylated hexosamine in a characteristic repeating disaccharide unit. The repeating structure of each disaccharide involves alternate 1,4- and 1,3-linkages consisting of either N-acetylglucosamine or N-acetylgalactosamine. [NIH]

Glycosidic: Formed by elimination of water between the anomeric hydroxyl of one sugar and a hydroxyl of another sugar molecule. [NIH]

Gonad: A sex organ, such as an ovary or a testicle, which produces the gametes in most multicellular animals. [NIH]

Gonadal: Pertaining to a gonad. [EU]

Gout: Hereditary metabolic disorder characterized by recurrent acute arthritis, hyperuricemia and deposition of sodium urate in and around the joints, sometimes with formation of uric acid calculi. [NIH]

Governing Board: The group in which legal authority is vested for the control of health-related institutions and organizations. [NIH]

Gp120: 120-kD HIV envelope glycoprotein which is involved in the binding of the virus to its membrane receptor, the CD4 molecule, found on the surface of certain cells in the body. [NIH]

Grade: The grade of a tumor depends on how abnormal the cancer cells look under a microscope and how quickly the tumor is likely to grow and spread. Grading systems are different for each type of cancer. [NIH]

Graft: Healthy skin, bone, or other tissue taken from one part of the body and used to replace diseased or injured tissue removed from another part of the body. [NIH]

Graft Rejection: An immune response with both cellular and humoral components, directed against an allogeneic transplant, whose tissue antigens are not compatible with those of the recipient. [NIH]

Grafting: The operation of transfer of tissue from one site to another. [NIH]

Graft-versus-host disease: GVHD. A reaction of donated bone marrow or peripheral stem cells against a person's tissue. [NIH]

Gram-negative: Losing the stain or decolorized by alcohol in Gram's method of staining, a primary characteristic of bacteria having a cell wall composed of a thin layer of peptidoglycan covered by an outer membrane of lipoprotein and lipopolysaccharide. [EU]

Granulocytes: Leukocytes with abundant granules in the cytoplasm. They are divided into three groups: neutrophils, eosinophils, and basophils. [NIH]

Granuloma: A relatively small nodular inflammatory lesion containing grouped mononuclear phagocytes, caused by infectious and noninfectious agents. [NIH]

Granulosa Cells: Cells of the membrana granulosa lining the vesicular ovarian follicle which become luteal cells after ovulation. [NIH]

Growth factors: Substances made by the body that function to regulate cell division and cell survival. Some growth factors are also produced in the laboratory and used in biological therapy. [NIH]

Guanine: One of the four DNA bases. [NIH]

Guanylate Cyclase: An enzyme that catalyzes the conversion of GTP to 3',5'-cyclic GMP and pyrophosphate. It also acts on ITP and dGTP. (From Enzyme Nomenclature, 1992) EC 4.6.1.2. [NIH]

Habituation: Decline in response of an organism to environmental or other stimuli with repeated or maintained exposure. [NIH]

Haematemesis: The vomiting of blood. [EU]

Health Care Costs: The actual costs of providing services related to the delivery of health care, including the costs of procedures, therapies, and medications. It is differentiated from health expenditures, which refers to the amount of money paid for the services, and from fees, which refers to the amount charged, regardless of cost. [NIH]

Health Expenditures: The amounts spent by individuals, groups, nations, or private or public organizations for total health care and/or its various components. These amounts may or may not be equivalent to the actual costs (health care costs) and may or may not be shared among the patient, insurers, and/or employers. [NIH]

Heart attack: A seizure of weak or abnormal functioning of the heart. [NIH]

Heart failure: Loss of pumping ability by the heart, often accompanied by fatigue, breathlessness, and excess fluid accumulation in body tissues. [NIH]

Heart Transplantation: The transference of a heart from one human or animal to another. [NIH]

Hematopoiesis: The development and formation of various types of blood cells. [NIH]

Hematopoietic Stem Cells: Progenitor cells from which all blood cells derive. [NIH]

Hemodialysis: The use of a machine to clean wastes from the blood after the kidneys have failed. The blood travels through tubes to a dialyzer, which removes wastes and extra fluid. The cleaned blood then flows through another set of tubes back into the body. [NIH]

Hemoglobin: One of the fractions of glycosylated hemoglobin A1c. Glycosylated hemoglobin is formed when linkages of glucose and related monosaccharides bind to hemoglobin A and its concentration represents the average blood glucose level over the previous several weeks. HbA1c levels are used as a measure of long-term control of plasma glucose (normal, 4 to 6 percent). In controlled diabetes mellitus, the concentration of glycosylated hemoglobin A is within the normal range, but in uncontrolled cases the level may be 3 to 4 times the normal conentration. Generally, complications are substantially lower among patients with Hb levels of 7 percent or less than in patients with HbA1c levels of 9 percent or more. [NIH]

Hemoglobinopathies: A group of inherited disorders characterized by structural alterations within the hemoglobin molecule. [NIH]

Hemorrhage: Bleeding or escape of blood from a vessel. [NIH]

Hemostasis: The process which spontaneously arrests the flow of blood from vessels carrying blood under pressure. It is accomplished by contraction of the vessels, adhesion and aggregation of formed blood elements, and the process of blood or plasma coagulation. [NIH]

Heparan Sulfate Proteoglycan: A substance released by astrocytes, which is critical in stopping nervous fibers in their tracks. [NIH]

Heparin: Heparinic acid. A highly acidic mucopolysaccharide formed of equal parts of sulfated D-glucosamine and D-glucuronic acid with sulfaminic bridges. The molecular weight ranges from six to twenty thousand. Heparin occurs in and is obtained from liver, lung, mast cells, etc., of vertebrates. Its function is unknown, but it is used to prevent blood clotting in vivo and vitro, in the form of many different salts. [NIH]

Hepatic: Refers to the liver. [NIH]

Hepatitis: Inflammation of the liver and liver disease involving degenerative or necrotic alterations of hepatocytes. [NIH]

Hepatobiliary: Pertaining to the liver and the bile or the biliary ducts. [EU]

Hepatocyte: A liver cell. [NIH]

Hepatocyte Growth Factor: Multifunctional growth factor which regulates both cell growth and cell motility. It exerts a strong mitogenic effect on hepatocytes and primary epithelial cells. Its receptor is proto-oncogene protein C-met. [NIH]

Hepatoma: A liver tumor. [NIH]

Hepatorenal Syndrome: Renal failure in those with liver disease, usually liver cirrhosis or obstructive jaundice. Historically called Heyd disease, urohepatic syndrome, or bile nephrosis. [NIH]

Hereditary: Of, relating to, or denoting factors that can be transmitted genetically from one generation to another. [NIH]

Hereditary mutation: A gene change in the body's reproductive cells (egg or sperm) that becomes incorporated into the DNA of every cell in the body of offspring; hereditary mutations are passed on from parents to offspring. Also called germline mutation. [NIH]

Heredity: 1. The genetic transmission of a particular quality or trait from parent to offspring. 2. The genetic constitution of an individual. [EU]

Hernia: Protrusion of a loop or knuckle of an organ or tissue through an abnormal opening. [NIH]

Histamine: 1H-Imidazole-4-ethanamine. A depressor amine derived by enzymatic decarboxylation of histidine. It is a powerful stimulant of gastric secretion, a constrictor of bronchial smooth muscle, a vasodilator, and also a centrally acting neurotransmitter. [NIH]

Histamine Release: The secretion of histamine from mast cell and basophil granules by exocytosis. This can be initiated by a number of factors, all of which involve binding of IgE, cross-linked by antigen, to the mast cell or basophil's Fc receptors. Once released, histamine binds to a number of different target cell receptors and exerts a wide variety of effects. [NIH]

Histidine: An essential amino acid important in a number of metabolic processes. It is required for the production of histamine. [NIH]

Histology: The study of tissues and cells under a microscope. [NIH]

Homeostasis: The processes whereby the internal environment of an organism tends to remain balanced and stable. [NIH]

Homeotic: Characterizes genes the mutations of which lead to inappropriate expressions of characteristics normally associated with another part of the organism (homeotic mutants). [NIH]

Homodimer: Protein-binding "activation domains" always combine with identical proteins. [NIH]

Homologous: Corresponding in structure, position, origin, etc., as (a) the feathers of a bird and the scales of a fish, (b) antigen and its specific antibody, (c) allelic chromosomes. [EU]

Hormonal: Pertaining to or of the nature of a hormone. [EU]

Hormonal therapy: Treatment of cancer by removing, blocking, or adding hormones. Also called hormone therapy or endocrine therapy. [NIH]

Hormone: A substance in the body that regulates certain organs. Hormones such as gastrin help in breaking down food. Some hormones come from cells in the stomach and small intestine. [NIH]

Hormone Replacement Therapy: Therapeutic use of hormones to alleviate the effects of hormone deficiency. [NIH]

Hormone therapy: Treatment of cancer by removing, blocking, or adding hormones. Also called endocrine therapy. [NIH]

Human growth hormone: A protein hormone, secreted by the anterior lobe of the pituitary, which promotes growth of the whole body by stimulating protein synthesis. The human gene has already been cloned and successfully expressed in bacteria. [NIH]

Humoral: Of, relating to, proceeding from, or involving a bodily humour - now often used of endocrine factors as opposed to neural or somatic. [EU]

Hybrid: Cross fertilization between two varieties or, more usually, two species of vines, see also crossing. [NIH]

Hybridization: The genetic process of crossbreeding to produce a hybrid. Hybrid nucleic acids can be formed by nucleic acid hybridization of DNA and RNA molecules. Protein hybridization allows for hybrid proteins to be formed from polypeptide chains. [NIH]

Hybridomas: Cells artificially created by fusion of activated lymphocytes with neoplastic cells. The resulting hybrid cells are cloned and produce pure or "monoclonal" antibodies or

T-cell products, identical to those produced by the immunologically competent parent, and continually grow and divide as the neoplastic parent. [NIH]

Hydrazine sulfate: A substance that has been studied as a treatment for cancer and as a treatment for cachexia (body wasting) associated with advanced cancer. [NIH]

Hydrogen: The first chemical element in the periodic table. It has the atomic symbol H, atomic number 1, and atomic weight 1. It exists, under normal conditions, as a colorless, odorless, tasteless, diatomic gas. Hydrogen ions are protons. Besides the common H1 isotope, hydrogen exists as the stable isotope deuterium and the unstable, radioactive isotope tritium. [NIH]

Hydrogen Peroxide: A strong oxidizing agent used in aqueous solution as a ripening agent, bleach, and topical anti-infective. It is relatively unstable and solutions deteriorate over time unless stabilized by the addition of acetanilide or similar organic materials. [NIH]

Hydrolysis: The process of cleaving a chemical compound by the addition of a molecule of water. [NIH]

Hydrophobic: Not readily absorbing water, or being adversely affected by water, as a hydrophobic colloid. [EU]

Hydroxamic Acids: A class of weak acids with the general formula R-conhoh. [NIH]

Hydroxides: Inorganic compounds that contain the OH- group. [NIH]

Hydroxyl Radical: The univalent radical OH that is present in hydroxides, alcohols, phenols, glycols. [NIH]

Hydroxylysine: A hydroxylated derivative of the amino acid lysine that is present in certain collagens. [NIH]

Hydroxyproline: A hydroxylated form of the imino acid proline. A deficiency in ascorbic acid can result in impaired hydroxyproline formation. [NIH]

Hypercalcemia: Abnormally high level of calcium in the blood. [NIH]

Hyperlipidemia: An excess of lipids in the blood. [NIH]

Hyperlipoproteinemia: Metabolic disease characterized by elevated plasma cholesterol and/or triglyceride levels. The inherited form is attributed to a single gene mechanism. [NIH]

Hyperphagia: Ingestion of a greater than optimal quantity of food. [NIH]

Hyperplasia: An increase in the number of cells in a tissue or organ, not due to tumor formation. It differs from hypertrophy, which is an increase in bulk without an increase in the number of cells. [NIH]

Hypersensitivity: Altered reactivity to an antigen, which can result in pathologic reactions upon subsequent exposure to that particular antigen. [NIH]

Hypertension: Persistently high arterial blood pressure. Currently accepted threshold levels are 140 mm Hg systolic and 90 mm Hg diastolic pressure. [NIH]

Hypertrophy: General increase in bulk of a part or organ, not due to tumor formation, nor to an increase in the number of cells. [NIH]

Hypnotic: A drug that acts to induce sleep. [EU]

Hypoglycaemia: An abnormally diminished concentration of glucose in the blood, which may lead to tremulousness, cold sweat, piloerection, hypothermia, and headache, accompanied by irritability, confusion, hallucinations, bizarre behaviour, and ultimately, convulsions and coma. [EU]

Hypoglycemic: An orally active drug that produces a fall in blood glucose concentration. [NIH]

Hypogonadism: Condition resulting from or characterized by abnormally decreased functional activity of the gonads, with retardation of growth and sexual development. [NIH]

Hypotension: Abnormally low blood pressure. [NIH]

Hypothalamic: Of or involving the hypothalamus. [EU]

Hypothalamus: Ventral part of the diencephalon extending from the region of the optic chiasm to the caudal border of the mammillary bodies and forming the inferior and lateral walls of the third ventricle. [NIH]

Hypoxia: Reduction of oxygen supply to tissue below physiological levels despite adequate perfusion of the tissue by blood. [EU]

Hypoxic: Having too little oxygen. [NIH]

Iatrogenic: Resulting from the activity of physicians. Originally applied to disorders induced in the patient by autosuggestion based on the physician's examination, manner, or discussion, the term is now applied to any adverse condition in a patient occurring as the result of treatment by a physician or surgeon, especially to infections acquired by the patient during the course of treatment. [EU]

Ibuprofen: A nonsteroidal anti-inflammatory agent with analgesic properties used in the therapy of rheumatism and arthritis. [NIH]

Imaging procedures: Methods of producing pictures of areas inside the body. [NIH]

Immune response: The activity of the immune system against foreign substances (antigens). [NIH]

Immune system: The organs, cells, and molecules responsible for the recognition and disposal of foreign ("non-self") material which enters the body. [NIH]

Immunity: Nonsusceptibility to the invasive or pathogenic effects of foreign microorganisms or to the toxic effect of antigenic substances. [NIH]

Immunocompromised: Having a weakened immune system caused by certain diseases or treatments. [NIH]

Immunodeficiency: The decreased ability of the body to fight infection and disease. [NIH]

Immunologic: The ability of the antibody-forming system to recall a previous experience with an antigen and to respond to a second exposure with the prompt production of large amounts of antibody. [NIH]

Immunology: The study of the body's immune system. [NIH]

Immunosuppressant: An agent capable of suppressing immune responses. [EU]

Immunosuppression: Deliberate prevention or diminution of the host's immune response. It may be nonspecific as in the administration of immunosuppressive agents (drugs or radiation) or by lymphocyte depletion or may be specific as in desensitization or the simultaneous administration of antigen and immunosuppressive drugs. [NIH]

Immunosuppressive: Describes the ability to lower immune system responses. [NIH]

Immunosuppressive Agents: Agents that suppress immune function by one of several mechanisms of action. Classical cytotoxic immunosuppressants act by inhibiting DNA synthesis. Others may act through activation of suppressor T-cell populations or by inhibiting the activation of helper cells. While immunosuppression has been brought about in the past primarily to prevent rejection of transplanted organs, new applications involving mediation of the effects of interleukins and other cytokines are emerging. [NIH]

Impairment: In the context of health experience, an impairment is any loss or abnormality of psychological, physiological, or anatomical structure or function. [NIH]

Implant radiation: A procedure in which radioactive material sealed in needles, seeds, wires, or catheters is placed directly into or near the tumor. Also called [NIH]

Implantation: The insertion or grafting into the body of biological, living, inert, or radioactive material. [EU]

Impotence: The inability to perform sexual intercourse. [NIH]

In situ: In the natural or normal place; confined to the site of origin without invasion of neighbouring tissues. [EU]

In Situ Hybridization: A technique that localizes specific nucleic acid sequences within intact chromosomes, eukaryotic cells, or bacterial cells through the use of specific nucleic acid-labeled probes. [NIH]

In vitro: In the laboratory (outside the body). The opposite of in vivo (in the body). [NIH]

In vivo: In the body. The opposite of in vitro (outside the body or in the laboratory). [NIH]

Incision: A cut made in the body during surgery. [NIH]

Incompetence: Physical or mental inadequacy or insufficiency. [EU]

Incubated: Grown in the laboratory under controlled conditions. (For instance, white blood cells can be grown in special conditions so that they attack specific cancer cells when returned to the body.) [NIH]

Induction: The act or process of inducing or causing to occur, especially the production of a specific morphogenetic effect in the developing embryo through the influence of evocators or organizers, or the production of anaesthesia or unconsciousness by use of appropriate agents. [EU]

Infancy: The period of complete dependency prior to the acquisition of competence in walking, talking, and self-feeding. [NIH]

Infantile: Pertaining to an infant or to infancy. [EU]

Infarction: A pathological process consisting of a sudden insufficient blood supply to an area, which results in necrosis of that area. It is usually caused by a thrombus, an embolus, or a vascular torsion. [NIH]

Infection: 1. Invasion and multiplication of microorganisms in body tissues, which may be clinically unapparent or result in local cellular injury due to competitive metabolism, toxins, intracellular replication, or antigen-antibody response. The infection may remain localized, subclinical, and temporary if the body's defensive mechanisms are effective. A local infection may persist and spread by extension to become an acute, subacute, or chronic clinical infection or disease state. A local infection may also become systemic when the microorganisms gain access to the lymphatic or vascular system. 2. An infectious disease. [EU]

Inflammation: A pathological process characterized by injury or destruction of tissues caused by a variety of cytologic and chemical reactions. It is usually manifested by typical signs of pain, heat, redness, swelling, and loss of function. [NIH]

Inflammatory bowel disease: A general term that refers to the inflammation of the colon and rectum. Inflammatory bowel disease includes ulcerative colitis and Crohn's disease. [NIH]

Infusion: A method of putting fluids, including drugs, into the bloodstream. Also called intravenous infusion. [NIH]

Ingestion: Taking into the body by mouth [NIH]

Inhalation: The drawing of air or other substances into the lungs. [EU]

Inhibin: Glyceroprotein hormone produced in the seminiferous tubules by the Sertoli cells in the male and by the granulosa cells in the female follicles. The hormone inhibits FSH and LH synthesis and secretion by the pituitary cells thereby affecting sexual maturation and fertility. [NIH]

Initiation: Mutation induced by a chemical reactive substance causing cell changes; being a step in a carcinogenic process. [NIH]

Innervation: 1. The distribution or supply of nerves to a part. 2. The supply of nervous energy or of nerve stimulus sent to a part. [EU]

Inorganic: Pertaining to substances not of organic origin. [EU]

Inotropic: Affecting the force or energy of muscular contractions. [EU]

Inpatients: Persons admitted to health facilities which provide board and room, for the purpose of observation, care, diagnosis or treatment. [NIH]

Insight: The capacity to understand one's own motives, to be aware of one's own psychodynamics, to appreciate the meaning of symbolic behavior. [NIH]

Institutionalization: The caring for individuals in institutions and their adaptation to routines characteristic of the institutional environment, and/or their loss of adaptation to life outside the institution. [NIH]

Insulator: Material covering the metal conductor of the lead. It is usually polyurethane or silicone. [NIH]

Insulin: A protein hormone secreted by beta cells of the pancreas. Insulin plays a major role in the regulation of glucose metabolism, generally promoting the cellular utilization of glucose. It is also an important regulator of protein and lipid metabolism. Insulin is used as a drug to control insulin-dependent diabetes mellitus. [NIH]

Insulin-dependent diabetes mellitus: A disease characterized by high levels of blood glucose resulting from defects in insulin secretion, insulin action, or both. Autoimmune, genetic, and environmental factors are involved in the development of type I diabetes. [NIH]

Insulin-like: Muscular growth factor. [NIH]

Intensive Care: Advanced and highly specialized care provided to medical or surgical patients whose conditions are life-threatening and require comprehensive care and constant monitoring. It is usually administered in specially equipped units of a health care facility. [NIH]

Interferon: A biological response modifier (a substance that can improve the body's natural response to disease). Interferons interfere with the division of cancer cells and can slow tumor growth. There are several types of interferons, including interferon-alpha, -beta, and -gamma. These substances are normally produced by the body. They are also made in the laboratory for use in treating cancer and other diseases. [NIH]

Interferon-alpha: One of the type I interferons produced by peripheral blood leukocytes or lymphoblastoid cells when exposed to live or inactivated virus, double-stranded RNA, or bacterial products. It is the major interferon produced by virus-induced leukocyte cultures and, in addition to its pronounced antiviral activity, it causes activation of NK cells. [NIH]

Interleukin-1: A soluble factor produced by monocytes, macrophages, and other cells which activates T-lymphocytes and potentiates their response to mitogens or antigens. IL-1 consists of two distinct forms, IL-1 alpha and IL-1 beta which perform the same functions but are distinct proteins. The biological effects of IL-1 include the ability to replace macrophage requirements for T-cell activation. The factor is distinct from interleukin-2. [NIH]

Interleukin-2: Chemical mediator produced by activated T lymphocytes and which regulates the proliferation of T cells, as well as playing a role in the regulation of NK cell activity. [NIH]

Interleukin-6: Factor that stimulates the growth and differentiation of human B-cells and is also a growth factor for hybridomas and plasmacytomas. It is produced by many different cells including T-cells, monocytes, and fibroblasts. [NIH]

Interleukin-8: A cytokine that activates neutrophils and attracts neutrophils and T-lymphocytes. It is released by several cell types including monocytes, macrophages, T-lymphocytes, fibroblasts, endothelial cells, and keratinocytes by an inflammatory stimulus. IL-8 is a member of the beta-thromboglobulin superfamily and structurally related to platelet factor 4. [NIH]

Interleukins: Soluble factors which stimulate growth-related activities of leukocytes as well as other cell types. They enhance cell proliferation and differentiation, DNA synthesis, secretion of other biologically active molecules and responses to immune and inflammatory stimuli. [NIH]

Internal Medicine: A medical specialty concerned with the diagnosis and treatment of diseases of the internal organ systems of adults. [NIH]

Internal radiation: A procedure in which radioactive material sealed in needles, seeds, wires, or catheters is placed directly into or near the tumor. Also called brachytherapy, implant radiation, or interstitial radiation therapy. [NIH]

Interneurons: Most generally any neurons which are not motor or sensory. Interneurons may also refer to neurons whose axons remain within a particular brain region as contrasted with projection neurons which have axons projecting to other brain regions. [NIH]

Interstitial: Pertaining to or situated between parts or in the interspaces of a tissue. [EU]

Interstitial Collagenase: A member of the metalloproteinase family of enzymes that is principally responsible for cleaving fibrillar collagen. It can degrade interstitial collagens, types I, II and III. EC 3.4.24.7. [NIH]

Intervertebral: Situated between two contiguous vertebrae. [EU]

Intestinal: Having to do with the intestines. [NIH]

Intestine: A long, tube-shaped organ in the abdomen that completes the process of digestion. There is both a large intestine and a small intestine. Also called the bowel. [NIH]

Intoxication: Poisoning, the state of being poisoned. [EU]

Intracellular: Inside a cell. [NIH]

Intramuscular: IM. Within or into muscle. [NIH]

Intraperitoneal: IP. Within the peritoneal cavity (the area that contains the abdominal organs). [NIH]

Intravascular: Within a vessel or vessels. [EU]

Intravenous: IV. Into a vein. [NIH]

Intrinsic: Situated entirely within or pertaining exclusively to a part. [EU]

Inulin: A starch found in the tubers and roots of many plants. Since it is hydrolyzable to fructose, it is classified as a fructosan. It has been used in physiologic investigation for determination of the rate of glomerular function. [NIH]

Invasive: 1. Having the quality of invasiveness. 2. Involving puncture or incision of the skin or insertion of an instrument or foreign material into the body; said of diagnostic techniques. [EU]

Investigative Techniques: Investigative techniques used in pre-clinical and clinical research, epidemiology, chemistry, immunology, genetics, etc. They do not include techniques specifically applied to diagnosis; therapeutics; anesthesia and analgesia, surgery, operative, and dentistry. [NIH]

Involuntary: Reaction occurring without intention or volition. [NIH]

Ionization: 1. Any process by which a neutral atom gains or loses electrons, thus acquiring a net charge, as the dissociation of a substance in solution into ions or ion production by the passage of radioactive particles. 2. Iontophoresis. [EU]

Ionizing: Radiation comprising charged particles, e. g. electrons, protons, alpha-particles, etc., having sufficient kinetic energy to produce ionization by collision. [NIH]

Ionophores: Chemical agents that increase the permeability of biological or artificial lipid membranes to specific ions. Most ionophores are relatively small organic molecules that act as mobile carriers within membranes or coalesce to form ion permeable channels across membranes. Many are antibiotics, and many act as uncoupling agents by short-circuiting the proton gradient across mitochondrial membranes. [NIH]

Ions: An atom or group of atoms that have a positive or negative electric charge due to a gain (negative charge) or loss (positive charge) of one or more electrons. Atoms with a positive charge are known as cations; those with a negative charge are anions. [NIH]

Ischemia: Deficiency of blood in a part, due to functional constriction or actual obstruction of a blood vessel. [EU]

Isoleucine: An essential branched-chain amino acid found in many proteins. It is an isomer of LEUCINE. It is important in hemoglobin synthesis and regulation of blood sugar and energy levels. [NIH]

Jaundice: A clinical manifestation of hyperbilirubinemia, consisting of deposition of bile pigments in the skin, resulting in a yellowish staining of the skin and mucous membranes. [NIH]

Kb: A measure of the length of DNA fragments, 1 Kb = 1000 base pairs. The largest DNA fragments are up to 50 kilobases long. [NIH]

Keratinocytes: Epidermal cells which synthesize keratin and undergo characteristic changes as they move upward from the basal layers of the epidermis to the cornified (horny) layer of the skin. Successive stages of differentiation of the keratinocytes forming the epidermal layers are basal cell, spinous or prickle cell, and the granular cell. [NIH]

Keratoconus: A disorder characterized by an irregular corneal surface (cone-shaped) resulting in blurred and distorted images. [NIH]

Ketoacidosis: Acidosis accompanied by the accumulation of ketone bodies (ketosis) in the body tissues and fluids, as in diabetic acidosis. [EU]

Ketone Bodies: Chemicals that the body makes when there is not enough insulin in the blood and it must break down fat for its energy. Ketone bodies can poison and even kill body cells. When the body does not have the help of insulin, the ketones build up in the blood and then "spill" over into the urine so that the body can get rid of them. The body can also rid itself of one type of ketone, called acetone, through the lungs. This gives the breath a fruity odor. Ketones that build up in the body for a long time lead to serious illness and coma. [NIH]

Ketosis: A condition of having ketone bodies build up in body tissues and fluids. The signs of ketosis are nausea, vomiting, and stomach pain. Ketosis can lead to ketoacidosis. [NIH]

Kidney Disease: Any one of several chronic conditions that are caused by damage to the cells of the kidney. People who have had diabetes for a long time may have kidney damage. Also called nephropathy. [NIH]

Kidney Failure: The inability of a kidney to excrete metabolites at normal plasma levels under conditions of normal loading, or the inability to retain electrolytes under conditions of normal intake. In the acute form (kidney failure, acute), it is marked by uremia and usually by oliguria or anuria, with hyperkalemia and pulmonary edema. The chronic form (kidney failure, chronic) is irreversible and requires hemodialysis. [NIH]

Kidney Failure, Acute: A clinical syndrome characterized by a sudden decrease in glomerular filtration rate, often to values of less than 1 to 2 ml per minute. It is usually associated with oliguria (urine volumes of less than 400 ml per day) and is always associated with biochemical consequences of the reduction in glomerular filtration rate such as a rise in blood urea nitrogen (BUN) and serum creatinine concentrations. [NIH]

Kidney Failure, Chronic: An irreversible and usually progressive reduction in renal function in which both kidneys have been damaged by a variety of diseases to the extent that they are unable to adequately remove the metabolic products from the blood and regulate the body's electrolyte composition and acid-base balance. Chronic kidney failure requires hemodialysis or surgery, usually kidney transplantation. [NIH]

Kinetics: The study of rate dynamics in chemical or physical systems. [NIH]

Laminin: Large, noncollagenous glycoprotein with antigenic properties. It is localized in the basement membrane lamina lucida and functions to bind epithelial cells to the basement membrane. Evidence suggests that the protein plays a role in tumor invasion. [NIH]

Large Intestine: The part of the intestine that goes from the cecum to the rectum. The large intestine absorbs water from stool and changes it from a liquid to a solid form. The large intestine is 5 feet long and includes the appendix, cecum, colon, and rectum. Also called colon. [NIH]

Latent: Phoria which occurs at one distance or another and which usually has no troublesome effect. [NIH]

Leishmaniasis: A disease caused by any of a number of species of protozoa in the genus Leishmania. There are four major clinical types of this infection: cutaneous (Old and New World), diffuse cutaneous, mucocutaneous, and visceral leishmaniasis. [NIH]

Lens: The transparent, double convex (outward curve on both sides) structure suspended between the aqueous and vitreous; helps to focus light on the retina. [NIH]

Leptin: A 16-kD peptide hormone secreted from white adipocytes and implicated in the regulation of food intake and energy balance. Leptin provides the key afferent signal from fat cells in the feedback system that controls body fat stores. [NIH]

Lesion: An area of abnormal tissue change. [NIH]

Lethal: Deadly, fatal. [EU]

Lethargy: Abnormal drowsiness or stupor; a condition of indifference. [EU]

Leucine: An essential branched-chain amino acid important for hemoglobin formation. [NIH]

Leukemia: Cancer of blood-forming tissue. [NIH]

Leukocytosis: A transient increase in the number of leukocytes in a body fluid. [NIH]

Leukotrienes: A family of biologically active compounds derived from arachidonic acid by oxidative metabolism through the 5-lipoxygenase pathway. They participate in host defense reactions and pathophysiological conditions such as immediate hypersensitivity and inflammation. They have potent actions on many essential organs and systems, including the cardiovascular, pulmonary, and central nervous system as well as the gastrointestinal tract and the immune system. [NIH]

Libido: The psychic drive or energy associated with sexual instinct in the broad sense (pleasure and love-object seeking). It may also connote the psychic energy associated with instincts in general that motivate behavior. [NIH]

Life Expectancy: A figure representing the number of years, based on known statistics, to which any person of a given age may reasonably expect to live. [NIH]

Ligament: A band of fibrous tissue that connects bones or cartilages, serving to support and strengthen joints. [EU]

Ligands: A RNA simulation method developed by the MIT. [NIH]

Ligase: An enzyme that repairs single stranded discontinuities in double-stranded DNA molecules in the cell. Purified DNA ligase is used in gene cloning to join DNA molecules together. [NIH]

Ligation: Application of a ligature to tie a vessel or strangulate a part. [NIH]

Linkages: The tendency of two or more genes in the same chromosome to remain together from one generation to the next more frequently than expected according to the law of independent assortment. [NIH]

Lipase: An enzyme of the hydrolase class that catalyzes the reaction of triacylglycerol and water to yield diacylglycerol and a fatty acid anion. It is produced by glands on the tongue and by the pancreas and initiates the digestion of dietary fats. (From Dorland, 27th ed) EC 3.1.1.3. [NIH]

Lipid: Fat. [NIH]

Lipid Mobilization: The breakdown of stored triglyceride in adipose tissue with the release of free fatty acids and glycerol. Depot fat hydrolysis is catalyzed by a lipase in response to pituitary lipid mobilization factors (LMF), various hormones, serotonin, or hepatotoxins such as carbon tetrachloride. [NIH]

Lipid Peroxidation: Peroxidase catalyzed oxidation of lipids using hydrogen peroxide as an electron acceptor. [NIH]

Lipodystrophy: A collection of rare conditions resulting from defective fat metabolism and characterized by atrophy of the subcutaneous fat. They include total, congenital or acquired, partial, abdominal infantile, and localized lipodystrophy. [NIH]

Lipolysis: The hydrolysis of lipids. [NIH]

Lipopolysaccharide: Substance consisting of polysaccaride and lipid. [NIH]

Lipoprotein: Any of the lipid-protein complexes in which lipids are transported in the blood; lipoprotein particles consist of a spherical hydrophobic core of triglycerides or cholesterol esters surrounded by an amphipathic monolayer of phospholipids, cholesterol, and apolipoproteins; the four principal classes are high-density, low-density, and very-low-density lipoproteins and chylomicrons. [EU]

Lipoprotein Lipase: An enzyme of the hydrolase class that catalyzes the reaction of triacylglycerol and water to yield diacylglycerol and a fatty acid anion. The enzyme hydrolyzes triacylglycerols in chylomicrons, very-low-density lipoproteins, low-density lipoproteins, and diacylglycerols. It occurs on capillary endothelial surfaces, especially in mammary, muscle, and adipose tissue. Genetic deficiency of the enzyme causes familial hyperlipoproteinemia Type I. (Dorland, 27th ed) EC 3.1.1.34. [NIH]

Liposarcoma: A rare cancer of the fat cells. [NIH]

Liver: A large, glandular organ located in the upper abdomen. The liver cleanses the blood and aids in digestion by secreting bile. [NIH]

Liver Cirrhosis: Liver disease in which the normal microcirculation, the gross vascular anatomy, and the hepatic architecture have been variably destroyed and altered with fibrous septa surrounding regenerated or regenerating parenchymal nodules. [NIH]

Lobe: A portion of an organ such as the liver, lung, breast, or brain. [NIH]

Localized: Cancer which has not metastasized yet. [NIH]

Loop: A wire usually of platinum bent at one end into a small loop (usually 4 mm inside diameter) and used in transferring microorganisms. [NIH]

Low-density lipoprotein: Lipoprotein that contains most of the cholesterol in the blood. LDL carries cholesterol to the tissues of the body, including the arteries. A high level of LDL increases the risk of heart disease. LDL typically contains 60 to 70 percent of the total serum cholesterol and both are directly correlated with CHD risk. [NIH]

Lower Esophageal Sphincter: The muscle between the esophagus and stomach. When a person swallows, this muscle relaxes to let food pass from the esophagus to the stomach. It stays closed at other times to keep stomach contents from flowing back into the esophagus. [NIH]

Lung Transplantation: The transference of either one or both of the lungs from one human or animal to another. [NIH]

Lupus: A form of cutaneous tuberculosis. It is seen predominantly in women and typically involves the nasal, buccal, and conjunctival mucosa. [NIH]

Lymph: The almost colorless fluid that travels through the lymphatic system and carries cells that help fight infection and disease. [NIH]

Lymph node: A rounded mass of lymphatic tissue that is surrounded by a capsule of connective tissue. Also known as a lymph gland. Lymph nodes are spread out along lymphatic vessels and contain many lymphocytes, which filter the lymphatic fluid (lymph). [NIH]

Lymphadenopathy: Disease or swelling of the lymph nodes. [NIH]

Lymphatic: The tissues and organs, including the bone marrow, spleen, thymus, and lymph nodes, that produce and store cells that fight infection and disease. [NIH]

Lymphatic system: The tissues and organs that produce, store, and carry white blood cells that fight infection and other diseases. This system includes the bone marrow, spleen, thymus, lymph nodes and a network of thin tubes that carry lymph and white blood cells. These tubes branch, like blood vessels, into all the tissues of the body. [NIH]

Lymphocyte Count: A count of the number of lymphocytes in the blood. [NIH]

Lymphocyte Depletion: Immunosuppression by reduction of circulating lymphocytes or by T-cell depletion of bone marrow. The former may be accomplished in vivo by thoracic duct drainage or administration of antilymphocyte serum. The latter is performed ex vivo on bone marrow before its transplantation. [NIH]

Lymphocytes: White blood cells formed in the body's lymphoid tissue. The nucleus is round or ovoid with coarse, irregularly clumped chromatin while the cytoplasm is typically pale blue with azurophilic (if any) granules. Most lymphocytes can be classified as either T or B (with subpopulations of each); those with characteristics of neither major class are called null cells. [NIH]

Lymphoid: Referring to lymphocytes, a type of white blood cell. Also refers to tissue in which lymphocytes develop. [NIH]

Lymphokines: Soluble protein factors generated by activated lymphocytes that affect other cells, primarily those involved in cellular immunity. [NIH]

Lymphoma: A general term for various neoplastic diseases of the lymphoid tissue. [NIH]

Lymphopenia: Reduction in the number of lymphocytes. [NIH]

Macrophage: A type of white blood cell that surrounds and kills microorganisms, removes dead cells, and stimulates the action of other immune system cells. [NIH]

Macula: A stain, spot, or thickening. Often used alone to refer to the macula retinae. [EU]

Macula Lutea: An oval area in the retina, 3 to 5 mm in diameter, usually located temporal to the superior pole of the eye and slightly below the level of the optic disk. [NIH]

Macular Degeneration: Degenerative changes in the macula lutea of the retina. [NIH]

Magnetic Resonance Imaging: Non-invasive method of demonstrating internal anatomy based on the principle that atomic nuclei in a strong magnetic field absorb pulses of radiofrequency energy and emit them as radiowaves which can be reconstructed into computerized images. The concept includes proton spin tomographic techniques. [NIH]

Malabsorption: Impaired intestinal absorption of nutrients. [EU]

Malaise: A vague feeling of bodily discomfort. [EU]

Malaria: A protozoan disease caused in humans by four species of the genus Plasmodium (P. falciparum (malaria, falciparum), P. vivax (malaria, vivax), P. ovale, and P. malariae) and transmitted by the bite of an infected female mosquito of the genus Anopheles. Malaria is endemic in parts of Asia, Africa, Central and South America, Oceania, and certain Caribbean islands. It is characterized by extreme exhaustion associated with paroxysms of high fever, sweating, shaking chills, and anemia. Malaria in animals is caused by other species of plasmodia. [NIH]

Malaria, Falciparum: Malaria caused by Plasmodium falciparum. This is the severest form of malaria and is associated with the highest levels of parasites in the blood. This disease is characterized by irregularly recurring febrile paroxysms that in extreme cases occur with acute cerebral, renal, or gastrointestinal manifestations. [NIH]

Malaria, Vivax: Malaria caused by Plasmodium vivax. This form of malaria is less severe than malaria, falciparum, but there is a higher probability for relapses to occur. Febrile paroxysms often occur every other day. [NIH]

Malformation: A morphologic defect resulting from an intrinsically abnormal developmental process. [EU]

Malignancy: A cancerous tumor that can invade and destroy nearby tissue and spread to other parts of the body. [NIH]

Malignant: Cancerous; a growth with a tendency to invade and destroy nearby tissue and spread to other parts of the body. [NIH]

Malignant mesothelioma: A rare type of cancer in which malignant cells are found in the sac lining the chest or abdomen. Exposure to airborne asbestos particles increases one's risk of developing malignant mesothelioma. [NIH]

Malnutrition: A condition caused by not eating enough food or not eating a balanced diet. [NIH]

Mammary: Pertaining to the mamma, or breast. [EU]

Mania: Excitement of psychotic proportions manifested by mental and physical hyperactivity, disorganization of behaviour, and elevation of mood. [EU]

Manic: Affected with mania. [EU]

Mastication: The act and process of chewing and grinding food in the mouth. [NIH]

Matrix metalloproteinase: A member of a group of enzymes that can break down proteins, such as collagen, that are normally found in the spaces between cells in tissues (i.e., extracellular matrix proteins). Because these enzymes need zinc or calcium atoms to work properly, they are called metalloproteinases. Matrix metalloproteinases are involved in wound healing, angiogenesis, and tumor cell metastasis. [NIH]

Maxillary: Pertaining to the maxilla : the irregularly shaped bone that with its fellow forms the upper jaw. [EU]

Maxillary Nerve: The intermediate sensory division of the trigeminal (5th cranial) nerve. The maxillary nerve carries general afferents from the intermediate region of the face including the lower eyelid, nose and upper lip, the maxillary teeth, and parts of the dura. [NIH]

Mediate: Indirect; accomplished by the aid of an intervening medium. [EU]

Mediator: An object or substance by which something is mediated, such as (1) a structure of the nervous system that transmits impulses eliciting a specific response; (2) a chemical substance (transmitter substance) that induces activity in an excitable tissue, such as nerve or muscle; or (3) a substance released from cells as the result of the interaction of antigen with antibody or by the action of antigen with a sensitized lymphocyte. [EU]

Medical Oncology: A subspecialty of internal medicine concerned with the study of neoplasms. [NIH]

MEDLINE: An online database of MEDLARS, the computerized bibliographic Medical Literature Analysis and Retrieval System of the National Library of Medicine. [NIH]

Medroxyprogesterone Acetate: An injectable contraceptive, generally marketed under the name Depo-Provera. [NIH]

Megestrol: 17-Hydroxy-6-methylpregna-3,6-diene-3,20-dione. A progestational hormone used most commonly as the acetate ester. As the acetate, it is more potent than progesterone both as a progestagen and as an ovulation inhibitor. It has also been used in the palliative treatment of breast cancer. [NIH]

Megestrol Acetate: A drug that belongs to the group of hormones called progestins, used as hormone therapy to block estrogen and to suppress the effects of estrogen and androgens. [NIH]

Melanin: The substance that gives the skin its color. [NIH]

Melanocytes: Epidermal dendritic pigment cells which control long-term morphological color changes by alteration in their number or in the amount of pigment they produce and store in the pigment containing organelles called melanosomes. Melanophores are larger cells which do not exist in mammals. [NIH]

Melanoma: A form of skin cancer that arises in melanocytes, the cells that produce pigment. Melanoma usually begins in a mole. [NIH]

Membrane: A very thin layer of tissue that covers a surface. [NIH]

Membrane Lipids: Lipids, predominantly phospholipids, cholesterol and small amounts of glycolipids found in membranes including cellular and intracellular membranes. These lipids may be arranged in bilayers in the membranes with integral proteins between the layers and peripheral proteins attached to the outside. Membrane lipids are required for active transport, several enzymatic activities and membrane formation. [NIH]

Memory: Complex mental function having four distinct phases: (1) memorizing or learning, (2) retention, (3) recall, and (4) recognition. Clinically, it is usually subdivided into immediate, recent, and remote memory. [NIH]

Meninges: The three membranes that cover and protect the brain and spinal cord. [NIH]

Meningitis: Inflammation of the meninges. When it affects the dura mater, the disease is termed pachymeningitis; when the arachnoid and pia mater are involved, it is called leptomeningitis, or meningitis proper. [EU]

Menstrual Cycle: The period of the regularly recurring physiologic changes in the endometrium occurring during the reproductive period in human females and some primates and culminating in partial sloughing of the endometrium (menstruation). [NIH]

Mental: Pertaining to the mind; psychic. 2. (L. mentum chin) pertaining to the chin. [EU]

Mental Health: The state wherein the person is well adjusted. [NIH]

Mental Retardation: Refers to sub-average general intellectual functioning which originated during the developmental period and is associated with impairment in adaptive behavior. [NIH]

Mesenchymal: Refers to cells that develop into connective tissue, blood vessels, and lymphatic tissue. [NIH]

Mesothelioma: A benign (noncancerous) or malignant (cancerous) tumor affecting the lining of the chest or abdomen. Exposure to asbestos particles in the air increases the risk of developing malignant mesothelioma. [NIH]

Metabolic disorder: A condition in which normal metabolic processes are disrupted, usually because of a missing enzyme. [NIH]

Metabolite: Any substance produced by metabolism or by a metabolic process. [EU]

Metastasis: The spread of cancer from one part of the body to another. Tumors formed from cells that have spread are called "secondary tumors" and contain cells that are like those in the original (primary) tumor. The plural is metastases. [NIH]

Metastatic: Having to do with metastasis, which is the spread of cancer from one part of the body to another. [NIH]

Metastatic cancer: Cancer that has spread from the place in which it started to other parts of the body. [NIH]

Microbe: An organism which cannot be observed with the naked eye; e. g. unicellular animals, lower algae, lower fungi, bacteria. [NIH]

Microbiology: The study of microorganisms such as fungi, bacteria, algae, archaea, and viruses. [NIH]

Microcirculation: The vascular network lying between the arterioles and venules; includes capillaries, metarterioles and arteriovenous anastomoses. Also, the flow of blood through this network. [NIH]

Microdialysis: A technique for measuring extracellular concentrations of substances in tissues, usually in vivo, by means of a small probe equipped with a semipermeable membrane. Substances may also be introduced into the extracellular space through the membrane. [NIH]

Micronutrients: Essential dietary elements or organic compounds that are required in only small quantities for normal physiologic processes to occur. [NIH]

Microorganism: An organism that can be seen only through a microscope. Microorganisms include bacteria, protozoa, algae, and fungi. Although viruses are not considered living organisms, they are sometimes classified as microorganisms. [NIH]

Micro-organism: An organism which cannot be observed with the naked eye; e. g. unicellular animals, lower algae, lower fungi, bacteria. [NIH]

Microscopy: The application of microscope magnification to the study of materials that cannot be properly seen by the unaided eye. [NIH]

Microsporidiosis: Infections with protozoa of the phylum Microspora. [NIH]

Microtubules: Slender, cylindrical filaments found in the cytoskeleton of plant and animal cells. They are composed of the protein tubulin. [NIH]

Mineralocorticoids: A group of corticosteroids primarily associated with the regulation of water and electrolyte balance. This is accomplished through the effect on ion transport in renal tubules, resulting in retention of sodium and loss of potassium. Mineralocorticoid secretion is itself regulated by plasma volume, serum potassium, and angiotensin II. [NIH]

Mitochondria: Parts of a cell where aerobic production (also known as cell respiration) takes place. [NIH]

Mitochondrial Swelling: Increase in volume of mitochondria due to an influx of fluid; it occurs in hypotonic solutions due to osmotic pressure and in isotonic solutions as a result of altered permeability of the membranes of respiring mitochondria. [NIH]

Mitosis: A method of indirect cell division by means of which the two daughter nuclei normally receive identical complements of the number of chromosomes of the somatic cells of the species. [NIH]

Mitotic: Cell resulting from mitosis. [NIH]

Mobility: Capability of movement, of being moved, or of flowing freely. [EU]

Mobilization: The process of making a fixed part or stored substance mobile, as by separating a part from surrounding structures to make it accessible for an operative procedure or by causing release into the circulation for body use of a substance stored in the body. [EU]

Modeling: A treatment procedure whereby the therapist presents the target behavior which the learner is to imitate and make part of his repertoire. [NIH]

Modification: A change in an organism, or in a process in an organism, that is acquired from its own activity or environment. [NIH]

Molecular: Of, pertaining to, or composed of molecules : a very small mass of matter. [EU]

Molecular Probes: A group of atoms or molecules attached to other molecules or cellular structures and used in studying the properties of these molecules and structures. Radioactive DNA or RNA sequences are used in molecular genetics to detect the presence of a complementary sequence by molecular hybridization. [NIH]

Molecule: A chemical made up of two or more atoms. The atoms in a molecule can be the same (an oxygen molecule has two oxygen atoms) or different (a water molecule has two hydrogen atoms and one oxygen atom). Biological molecules, such as proteins and DNA, can be made up of many thousands of atoms. [NIH]

Monitor: An apparatus which automatically records such physiological signs as respiration, pulse, and blood pressure in an anesthetized patient or one undergoing surgical or other procedures. [NIH]

Monoclonal: An antibody produced by culturing a single type of cell. It therefore consists of a single species of immunoglobulin molecules. [NIH]

Monocytes: Large, phagocytic mononuclear leukocytes produced in the vertebrate bone marrow and released into the blood; contain a large, oval or somewhat indented nucleus surrounded by voluminous cytoplasm and numerous organelles. [NIH]

Monokines: Soluble mediators of the immune response that are neither antibodies nor complement. They are produced largely, but not exclusively, by monocytes and macrophages. [NIH]

Mononuclear: A cell with one nucleus. [NIH]

Morphine: The principal alkaloid in opium and the prototype opiate analgesic and narcotic. Morphine has widespread effects in the central nervous system and on smooth muscle. [NIH]

Morphology: The science of the form and structure of organisms (plants, animals, and other forms of life). [NIH]

Motility: The ability to move spontaneously. [EU]

Motion Sickness: Sickness caused by motion, as sea sickness, train sickness, car sickness, and air sickness. [NIH]

Movement Disorders: Syndromes which feature dyskinesias as a cardinal manifestation of the disease process. Included in this category are degenerative, hereditary, post-infectious, medication-induced, post-inflammatory, and post-traumatic conditions. [NIH]

Mucocutaneous: Pertaining to or affecting the mucous membrane and the skin. [EU]

Mucolytic: Destroying or dissolving mucin; an agent that so acts : a mucopolysaccharide or glycoprotein, the chief constituent of mucus. [EU]

Mucosa: A mucous membrane, or tunica mucosa. [EU]

Mucositis: A complication of some cancer therapies in which the lining of the digestive system becomes inflamed. Often seen as sores in the mouth. [NIH]

Mucus: The viscous secretion of mucous membranes. It contains mucin, white blood cells, water, inorganic salts, and exfoliated cells. [NIH]

Multiple Organ Failure: A progressive condition usually characterized by combined failure of several organs such as the lungs, liver, kidney, along with some clotting mechanisms, usually postinjury or postoperative. [NIH]

Multiple sclerosis: A disorder of the central nervous system marked by weakness, numbness, a loss of muscle coordination, and problems with vision, speech, and bladder control. Multiple sclerosis is thought to be an autoimmune disease in which the body's immune system destroys myelin. Myelin is a substance that contains both protein and fat (lipid) and serves as a nerve insulator and helps in the transmission of nerve signals. [NIH]

Muscle Fibers: Large single cells, either cylindrical or prismatic in shape, that form the basic unit of muscle tissue. They consist of a soft contractile substance enclosed in a tubular sheath. [NIH]

Muscle Proteins: The protein constituents of muscle, the major ones being ACTINS and MYOSIN. More than a dozen accessary proteins exist including troponin, tropomyosin, and dystrophin. [NIH]

Muscle relaxant: An agent that specifically aids in reducing muscle tension, as those acting at the polysynaptic neurons of motor nerves (e.g. meprobamate) or at the myoneural junction (curare and related compounds). [EU]

Musculature: The muscular apparatus of the body, or of any part of it. [EU]

Myasthenia: Muscular debility; any constitutional anomaly of muscle. [EU]

Myelin: The fatty substance that covers and protects nerves. [NIH]

Myeloid Cells: Cells which include the monocytes and the granulocytes. [NIH]

Myeloid Progenitor Cells: One of the two stem cells derived from hematopoietic stem cells - the other being the lymphoid progenitor cell. Derived from these myeloid progenitor cells are the erythroid progenitor cells and the myeloid cells (monocytes and granulocytes). [NIH]

Myelosuppression: A condition in which bone marrow activity is decreased, resulting in fewer red blood cells, white blood cells, and platelets. Myelosuppression is a side effect of some cancer treatments. [NIH]

Myocardial infarction: Gross necrosis of the myocardium as a result of interruption of the blood supply to the area; it is almost always caused by atherosclerosis of the coronary arteries, upon which coronary thrombosis is usually superimposed. [NIH]

Myocardial Ischemia: A disorder of cardiac function caused by insufficient blood flow to the muscle tissue of the heart. The decreased blood flow may be due to narrowing of the coronary arteries (coronary arteriosclerosis), to obstruction by a thrombus (coronary thrombosis), or less commonly, to diffuse narrowing of arterioles and other small vessels within the heart. Severe interruption of the blood supply to the myocardial tissue may result in necrosis of cardiac muscle (myocardial infarction). [NIH]

Myocardial Reperfusion: Generally, restoration of blood supply to heart tissue which is ischemic due to decrease in normal blood supply. The decrease may result from any source including atherosclerotic obstruction, narrowing of the artery, or surgical clamping. Reperfusion can be induced to treat ischemia. Methods include chemical dissolution of an occluding thrombus, administration of vasodilator drugs, angioplasty, catheterization, and artery bypass graft surgery. However, it is thought that reperfusion can itself further damage the ischemic tissue, causing myocardial reperfusion injury. [NIH]

Myocardial Reperfusion Injury: Functional, metabolic, or structural changes in ischemic heart muscle thought to result from reperfusion to the ischemic areas. Changes can be fatal to muscle cells and may include edema with explosive cell swelling and disintegration, sarcolemma disruption, fragmentation of mitochondria, contraction band necrosis, enzyme washout, and calcium overload. Other damage may include hemorrhage and ventricular arrhythmias. One possible mechanism of damage is thought to be oxygen free radicals. Treatment currently includes the introduction of scavengers of oxygen free radicals, and injury is thought to be prevented by warm blood cardioplegic infusion prior to reperfusion. [NIH]

Myocardium: The muscle tissue of the heart composed of striated, involuntary muscle known as cardiac muscle. [NIH]

Myofibrils: Highly organized bundles of actin, myosin, and other proteins in the cytoplasm of skeletal and cardiac muscle cells that contract by a sliding filament mechanism. [NIH]

Myopathy: Any disease of a muscle. [EU]

Myopia: That error of refraction in which rays of light entering the eye parallel to the optic axis are brought to a focus in front of the retina, as a result of the eyeball being too long from front to back (axial m.) or of an increased strength in refractive power of the media of the eye (index m.). Called also nearsightedness, because the near point is less distant than it is in emmetropia with an equal amplitude of accommodation. [EU]

Myosin: Chief protein in muscle and the main constituent of the thick filaments of muscle fibers. In conjunction with actin, it is responsible for the contraction and relaxation of muscles. [NIH]

Naproxen: An anti-inflammatory agent with analgesic and antipyretic properties. Both the acid and its sodium salt are used in the treatment of rheumatoid arthritis and other rheumatic or musculoskeletal disorders, dysmenorrhea, and acute gout. [NIH]

Narcosis: A general and nonspecific reversible depression of neuronal excitability, produced by a number of physical and chemical aspects, usually resulting in stupor. [NIH]

Narcotic: 1. Pertaining to or producing narcosis. 2. An agent that produces insensibility or stupor, applied especially to the opioids, i.e. to any natural or synthetic drug that has morphine-like actions. [EU]

Natural selection: A part of the evolutionary process resulting in the survival and reproduction of the best adapted individuals. [NIH]

Nausea: An unpleasant sensation in the stomach usually accompanied by the urge to vomit. Common causes are early pregnancy, sea and motion sickness, emotional stress, intense pain, food poisoning, and various enteroviruses. [NIH]

NCI: National Cancer Institute. NCI, part of the National Institutes of Health of the United States Department of Health and Human Services, is the federal government's principal agency for cancer research. NCI conducts, coordinates, and funds cancer research, training, health information dissemination, and other programs with respect to the cause, diagnosis, prevention, and treatment of cancer. Access the NCI Web site at http://cancer.gov. [NIH]

Nearsightedness: The common term for myopia. [NIH]

Necrosis: A pathological process caused by the progressive degradative action of enzymes that is generally associated with severe cellular trauma. It is characterized by mitochondrial swelling, nuclear flocculation, uncontrolled cell lysis, and ultimately cell death. [NIH]

Neonatal: Pertaining to the first four weeks after birth. [EU]

Neonatal period: The first 4 weeks after birth. [NIH]

Neoplasm: A new growth of benign or malignant tissue. [NIH]

Neopterin: A pteridine derivative present in body fluids; elevated levels result from immune system activation, malignant disease, allograft rejection, and viral infections. (From Stedman, 26th ed) Neopterin also serves as a precursor in the biosynthesis of biopterin. [NIH]

Nephropathy: Disease of the kidneys. [EU]

Nephrosis: Descriptive histopathologic term for renal disease without an inflammatory component. [NIH]

Nerve Growth Factor: Nerve growth factor is the first of a series of neurotrophic factors that were found to influence the growth and differentiation of sympathetic and sensory neurons. It is comprised of alpha, beta, and gamma subunits. The beta subunit is responsible for its growth stimulating activity. [NIH]

Nervous System: The entire nerve apparatus composed of the brain, spinal cord, nerves and ganglia. [NIH]

Neural: 1. Pertaining to a nerve or to the nerves. 2. Situated in the region of the spinal axis, as the neutral arch. [EU]

Neuralgia: Intense or aching pain that occurs along the course or distribution of a peripheral or cranial nerve. [NIH]

Neurodegenerative Diseases: Hereditary and sporadic conditions which are characterized by progressive nervous system dysfunction. These disorders are often associated with atrophy of the affected central or peripheral nervous system structures. [NIH]

Neuroendocrine: Having to do with the interactions between the nervous system and the endocrine system. Describes certain cells that release hormones into the blood in response to stimulation of the nervous system. [NIH]

Neurogenic: Loss of bladder control caused by damage to the nerves controlling the bladder. [NIH]

Neurologic: Having to do with nerves or the nervous system. [NIH]

Neuromuscular: Pertaining to muscles and nerves. [EU]

Neuronal: Pertaining to a neuron or neurons (= conducting cells of the nervous system). [EU]

Neurons: The basic cellular units of nervous tissue. Each neuron consists of a body, an axon, and dendrites. Their purpose is to receive, conduct, and transmit impulses in the nervous system. [NIH]

Neuropathy: A problem in any part of the nervous system except the brain and spinal cord. Neuropathies can be caused by infection, toxic substances, or disease. [NIH]

Neuropeptide: A member of a class of protein-like molecules made in the brain. Neuropeptides consist of short chains of amino acids, with some functioning as neurotransmitters and some functioning as hormones. [NIH]

Neuropeptide Y: A 36-amino acid peptide present in many organs and in many sympathetic noradrenergic neurons. It has vasoconstrictor and natriuretic activity and regulates local blood flow, glandular secretion, and smooth muscle activity. The peptide also stimulates feeding and drinking behavior and influences secretion of pituitary hormones. [NIH]

Neurotoxicity: The tendency of some treatments to cause damage to the nervous system. [NIH]

Neurotransmitter: Any of a group of substances that are released on excitation from the axon terminal of a presynaptic neuron of the central or peripheral nervous system and travel across the synaptic cleft to either excite or inhibit the target cell. Among the many substances that have the properties of a neurotransmitter are acetylcholine, norepinephrine, epinephrine, dopamine, glycine, y-aminobutyrate, glutamic acid, substance P, enkephalins, endorphins, and serotonin. [EU]

Neurotrophins: A nerve growth factor. [NIH]

Neutrons: Electrically neutral elementary particles found in all atomic nuclei except light hydrogen; the mass is equal to that of the proton and electron combined and they are unstable when isolated from the nucleus, undergoing beta decay. Slow, thermal, epithermal, and fast neutrons refer to the energy levels with which the neutrons are ejected from heavier nuclei during their decay. [NIH]

Neutropenia: An abnormal decrease in the number of neutrophils, a type of white blood cell. [NIH]

Neutrophils: Granular leukocytes having a nucleus with three to five lobes connected by slender threads of chromatin, and cytoplasm containing fine inconspicuous granules and stainable by neutral dyes. [NIH]

Niacin: Water-soluble vitamin of the B complex occurring in various animal and plant tissues. Required by the body for the formation of coenzymes NAD and NADP. Has pellagra-curative, vasodilating, and antilipemic properties. [NIH]

Nitric Oxide: A free radical gas produced endogenously by a variety of mammalian cells. It is synthesized from arginine by a complex reaction, catalyzed by nitric oxide synthase. Nitric oxide is endothelium-derived relaxing factor. It is released by the vascular endothelium and mediates the relaxation induced by some vasodilators such as acetylcholine and bradykinin. It also inhibits platelet aggregation, induces disaggregation of aggregated platelets, and inhibits platelet adhesion to the vascular endothelium. Nitric oxide activates cytosolic guanylate cyclase and thus elevates intracellular levels of cyclic GMP. [NIH]

Nitrogen: An element with the atomic symbol N, atomic number 7, and atomic weight 14. Nitrogen exists as a diatomic gas and makes up about 78% of the earth's atmosphere by volume. It is a constituent of proteins and nucleic acids and found in all living cells. [NIH]

Non-small cell lung cancer: A group of lung cancers that includes squamous cell carcinoma, adenocarcinoma, and large cell carcinoma. [NIH]

Norepinephrine: Precursor of epinephrine that is secreted by the adrenal medulla and is a widespread central and autonomic neurotransmitter. Norepinephrine is the principal transmitter of most postganglionic sympathetic fibers and of the diffuse projection system in the brain arising from the locus ceruleus. It is also found in plants and is used pharmacologically as a sympathomimetic. [NIH]

Nuclear: A test of the structure, blood flow, and function of the kidneys. The doctor injects a mildly radioactive solution into an arm vein and uses x-rays to monitor its progress through the kidneys. [NIH]

Nuclei: A body of specialized protoplasm found in nearly all cells and containing the chromosomes. [NIH]

Nucleic acid: Either of two types of macromolecule (DNA or RNA) formed by polymerization of nucleotides. Nucleic acids are found in all living cells and contain the information (genetic code) for the transfer of genetic information from one generation to the next. [NIH]

Nucleic Acid Hybridization: The process whereby two single-stranded polynucleotides form a double-stranded molecule, with hydrogen bonding between the complementary bases in the two strains. [NIH]

Nucleus: A body of specialized protoplasm found in nearly all cells and containing the chromosomes. [NIH]

Nutritional Status: State of the body in relation to the consumption and utilization of nutrients. [NIH]

Nutritional Support: The administration of nutrients for assimilation and utilization by a patient by means other than normal eating. It does not include fluid therapy which normalizes body fluids to restore water-electrolyte balance. [NIH]

Nystagmus: An involuntary, rapid, rhythmic movement of the eyeball, which may be horizontal, vertical, rotatory, or mixed, i.e., of two varieties. [EU]

Occult: Obscure; concealed from observation, difficult to understand. [EU]

Ocular: 1. Of, pertaining to, or affecting the eye. 2. Eyepiece. [EU]

Odds Ratio: The ratio of two odds. The exposure-odds ratio for case control data is the ratio of the odds in favor of exposure among cases to the odds in favor of exposure among noncases. The disease-odds ratio for a cohort or cross section is the ratio of the odds in favor of disease among the exposed to the odds in favor of disease among the unexposed. The prevalence-odds ratio refers to an odds ratio derived cross-sectionally from studies of prevalent cases. [NIH]

Olfactory Bulb: Ovoid body resting on the cribriform plate of the ethmoid bone where the olfactory nerve terminates. The olfactory bulb contains several types of nerve cells including the mitral cells, on whose dendrites the olfactory nerve synapses, forming the olfactory glomeruli. The accessory olfactory bulb, which receives the projection from the vomeronasal organ via the vomeronasal nerve, is also included here. [NIH]

Olfactory Nerve: The 1st cranial nerve. The olfactory nerve conveys the sense of smell. It is formed by the axons of olfactory receptor neurons which project from the olfactory epithelium (in the nasal epithelium) to the olfactory bulb. [NIH]

Oligo: Chemical and mineral elements that exist in minimal (oligo) quantities in the body, in foods, in the air, in soil; name applied to any element observed as a microconstituent of plant or animal tissue and of beneficial, harmful, or even doubtful significance. [NIH]

Oligomenorrhea: Abnormally infrequent menstruation. [NIH]

Oliguria: Clinical manifestation of the urinary system consisting of a decrease in the amount of urine secreted. [NIH]

Omega-3 fatty acid: A type of fat obtained in the diet and involved in immunity. [NIH]

Oncogene: A gene that normally directs cell growth. If altered, an oncogene can promote or allow the uncontrolled growth of cancer. Alterations can be inherited or caused by an environmental exposure to carcinogens. [NIH]

Oncologist: A doctor who specializes in treating cancer. Some oncologists specialize in a particular type of cancer treatment. For example, a radiation oncologist specializes in treating cancer with radiation. [NIH]

Oncology: The study of cancer. [NIH]

Oncology nurse: A nurse who specializes in treating and caring for people who have cancer. [NIH]

Oncolysis: The destruction of or disposal by absorption of any neoplastic cells. [NIH]

Opacity: Degree of density (area most dense taken for reading). [NIH]

Ophthalmic: Pertaining to the eye. [EU]

Opportunistic Infections: An infection caused by an organism which becomes pathogenic under certain conditions, e.g., during immunosuppression. [NIH]

Optic Chiasm: The X-shaped structure formed by the meeting of the two optic nerves. At the optic chiasm the fibers from the medial part of each retina cross to project to the other side of the brain while the lateral retinal fibers continue on the same side. As a result each half of the brain receives information about the contralateral visual field from both eyes. [NIH]

Optic Disk: The portion of the optic nerve seen in the fundus with the ophthalmoscope. It is formed by the meeting of all the retinal ganglion cell axons as they enter the optic nerve. [NIH]

Optic Nerve: The 2nd cranial nerve. The optic nerve conveys visual information from the retina to the brain. The nerve carries the axons of the retinal ganglion cells which sort at the optic chiasm and continue via the optic tracts to the brain. The largest projection is to the lateral geniculate nuclei; other important targets include the superior colliculi and the suprachiasmatic nuclei. Though known as the second cranial nerve, it is considered part of the central nervous system. [NIH]

Organ Culture: The growth in aseptic culture of plant organs such as roots or shoots, beginning with organ primordia or segments and maintaining the characteristics of the organ. [NIH]

Organelles: Specific particles of membrane-bound organized living substances present in eukaryotic cells, such as the mitochondria; the golgi apparatus; endoplasmic reticulum; lysomomes; plastids; and vacuoles. [NIH]

Osmotic: Pertaining to or of the nature of osmosis (= the passage of pure solvent from a solution of lesser to one of greater solute concentration when the two solutions are separated by a membrane which selectively prevents the passage of solute molecules, but is permeable to the solvent). [EU]

Osteoarthritis: A progressive, degenerative joint disease, the most common form of arthritis, especially in older persons. The disease is thought to result not from the aging process but from biochemical changes and biomechanical stresses affecting articular cartilage. In the foreign literature it is often called osteoarthrosis deformans. [NIH]

Osteoclasts: A large multinuclear cell associated with the absorption and removal of bone. An odontoclast, also called cementoclast, is cytomorphologically the same as an osteoclast and is involved in cementum resorption. [NIH]

Osteoporosis: Reduction of bone mass without alteration in the composition of bone, leading to fractures. Primary osteoporosis can be of two major types: postmenopausal osteoporosis and age-related (or senile) osteoporosis. [NIH]

Outpatient: A patient who is not an inmate of a hospital but receives diagnosis or treatment in a clinic or dispensary connected with the hospital. [NIH]

Ovaries: The pair of female reproductive glands in which the ova, or eggs, are formed. The ovaries are located in the pelvis, one on each side of the uterus. [NIH]

Ovary: Either of the paired glands in the female that produce the female germ cells and secrete some of the female sex hormones. [NIH]

Overweight: An excess of body weight but not necessarily body fat; a body mass index of 25 to 29.9 kg/m2. [NIH]

Ovulation: The discharge of a secondary oocyte from a ruptured graafian follicle. [NIH]

Ovum: A female germ cell extruded from the ovary at ovulation. [NIH]

Oxidation: The act of oxidizing or state of being oxidized. Chemically it consists in the increase of positive charges on an atom or the loss of negative charges. Most biological oxidations are accomplished by the removal of a pair of hydrogen atoms (dehydrogenation) from a molecule. Such oxidations must be accompanied by reduction of an acceptor molecule. Univalent o. indicates loss of one electron; divalent o., the loss of two electrons. [EU]

Oxidative metabolism: A chemical process in which oxygen is used to make energy from carbohydrates (sugars). Also known as aerobic respiration, cell respiration, or aerobic metabolism. [NIH]

Oxidative Phosphorylation: Electron transfer through the cytochrome system liberating free energy which is transformed into high-energy phosphate bonds. [NIH]

Oxidative Stress: A disturbance in the prooxidant-antioxidant balance in favor of the former, leading to potential damage. Indicators of oxidative stress include damaged DNA bases, protein oxidation products, and lipid peroxidation products (Sies, Oxidative Stress, 1991, pxv-xvi). [NIH]

Oxygen Consumption: The oxygen consumption is determined by calculating the difference between the amount of oxygen inhaled and exhaled. [NIH]

Oxygenase: Enzyme which breaks down heme, the iron-containing oxygen-carrying constituent of the red blood cells. [NIH]

Pachymeningitis: Inflammation of the dura mater of the brain, the spinal cord or the optic nerve. [NIH]

Paclitaxel: Antineoplastic agent isolated from the bark of the Pacific yew tree, Taxus brevifolia. Paclitaxel stabilizes microtubules in their polymerized form and thus mimics the action of the proto-oncogene proteins c-mos. [NIH]

Palate: The structure that forms the roof of the mouth. It consists of the anterior hard palate and the posterior soft palate. [NIH]

Palliative: 1. Affording relief, but not cure. 2. An alleviating medicine. [EU]

Pancreas: A mixed exocrine and endocrine gland situated transversely across the posterior abdominal wall in the epigastric and hypochondriac regions. The endocrine portion is comprised of the Islets of Langerhans, while the exocrine portion is a compound acinar gland that secretes digestive enzymes. [NIH]

Pancreatic: Having to do with the pancreas. [NIH]

Pancreatic cancer: Cancer of the pancreas, a salivary gland of the abdomen. [NIH]

Pancreatic Juice: The fluid containing digestive enzymes secreted by the pancreas in response to food in the duodenum. [NIH]

Pancreatitis: Acute or chronic inflammation of the pancreas, which may be asymptomatic or symptomatic, and which is due to autodigestion of a pancreatic tissue by its own enzymes. It is caused most often by alcoholism or biliary tract disease; less commonly it may be associated with hyperlipaemia, hyperparathyroidism, abdominal trauma (accidental or operative injury), vasculitis, or uraemia. [EU]

Paralysis: Loss of ability to move all or part of the body. [NIH]

Paraneoplastic Syndromes: In patients with neoplastic diseases a wide variety of clinical pictures which are indirect and usually remote effects produced by tumor cell metabolites or other products. [NIH]

Parasite: An animal or a plant that lives on or in an organism of another species and gets at least some of its nutrition from that other organism. [NIH]

Parasitic: Having to do with or being a parasite. A parasite is an animal or a plant that lives on or in an organism of another species and gets at least some of its nutrients from it. [NIH]

Parathyroid: 1. Situated beside the thyroid gland. 2. One of the parathyroid glands. 3. A sterile preparation of the water-soluble principle(s) of the parathyroid glands, ad-ministered parenterally as an antihypocalcaemic, especially in the treatment of acute hypoparathyroidism with tetany. [EU]

Parathyroid Glands: Two small paired endocrine glands in the region of the thyroid gland. They secrete parathyroid hormone and are concerned with the metabolism of calcium and phosphorus. [NIH]

Parathyroid hormone: A substance made by the parathyroid gland that helps the body store and use calcium. Also called parathormone, parathyrin, or PTH. [NIH]

Parenteral: Not through the alimentary canal but rather by injection through some other route, as subcutaneous, intramuscular, intraorbital, intracapsular, intraspinal, intrasternal, intravenous, etc. [EU]

Parenteral Nutrition: The administering of nutrients for assimilation and utilization by a patient who cannot maintain adequate nutrition by enteral feeding alone. Nutrients are administered by a route other than the alimentary canal (e.g., intravenously, subcutaneously). [NIH]

Paroxysmal: Recurring in paroxysms (= spasms or seizures). [EU]

Particle: A tiny mass of material. [EU]

Pathogen: Any disease-producing microorganism. [EU]

Pathologic: 1. Indicative of or caused by a morbid condition. 2. Pertaining to pathology (= branch of medicine that treats the essential nature of the disease, especially the structural and functional changes in tissues and organs of the body caused by the disease). [EU]

Pathologic Processes: The abnormal mechanisms and forms involved in the dysfunctions of tissues and organs. [NIH]

Pathologies: The study of abnormality, especially the study of diseases. [NIH]

Pathophysiology: Altered functions in an individual or an organ due to disease. [NIH]

Patient Education: The teaching or training of patients concerning their own health needs. [NIH]

Pelvic: Pertaining to the pelvis. [EU]

Pelvis: The lower part of the abdomen, located between the hip bones. [NIH]

Penicillin: An antibiotic drug used to treat infection. [NIH]

Peptide: Any compound consisting of two or more amino acids, the building blocks of proteins. Peptides are combined to make proteins. [NIH]

Peptide T: N-(N-(N(2)-(N-(N-(N-(N-D-Alanyl L-seryl)-L-threonyl)-L-threonyl) L-threonyl)-L-asparaginyl)-L-tyrosyl) L-threonine. Octapeptide sharing sequence homology with HIV envelope protein gp120. It is potentially useful as antiviral agent in AIDS therapy. The core pentapeptide sequence, TTNYT, consisting of amino acids 4-8 in peptide T, is the HIV envelope sequence required for attachment to the CD4 receptor. [NIH]

Perception: The ability quickly and accurately to recognize similarities and differences among presented objects, whether these be pairs of words, pairs of number series, or multiple sets of these or other symbols such as geometric figures. [NIH]

Perfusion: Bathing an organ or tissue with a fluid. In regional perfusion, a specific area of the body (usually an arm or a leg) receives high doses of anticancer drugs through a blood vessel. Such a procedure is performed to treat cancer that has not spread. [NIH]

Pericardial Effusion: Presence of fluid within the pericardium. [NIH]

Pericardium: The fibroserous sac surrounding the heart and the roots of the great vessels. [NIH]

Periodontal disease: Disease involving the supporting structures of the teeth (as the gums and periodontal membranes). [NIH]

Periodontal disease: Disease involving the supporting structures of the teeth (as the gums and periodontal membranes). [NIH]

Peripheral blood: Blood circulating throughout the body. [NIH]

Peripheral Nervous System: The nervous system outside of the brain and spinal cord. The peripheral nervous system has autonomic and somatic divisions. The autonomic nervous system includes the enteric, parasympathetic, and sympathetic subdivisions. The somatic nervous system includes the cranial and spinal nerves and their ganglia and the peripheral sensory receptors. [NIH]

Peripheral Neuropathy: Nerve damage, usually affecting the feet and legs; causing pain, numbness, or a tingling feeling. Also called "somatic neuropathy" or "distal sensory polyneuropathy." [NIH]

Peripheral stem cells: Immature cells found circulating in the bloodstream. New blood cells develop from peripheral stem cells. [NIH]

Peritoneal: Having to do with the peritoneum (the tissue that lines the abdominal wall and covers most of the organs in the abdomen). [NIH]

Peritoneal Cavity: The space enclosed by the peritoneum. It is divided into two portions, the greater sac and the lesser sac or omental bursa, which lies behind the stomach. The two sacs are connected by the foramen of Winslow, or epiploic foramen. [NIH]

Peroxide: Chemical compound which contains an atom group with two oxygen atoms tied to each other. [NIH]

Petrolatum: A colloidal system of semisolid hydrocarbons obtained from petroleum. It is used as an ointment base, topical protectant, and lubricant. [NIH]

Pharmacologic: Pertaining to pharmacology or to the properties and reactions of drugs. [EU]

Pharynx: The hollow tube about 5 inches long that starts behind the nose and ends at the top of the trachea (windpipe) and esophagus (the tube that goes to the stomach). [NIH]

Phenolphthalein: An acid-base indicator which is colorless in acid solution, but turns pink to red as the solution becomes alkaline. It is used medicinally as a cathartic. [NIH]

Phenotype: The outward appearance of the individual. It is the product of interactions between genes and between the genotype and the environment. This includes the killer phenotype, characteristic of yeasts. [NIH]

Phenylalanine: An aromatic amino acid that is essential in the animal diet. It is a precursor of melanin, dopamine, noradrenalin, and thyroxine. [NIH]

Phorbol: Class of chemicals that promotes the development of tumors. [NIH]

Phorbol Esters: Tumor-promoting compounds obtained from croton oil (Croton tiglium). Some of these are used in cell biological experiments as activators of protein kinase C. [NIH]

Phosphodiesterase: Effector enzyme that regulates the levels of a second messenger, the cyclic GMP. [NIH]

Phospholipases: A class of enzymes that catalyze the hydrolysis of phosphoglycerides or glycerophosphatidates. EC 3.1.-. [NIH]

Phospholipids: Lipids containing one or more phosphate groups, particularly those derived from either glycerol (phosphoglycerides; glycerophospholipids) or sphingosine (sphingolipids). They are polar lipids that are of great importance for the structure and function of cell membranes and are the most abundant of membrane lipids, although not stored in large amounts in the system. [NIH]

Phosphorus: A non-metallic element that is found in the blood, muscles, nevers, bones, and teeth, and is a component of adenosine triphosphate (ATP; the primary energy source for the body's cells.) [NIH]

Phosphorylase: An enzyme of the transferase class that catalyzes the phosphorylysis of a terminal alpha-1,4-glycosidic bond at the non-reducing end of a glycogen molecule, releasing a glucose 1-phosphate residue. Phosphorylase should be qualified by the natural substance acted upon. EC 2.4.1.1. [NIH]

Phosphorylated: Attached to a phosphate group. [NIH]

Phosphorylates: Attached to a phosphate group. [NIH]

Phosphorylation: The introduction of a phosphoryl group into a compound through the formation of an ester bond between the compound and a phosphorus moiety. [NIH]

Phosphorylcholine: Calcium and magnesium salts used therapeutically in hepatobiliary dysfunction. [NIH]

Photocoagulation: Using a special strong beam of light (laser) to seal off bleeding blood vessels such as in the eye. The laser can also burn away blood vessels that should not have grown in the eye. This is the main treatment for diabetic retinopathy. [NIH]

Physical Examination: Systematic and thorough inspection of the patient for physical signs of disease or abnormality. [NIH]

Physiologic: Having to do with the functions of the body. When used in the phrase "physiologic age," it refers to an age assigned by general health, as opposed to calendar age. [NIH]

Physiology: The science that deals with the life processes and functions of organismus, their cells, tissues, and organs. [NIH]

Pigment: A substance that gives color to tissue. Pigments are responsible for the color of skin, eyes, and hair. [NIH]

Pilot study: The initial study examining a new method or treatment. [NIH]

Pineal Body: A small conical midline body attached to the posterior part of the third ventricle and lying between the superior colliculi, below the splenium of the corpus callosum. [NIH]

Pineal gland: A tiny organ located in the cerebrum that produces melatonin. Also called pineal body or pineal organ. [NIH]

Pituitary Gland: A small, unpaired gland situated in the sella turcica tissue. It is connected to the hypothalamus by a short stalk. [NIH]

Pituitary Hormones: Hormones secreted by the anterior and posterior lobes of the pituitary gland and the pars intermedia, an ill-defined region between the two. Their secretion is regulated by the hypothalamus. [NIH]

Placenta: A highly vascular fetal organ through which the fetus absorbs oxygen and other nutrients and excretes carbon dioxide and other wastes. It begins to form about the eighth day of gestation when the blastocyst adheres to the decidua. [NIH]

Plants: Multicellular, eukaryotic life forms of the kingdom Plantae. They are characterized by a mainly photosynthetic mode of nutrition; essentially unlimited growth at localized regions of cell divisions (meristems); cellulose within cells providing rigidity; the absence of organs of locomotion; absense of nervous and sensory systems; and an alteration of haploid and diploid generations. [NIH]

Plaque: A clear zone in a bacterial culture grown on an agar plate caused by localized destruction of bacterial cells by a bacteriophage. The concentration of infective virus in a fluid can be estimated by applying the fluid to a culture and counting the number of. [NIH]

Plasma: The clear, yellowish, fluid part of the blood that carries the blood cells. The proteins that form blood clots are in plasma. [NIH]

Plasma cells: A type of white blood cell that produces antibodies. [NIH]

Plasma protein: One of the hundreds of different proteins present in blood plasma, including carrier proteins (such albumin, transferrin, and haptoglobin), fibrinogen and other coagulation factors, complement components, immunoglobulins, enzyme inhibitors, precursors of substances such as angiotension and bradykinin, and many other types of proteins. [EU]

Plasmapheresis: Procedure whereby plasma is separated and extracted from anticoagulated whole blood and the red cells retransfused to the donor. Plasmapheresis is also employed for therapeutic use. [NIH]

Plasmid: An autonomously replicating, extra-chromosomal DNA molecule found in many bacteria. Plasmids are widely used as carriers of cloned genes. [NIH]

Plastids: Self-replicating cytoplasmic organelles of plant and algal cells that contain pigments and may synthesize and accumulate various substances. Plastids are used in phylogenetic studies. [NIH]

Platelet Activation: A series of progressive, overlapping events triggered by exposure of the platelets to subendothelial tissue. These events include shape change, adhesiveness, aggregation, and release reactions. When carried through to completion, these events lead to the formation of a stable hemostatic plug. [NIH]

Platelet Aggregation: The attachment of platelets to one another. This clumping together can be induced by a number of agents (e.g., thrombin, collagen) and is part of the mechanism leading to the formation of a thrombus. [NIH]

Platelet Factor 4: A high-molecular-weight proteoglycan-platelet factor complex which is released from blood platelets by thrombin. It acts as a mediator in the heparin-neutralizing capacity of the blood and plays a role in platelet aggregation. At high ionic strength (I=0.75), the complex dissociates into the active component (molecular weight 29,000) and the proteoglycan carrier (chondroitin 4-sulfate, molecular weight 350,000). The molecule exists in the form of a dimer consisting of 8 moles of platelet factor 4 and 2 moles of proteoglycan. [NIH]

Platelets: A type of blood cell that helps prevent bleeding by causing blood clots to form. Also called thrombocytes. [NIH]

Plicamycin: A tricyclic pentaglycosidic antibiotic from Streptomyces strains that inhibits RNA and protein synthesis by adhering to DNA. It is used as a fluorescent dye and as an antineoplastic agent, especially in bone and testicular tumors. Plicamycin is also used to reduce hypercalcemia, especially that due to malignancies. [NIH]

Pneumonia: Inflammation of the lungs. [NIH]

Podophyllotoxin: The main active constituent of the resin from the roots of may apple or mandrake (Podophyllum peltatum and P. emodi). It is a potent spindle poison, toxic if taken internally, and has been used as a cathartic. It is very irritating to skin and mucous membranes, has keratolytic actions, has been used to treat warts and keratoses, and may have antineoplastic properties, as do some of its congeners and derivatives. [NIH]

Point Mutation: A mutation caused by the substitution of one nucleotide for another. This results in the DNA molecule having a change in a single base pair. [NIH]

Poisoning: A condition or physical state produced by the ingestion, injection or inhalation of, or exposure to a deleterious agent. [NIH]

Polycystic: An inherited disorder characterized by many grape-like clusters of fluid-filled cysts that make both kidneys larger over time. These cysts take over and destroy working kidney tissue. PKD may cause chronic renal failure and end-stage renal disease. [NIH]

Polycystic Ovary Syndrome: Clinical symptom complex characterized by oligomenorrhea or amenorrhea, anovulation, and regularly associated with bilateral polycystic ovaries. [NIH]

Polyp: A growth that protrudes from a mucous membrane. [NIH]

Polypeptide: A peptide which on hydrolysis yields more than two amino acids; called tripeptides, tetrapeptides, etc. according to the number of amino acids contained. [EU]

Polyunsaturated fat: An unsaturated fat found in greatest amounts in foods derived from plants, including safflower, sunflower, corn, and soybean oils. [NIH]

Port: An implanted device through which blood may be withdrawn and drugs may be infused without repeated needle sticks. Also called a port-a-cath. [NIH]

Port-a-cath: An implanted device through which blood may be withdrawn and drugs may be infused without repeated needle sticks. Also called a port. [NIH]

Posterior: Situated in back of, or in the back part of, or affecting the back or dorsal surface of the body. In lower animals, it refers to the caudal end of the body. [EU]

Postmenopausal: Refers to the time after menopause. Menopause is the time in a woman's life when menstrual periods stop permanently; also called "change of life." [NIH]

Postnatal: Occurring after birth, with reference to the newborn. [EU]

Postoperative: After surgery. [NIH]

Postprandial: Occurring after dinner, or after a meal; postcibal. [EU]

Postsynaptic: Nerve potential generated by an inhibitory hyperpolarizing stimulation. [NIH]

Potentiates: A degree of synergism which causes the exposure of the organism to a harmful substance to worsen a disease already contracted. [NIH]

Potentiating: A degree of synergism which causes the exposure of the organism to a harmful substance to worsen a disease already contracted. [NIH]

Potentiation: An overall effect of two drugs taken together which is greater than the sum of the effects of each drug taken alone. [NIH]

Practice Guidelines: Directions or principles presenting current or future rules of policy for the health care practitioner to assist him in patient care decisions regarding diagnosis, therapy, or related clinical circumstances. The guidelines may be developed by government agencies at any level, institutions, professional societies, governing boards, or by the convening of expert panels. The guidelines form a basis for the evaluation of all aspects of health care and delivery. [NIH]

Preclinical: Before a disease becomes clinically recognizable. [EU]

Precursor: Something that precedes. In biological processes, a substance from which another, usually more active or mature substance is formed. In clinical medicine, a sign or symptom that heralds another. [EU]

Predisposition: A latent susceptibility to disease which may be activated under certain conditions, as by stress. [EU]

Premarin: A hormone replacement therapy drug developed by AHP (USA). [NIH]

Preoperative: Preceding an operation. [EU]

Presynaptic: Situated proximal to a synapse, or occurring before the synapse is crossed. [EU]

Prevalence: The total number of cases of a given disease in a specified population at a designated time. It is differentiated from incidence, which refers to the number of new cases in the population at a given time. [NIH]

Probe: An instrument used in exploring cavities, or in the detection and dilatation of strictures, or in demonstrating the potency of channels; an elongated instrument for exploring or sounding body cavities. [NIH]

Progeny: The offspring produced in any generation. [NIH]

Progesterone: Pregn-4-ene-3,20-dione. The principal progestational hormone of the body, secreted by the corpus luteum, adrenal cortex, and placenta. Its chief function is to prepare the uterus for the reception and development of the fertilized ovum. It acts as an antiovulatory agent when administered on days 5-25 of the menstrual cycle. [NIH]

Progression: Increase in the size of a tumor or spread of cancer in the body. [NIH]

Progressive: Advancing; going forward; going from bad to worse; increasing in scope or severity. [EU]

Projection: A defense mechanism, operating unconsciously, whereby that which is emotionally unacceptable in the self is rejected and attributed (projected) to others. [NIH]

Proline: A non-essential amino acid that is synthesized from glutamic acid. It is an essential component of collagen and is important for proper functioning of joints and tendons. [NIH]

Promoter: A chemical substance that increases the activity of a carcinogenic process. [NIH]

Prophylaxis: An attempt to prevent disease. [NIH]

Prostaglandin: Any of a group of components derived from unsaturated 20-carbon fatty acids, primarily arachidonic acid, via the cyclooxygenase pathway that are extremely potent mediators of a diverse group of physiologic processes. The abbreviation for prostaglandin is PG; specific compounds are designated by adding one of the letters A through I to indicate the type of substituents found on the hydrocarbon skeleton and a subscript (1, 2 or 3) to indicate the number of double bonds in the hydrocarbon skeleton e.g., PGE2. The predominant naturally occurring prostaglandins all have two double bonds and are synthesized from arachidonic acid (5,8,11,14-eicosatetraenoic acid) by the pathway shown in the illustration. The 1 series and 3 series are produced by the same pathway with fatty acids having one fewer double bond (8,11,14-eicosatrienoic acid or one more double bond (5,8,11,14,17-eicosapentaenoic acid) than arachidonic acid. The subscript a or ß indicates the configuration at C-9 (a denotes a substituent below the plane of the ring, ß, above the plane). The naturally occurring PGF's have the a configuration, e.g., PGF2a. All of the prostaglandins act by binding to specific cell-surface receptors causing an increase in the level of the intracellular second messenger cyclic AMP (and in some cases cyclic GMP also). The effect produced by the cyclic AMP increase depends on the specific cell type. In some cases there is also a positive feedback effect. Increased cyclic AMP increases prostaglandin synthesis leading to further increases in cyclic AMP. [EU]

Prostaglandins A: (13E,15S)-15-Hydroxy-9-oxoprosta-10,13-dien-1-oic acid (PGA(1));

(5Z,13E,15S)-15-hydroxy-9-oxoprosta-5,10,13-trien-1-oic acid (PGA(2)); (5Z,13E,15S,17Z)-15-hydroxy-9-oxoprosta-5,10,13,17-tetraen-1-oic acid (PGA(3)). A group of naturally occurring secondary prostaglandins derived from PGE. PGA(1) and PGA(2) as well as their 19-hydroxy derivatives are found in many organs and tissues. [NIH]

Prostate: A gland in males that surrounds the neck of the bladder and the urethra. It secretes a substance that liquifies coagulated semen. It is situated in the pelvic cavity behind the lower part of the pubic symphysis, above the deep layer of the triangular ligament, and rests upon the rectum. [NIH]

Protease: Proteinase (= any enzyme that catalyses the splitting of interior peptide bonds in a protein). [EU]

Protein C: A vitamin-K dependent zymogen present in the blood, which, upon activation by thrombin and thrombomodulin exerts anticoagulant properties by inactivating factors Va and VIIIa at the rate-limiting steps of thrombin formation. [NIH]

Protein Conformation: The characteristic 3-dimensional shape of a protein, including the secondary, supersecondary (motifs), tertiary (domains) and quaternary structure of the peptide chain. Quaternary protein structure describes the conformation assumed by multimeric proteins (aggregates of more than one polypeptide chain). [NIH]

Protein Folding: A rapid biochemical reaction involved in the formation of proteins. It begins even before a protein has been completely synthesized and proceeds through discrete intermediates (primary, secondary, and tertiary structures) before the final structure (quaternary structure) is developed. [NIH]

Protein S: The vitamin K-dependent cofactor of activated protein C. Together with protein C, it inhibits the action of factors VIIIa and Va. A deficiency in protein S can lead to recurrent venous and arterial thrombosis. [NIH]

Protein Subunits: Single chains of amino acids that are the units of a multimeric protein. They can be identical or non-identical subunits. [NIH]

Proteins: Polymers of amino acids linked by peptide bonds. The specific sequence of amino acids determines the shape and function of the protein. [NIH]

Proteinuria: The presence of protein in the urine, indicating that the kidneys are not working properly. [NIH]

Proteoglycans: Glycoproteins which have a very high polysaccharide content. [NIH]

Proteolytic: 1. Pertaining to, characterized by, or promoting proteolysis. 2. An enzyme that promotes proteolysis (= the splitting of proteins by hydrolysis of the peptide bonds with formation of smaller polypeptides). [EU]

Protocol: The detailed plan for a clinical trial that states the trial's rationale, purpose, drug or vaccine dosages, length of study, routes of administration, who may participate, and other aspects of trial design. [NIH]

Protons: Stable elementary particles having the smallest known positive charge, found in the nuclei of all elements. The proton mass is less than that of a neutron. A proton is the nucleus of the light hydrogen atom, i.e., the hydrogen ion. [NIH]

Proto-Oncogene Proteins: Products of proto-oncogenes. Normally they do not have oncogenic or transforming properties, but are involved in the regulation or differentiation of cell growth. They often have protein kinase activity. [NIH]

Proto-Oncogene Proteins c-mos: Cellular proteins encoded by the c-mos genes. They function in the cell cycle to maintain maturation promoting factor in the active state and have protein-serine/threonine kinase activity. Oncogenic transformation can take place when c-mos proteins are expressed at the wrong time. [NIH]

Protozoa: A subkingdom consisting of unicellular organisms that are the simplest in the animal kingdom. Most are free living. They range in size from submicroscopic to macroscopic. Protozoa are divided into seven phyla: Sarcomastigophora, Labyrinthomorpha, Apicomplexa, Microspora, Ascetospora, Myxozoa, and Ciliophora. [NIH]

Protozoal: Having to do with the simplest organisms in the animal kingdom. Protozoa are single-cell organisms, such as ameba, and are different from bacteria, which are not members of the animal kingdom. Some protozoa can be seen without a microscope. [NIH]

Protozoan: 1. Any individual of the protozoa; protozoon. 2. Of or pertaining to the protozoa; protozoal. [EU]

Proximal: Nearest; closer to any point of reference; opposed to distal. [EU]

Psoriasis: A common genetically determined, chronic, inflammatory skin disease characterized by rounded erythematous, dry, scaling patches. The lesions have a predilection for nails, scalp, genitalia, extensor surfaces, and the lumbosacral region. Accelerated epidermopoiesis is considered to be the fundamental pathologic feature in psoriasis. [NIH]

Psychic: Pertaining to the psyche or to the mind; mental. [EU]

Psychoactive: Those drugs which alter sensation, mood, consciousness or other psychological or behavioral functions. [NIH]

Psychogenic: Produced or caused by psychic or mental factors rather than organic factors. [EU]

Psychotherapy: A generic term for the treatment of mental illness or emotional disturbances primarily by verbal or nonverbal communication. [NIH]

Ptosis: 1. Prolapse of an organ or part. 2. Drooping of the upper eyelid from paralysis of the third nerve or from sympathetic innervation. [EU]

Puberty: The period during which the secondary sex characteristics begin to develop and the capability of sexual reproduction is attained. [EU]

Public Health: Branch of medicine concerned with the prevention and control of disease and disability, and the promotion of physical and mental health of the population on the international, national, state, or municipal level. [NIH]

Public Policy: A course or method of action selected, usually by a government, from among alternatives to guide and determine present and future decisions. [NIH]

Publishing: "The business or profession of the commercial production and issuance of literature" (Webster's 3d). It includes the publisher, publication processes, editing and editors. Production may be by conventional printing methods or by electronic publishing. [NIH]

Pulmonary: Relating to the lungs. [NIH]

Pulmonary Artery: The short wide vessel arising from the conus arteriosus of the right ventricle and conveying unaerated blood to the lungs. [NIH]

Pulmonary Edema: An accumulation of an excessive amount of watery fluid in the lungs, may be caused by acute exposure to dangerous concentrations of irritant gasses. [NIH]

Pulse: The rhythmical expansion and contraction of an artery produced by waves of pressure caused by the ejection of blood from the left ventricle of the heart as it contracts. [NIH]

Purines: A series of heterocyclic compounds that are variously substituted in nature and are known also as purine bases. They include adenine and guanine, constituents of nucleic acids, as well as many alkaloids such as caffeine and theophylline. Uric acid is the metabolic end product of purine metabolism. [NIH]

Pyogenic: Producing pus; pyopoietic (= liquid inflammation product made up of cells and a thin fluid called liquor puris). [EU]

Pyramidal Tracts: Fibers that arise from cells within the cerebral cortex, pass through the medullary pyramid, and descend in the spinal cord. Many authorities say the pyramidal tracts include both the corticospinal and corticobulbar tracts. [NIH]

Pyrimidines: A family of 6-membered heterocyclic compounds occurring in nature in a wide variety of forms. They include several nucleic acid constituents (cytosine, thymine, and uracil) and form the basic structure of the barbiturates. [NIH]

Quality of Life: A generic concept reflecting concern with the modification and enhancement of life attributes, e.g., physical, political, moral and social environment. [NIH]

Quaternary: 1. Fourth in order. 2. Containing four elements or groups. [EU]

Quiescent: Marked by a state of inactivity or repose. [EU]

Radiation: Emission or propagation of electromagnetic energy (waves/rays), or the waves/rays themselves; a stream of electromagnetic particles (electrons, neutrons, protons, alpha particles) or a mixture of these. The most common source is the sun. [NIH]

Radiation oncologist: A doctor who specializes in using radiation to treat cancer. [NIH]

Radiation therapy: The use of high-energy radiation from x-rays, gamma rays, neutrons, and other sources to kill cancer cells and shrink tumors. Radiation may come from a machine outside the body (external-beam radiation therapy), or it may come from radioactive material placed in the body in the area near cancer cells (internal radiation therapy, implant radiation, or brachytherapy). Systemic radiation therapy uses a radioactive substance, such as a radiolabeled monoclonal antibody, that circulates throughout the body. Also called radiotherapy. [NIH]

Radioactive: Giving off radiation. [NIH]

Radioimmunotherapy: Radiotherapy where cytotoxic radionuclides are linked to antibodies in order to deliver toxins directly to tumor targets. Therapy with targeted radiation rather than antibody-targeted toxins (immunotoxins) has the advantage that adjacent tumor cells, which lack the appropriate antigenic determinants, can be destroyed by radiation cross-fire. Radioimmunotherapy is sometimes called targeted radiotherapy, but this latter term can also refer to radionuclides linked to non-immune molecules (radiotherapy). [NIH]

Radioisotope: An unstable element that releases radiation as it breaks down. Radioisotopes can be used in imaging tests or as a treatment for cancer. [NIH]

Radiolabeled: Any compound that has been joined with a radioactive substance. [NIH]

Radiotherapy: The use of ionizing radiation to treat malignant neoplasms and other benign conditions. The most common forms of ionizing radiation used as therapy are x-rays, gamma rays, and electrons. A special form of radiotherapy, targeted radiotherapy, links a cytotoxic radionuclide to a molecule that targets the tumor. When this molecule is an antibody or other immunologic molecule, the technique is called radioimmunotherapy. [NIH]

Randomized: Describes an experiment or clinical trial in which animal or human subjects are assigned by chance to separate groups that compare different treatments. [NIH]

Randomized clinical trial: A study in which the participants are assigned by chance to separate groups that compare different treatments; neither the researchers nor the participants can choose which group. Using chance to assign people to groups means that the groups will be similar and that the treatments they receive can be compared objectively. At the time of the trial, it is not known which treatment is best. It is the patient's choice to be in a randomized trial. [NIH]

Reactive Oxygen Species: Reactive intermediate oxygen species including both radicals and non-radicals. These substances are constantly formed in the human body and have been shown to kill bacteria and inactivate proteins, and have been implicated in a number of diseases. Scientific data exist that link the reactive oxygen species produced by inflammatory phagocytes to cancer development. [NIH]

Reassurance: A procedure in psychotherapy that seeks to give the client confidence in a favorable outcome. It makes use of suggestion, of the prestige of the therapist. [NIH]

Receptor: A molecule inside or on the surface of a cell that binds to a specific substance and causes a specific physiologic effect in the cell. [NIH]

Receptors, Serotonin: Cell-surface proteins that bind serotonin and trigger intracellular changes which influence the behavior of cells. Several types of serotonin receptors have been recognized which differ in their pharmacology, molecular biology, and mode of action. [NIH]

Recombinant: A cell or an individual with a new combination of genes not found together in either parent; usually applied to linked genes. [EU]

Recombination: The formation of new combinations of genes as a result of segregation in crosses between genetically different parents; also the rearrangement of linked genes due to crossing-over. [NIH]

Rectum: The last 8 to 10 inches of the large intestine. [NIH]

Recurrence: The return of a sign, symptom, or disease after a remission. [NIH]

Red blood cells: RBCs. Cells that carry oxygen to all parts of the body. Also called erythrocytes. [NIH]

Reductase: Enzyme converting testosterone to dihydrotestosterone. [NIH]

Refer: To send or direct for treatment, aid, information, de decision. [NIH]

Refraction: A test to determine the best eyeglasses or contact lenses to correct a refractive error (myopia, hyperopia, or astigmatism). [NIH]

Refractive Power: The ability of an object, such as the eye, to bend light as light passes through it. [NIH]

Regeneration: The natural renewal of a structure, as of a lost tissue or part. [EU]

Regimen: A treatment plan that specifies the dosage, the schedule, and the duration of treatment. [NIH]

Regurgitation: A backward flowing, as the casting up of undigested food, or the backward flowing of blood into the heart, or between the chambers of the heart when a valve is incompetent. [EU]

Reinfection: A second infection by the same pathogenic agent, or a second infection of an organ such as the kidney by a different pathogenic agent. [EU]

Relapse: The return of signs and symptoms of cancer after a period of improvement. [NIH]

Relative risk: The ratio of the incidence rate of a disease among individuals exposed to a specific risk factor to the incidence rate among unexposed individuals; synonymous with risk ratio. Alternatively, the ratio of the cumulative incidence rate in the exposed to the cumulative incidence rate in the unexposed (cumulative incidence ratio). The term relative risk has also been used synonymously with odds ratio. This is because the odds ratio and relative risk approach each other if the disease is rare (5 percent of population) and the number of subjects is large. [NIH]

Remission: A decrease in or disappearance of signs and symptoms of cancer. In partial remission, some, but not all, signs and symptoms of cancer have disappeared. In complete remission, all signs and symptoms of cancer have disappeared, although there still may be cancer in the body. [NIH]

Renal cell carcinoma: A type of kidney cancer. [NIH]

Renal failure: Progressive renal insufficiency and uremia, due to irreversible and progressive renal glomerular tubular or interstitial disease. [NIH]

Renal Osteodystrophy: Decalcification of bone due to hyperparathyroidism secondary to chronic kidney disease. [NIH]

Reperfusion: Restoration of blood supply to tissue which is ischemic due to decrease in normal blood supply. The decrease may result from any source including atherosclerotic obstruction, narrowing of the artery, or surgical clamping. It is primarily a procedure for treating infarction or other ischemia, by enabling viable ischemic tissue to recover, thus limiting further necrosis. However, it is thought that reperfusion can itself further damage the ischemic tissue, causing reperfusion injury. [NIH]

Reperfusion Injury: Functional, metabolic, or structural changes, including necrosis, in ischemic tissues thought to result from reperfusion to ischemic areas of the tissue. The most common instance is myocardial reperfusion injury. [NIH]

Reproductive cells: Egg and sperm cells. Each mature reproductive cell carries a single set of 23 chromosomes. [NIH]

Respiration: The act of breathing with the lungs, consisting of inspiration, or the taking into the lungs of the ambient air, and of expiration, or the expelling of the modified air which contains more carbon dioxide than the air taken in (Blakiston's Gould Medical Dictionary, 4th ed.). This does not include tissue respiration (= oxygen consumption) or cell respiration (= cell respiration). [NIH]

Retina: The ten-layered nervous tissue membrane of the eye. It is continuous with the optic nerve and receives images of external objects and transmits visual impulses to the brain. Its outer surface is in contact with the choroid and the inner surface with the vitreous body. The outer-most layer is pigmented, whereas the inner nine layers are transparent. [NIH]

Retinal: 1. Pertaining to the retina. 2. The aldehyde of retinol, derived by the oxidative enzymatic splitting of absorbed dietary carotene, and having vitamin A activity. In the retina, retinal combines with opsins to form visual pigments. One isomer, 11-cis retinal combines with opsin in the rods (scotopsin) to form rhodopsin, or visual purple. Another, all-trans retinal (trans-r.); visual yellow; xanthopsin) results from the bleaching of rhodopsin by light, in which the 11-cis form is converted to the all-trans form. Retinal also combines with opsins in the cones (photopsins) to form the three pigments responsible for colour vision. Called also retinal, and retinene1. [EU]

Retinal Ganglion Cells: Cells of the innermost nuclear layer of the retina, the ganglion cell layer, which project axons through the optic nerve to the brain. They are quite variable in size and in the shapes of their dendritic arbors, which are generally confined to the inner plexiform layer. [NIH]

Retinopathy: 1. Retinitis (= inflammation of the retina). 2. Retinosis (= degenerative, noninflammatory condition of the retina). [EU]

Retrospective: Looking back at events that have already taken place. [NIH]

Retroviral vector: RNA from a virus that is used to insert genetic material into cells. [NIH]

Retrovirus: A member of a group of RNA viruses, the RNA of which is copied during viral replication into DNA by reverse transcriptase. The viral DNA is then able to be integrated into the host chromosomal DNA. [NIH]

Rheumatoid: Resembling rheumatism. [EU]

Rheumatoid arthritis: A form of arthritis, the cause of which is unknown, although infection, hypersensitivity, hormone imbalance and psychologic stress have been suggested as possible causes. [NIH]

Ribose: A pentose active in biological systems usually in its D-form. [NIH]

Ribosome: A granule of protein and RNA, synthesized in the nucleolus and found in the cytoplasm of cells. Ribosomes are the main sites of protein synthesis. Messenger RNA attaches to them and there receives molecules of transfer RNA bearing amino acids. [NIH]

Risk factor: A habit, trait, condition, or genetic alteration that increases a person's chance of developing a disease. [NIH]

Rod: A reception for vision, located in the retina. [NIH]

Salivary: The duct that convey saliva to the mouth. [NIH]

Saponins: Sapogenin glycosides. A type of glycoside widely distributed in plants. Each consists of a sapogenin as the aglycon moiety, and a sugar. The sapogenin may be a steroid or a triterpene and the sugar may be glucose, galactose, a pentose, or a methylpentose. Sapogenins are poisonous towards the lower forms of life and are powerful hemolytics when injected into the blood stream able to dissolve red blood cells at even extreme dilutions. [NIH]

Sarcoma: A connective tissue neoplasm formed by proliferation of mesodermal cells; it is usually highly malignant. [NIH]

Sarcomere: The repeating structural unit of a striated muscle fiber. [NIH]

Satiation: Full gratification of a need or desire followed by a state of relative insensitivity to that particular need or desire. [NIH]

Schistosome: Dermatitis caused by the snail parasite, Schistosoma cercariae. [NIH]

Schizoid: Having qualities resembling those found in greater degree in schizophrenics; a person of schizoid personality. [NIH]

Schizophrenia: A mental disorder characterized by a special type of disintegration of the personality. [NIH]

Schizotypal Personality Disorder: A personality disorder in which there are oddities of thought (magical thinking, paranoid ideation, suspiciousness), perception (illusions, depersonalization), speech (digressive, vague, overelaborate), and behavior (inappropriate affect in social interactions, frequently social isolation) that are not severe enough to characterize schizophrenia. [NIH]

Sclerosis: A pathological process consisting of hardening or fibrosis of an anatomical structure, often a vessel or a nerve. [NIH]

Screening: Checking for disease when there are no symptoms. [NIH]

Secondary tumor: Cancer that has spread from the organ in which it first appeared to another organ. For example, breast cancer cells may spread (metastasize) to the lungs and cause the growth of a new tumor. When this happens, the disease is called metastatic breast cancer, and the tumor in the lungs is called a secondary tumor. Also called secondary cancer. [NIH]

Secretion: 1. The process of elaborating a specific product as a result of the activity of a gland; this activity may range from separating a specific substance of the blood to the elaboration of a new chemical substance. 2. Any substance produced by secretion. [EU]

Secretory: Secreting; relating to or influencing secretion or the secretions. [NIH]

Sedative: 1. Allaying activity and excitement. 2. An agent that allays excitement. [EU]

Seizures: Clinical or subclinical disturbances of cortical function due to a sudden, abnormal, excessive, and disorganized discharge of brain cells. Clinical manifestations include abnormal motor, sensory and psychic phenomena. Recurrent seizures are usually referred to as epilepsy or "seizure disorder." [NIH]

Selective estrogen receptor modulator: SERM. A drug that acts like estrogen on some tissues, but blocks the effect of estrogen on other tissues. Tamoxifen and raloxifene are SERMs. [NIH]

Selenium: An element with the atomic symbol Se, atomic number 34, and atomic weight 78.96. It is an essential micronutrient for mammals and other animals but is toxic in large amounts. Selenium protects intracellular structures against oxidative damage. It is an essential component of glutathione peroxidase. [NIH]

Self Care: Performance of activities or tasks traditionally performed by professional health care providers. The concept includes care of oneself or one's family and friends. [NIH]

Semen: The thick, yellowish-white, viscid fluid secretion of male reproductive organs discharged upon ejaculation. In addition to reproductive organ secretions, it contains spermatozoa and their nutrient plasma. [NIH]

Seminiferous tubule: Tube used to transport sperm made in the testes. [NIH]

Semisynthetic: Produced by chemical manipulation of naturally occurring substances. [EU]

Senile: Relating or belonging to old age; characteristic of old age; resulting from infirmity of old age. [NIH]

Sepsis: The presence of bacteria in the bloodstream. [NIH]

Septic: Produced by or due to decomposition by microorganisms; putrefactive. [EU]

Septicaemia: A term originally used to denote a putrefactive process in the body, but now usually referring to infection with pyogenic micro-organisms; a genus of Diptera; the severe type of infection in which the blood stream is invaded by large numbers of the causal. [NIH]

Sequence Homology: The degree of similarity between sequences. Studies of amino acid and nucleotide sequences provide useful information about the genetic relatedness of certain species. [NIH]

Serine: A non-essential amino acid occurring in natural form as the L-isomer. It is synthesized from glycine or threonine. It is involved in the biosynthesis of purines, pyrimidines, and other amino acids. [NIH]

Serotonin: A biochemical messenger and regulator, synthesized from the essential amino acid L-tryptophan. In humans it is found primarily in the central nervous system, gastrointestinal tract, and blood platelets. Serotonin mediates several important physiological functions including neurotransmission, gastrointestinal motility, hemostasis, and cardiovascular integrity. Multiple receptor families (receptors, serotonin) explain the broad physiological actions and distribution of this biochemical mediator. [NIH]

Serum: The clear liquid part of the blood that remains after blood cells and clotting proteins have been removed. [NIH]

Sex Characteristics: Those characteristics that distinguish one sex from the other. The primary sex characteristics are the ovaries and testes and their related hormones. Secondary sex characteristics are those which are masculine or feminine but not directly related to reproduction. [NIH]

Shivering: Involuntary contraction or twitching of the muscles. It is a physiologic method of heat production in man and other mammals. [NIH]

Shock: The general bodily disturbance following a severe injury; an emotional or moral upset occasioned by some disturbing or unexpected experience; disruption of the circulation, which can upset all body functions: sometimes referred to as circulatory shock. [NIH]

Side effect: A consequence other than the one(s) for which an agent or measure is used, as the adverse effects produced by a drug, especially on a tissue or organ system other than the one sought to be benefited by its administration. [EU]

Signal Transduction: The intercellular or intracellular transfer of information (biological activation/inhibition) through a signal pathway. In each signal transduction system, an activation/inhibition signal from a biologically active molecule (hormone, neurotransmitter) is mediated via the coupling of a receptor/enzyme to a second messenger system or to an ion channel. Signal transduction plays an important role in activating cellular functions, cell differentiation, and cell proliferation. Examples of signal transduction systems are the GABA-postsynaptic receptor-calcium ion channel system, the receptor-mediated T-cell activation pathway, and the receptor-mediated activation of phospholipases. Those coupled to membrane depolarization or intracellular release of calcium include the receptor-mediated activation of cytotoxic functions in granulocytes and the synaptic potentiation of protein kinase activation. Some signal transduction pathways may be part of larger signal transduction pathways; for example, protein kinase activation is part of the platelet activation signal pathway. [NIH]

Signs and Symptoms: Clinical manifestations that can be either objective when observed by a physician, or subjective when perceived by the patient. [NIH]

Skeletal: Having to do with the skeleton (boney part of the body). [NIH]

Skeleton: The framework that supports the soft tissues of vertebrate animals and protects many of their internal organs. The skeletons of vertebrates are made of bone and/or cartilage. [NIH]

Skin Aging: The process of aging due to changes in the structure and elasticity of the skin over time. It may be a part of physiological aging or it may be due to the effects of ultraviolet radiation, usually through exposure to sunlight. [NIH]

Small cell lung cancer: A type of lung cancer in which the cells appear small and round when viewed under the microscope. Also called oat cell lung cancer. [NIH]

Small intestine: The part of the digestive tract that is located between the stomach and the large intestine. [NIH]

Smooth muscle: Muscle that performs automatic tasks, such as constricting blood vessels. [NIH]

Social Environment: The aggregate of social and cultural institutions, forms, patterns, and processes that influence the life of an individual or community. [NIH]

Sodium: An element that is a member of the alkali group of metals. It has the atomic symbol Na, atomic number 11, and atomic weight 23. With a valence of 1, it has a strong affinity for oxygen and other nonmetallic elements. Sodium provides the chief cation of the extracellular body fluids. Its salts are the most widely used in medicine. (From Dorland, 27th ed) Physiologically the sodium ion plays a major role in blood pressure regulation, maintenance of fluid volume, and electrolyte balance. [NIH]

Soft tissue: Refers to muscle, fat, fibrous tissue, blood vessels, or other supporting tissue of the body. [NIH]

Soft tissue sarcoma: A sarcoma that begins in the muscle, fat, fibrous tissue, blood vessels, or other supporting tissue of the body. [NIH]

Solid tumor: Cancer of body tissues other than blood, bone marrow, or the lymphatic system. [NIH]

Solitary Nucleus: Gray matter located in the dorsomedial part of the medulla oblongata associated with the solitary tract. The solitary nucleus receives inputs from most organ systems including the terminations of the facial, glossopharyngeal, and vagus nerves. It is a major coordinator of autonomic nervous system regulation of cardiovascular, respiratory, gustatory, gastrointestinal, and chemoreceptive aspects of homeostasis. The solitary nucleus is also notable for the large number of neurotransmitters which are found therein. [NIH]

Solvent: 1. Dissolving; effecting a solution. 2. A liquid that dissolves or that is capable of dissolving; the component of a solution that is present in greater amount. [EU]

Soma: The body as distinct from the mind; all the body tissue except the germ cells; all the axial body. [NIH]

Somatic: 1. Pertaining to or characteristic of the soma or body. 2. Pertaining to the body wall in contrast to the viscera. [EU]

Somatic cells: All the body cells except the reproductive (germ) cells. [NIH]

Soybean Oil: Oil from soybean or soybean plant. [NIH]

Spasticity: A state of hypertonicity, or increase over the normal tone of a muscle, with heightened deep tendon reflexes. [EU]

Specialist: In medicine, one who concentrates on 1 special branch of medical science. [NIH]

Species: A taxonomic category subordinate to a genus (or subgenus) and superior to a subspecies or variety, composed of individuals possessing common characters distinguishing them from other categories of individuals of the same taxonomic level. In taxonomic nomenclature, species are designated by the genus name followed by a Latin or Latinized adjective or noun. [EU]

Specificity: Degree of selectivity shown by an antibody with respect to the number and types of antigens with which the antibody combines, as well as with respect to the rates and the extents of these reactions. [NIH]

Spectroscopic: The recognition of elements through their emission spectra. [NIH]

Sperm: The fecundating fluid of the male. [NIH]

Sperm Motility: Ability of the spermatozoon to move by flagellate swimming. [NIH]

Spermatozoon: The mature male germ cell. [NIH]

Spinal cord: The main trunk or bundle of nerves running down the spine through holes in the spinal bone (the vertebrae) from the brain to the level of the lower back. [NIH]

Sporadic: Neither endemic nor epidemic; occurring occasionally in a random or isolated manner. [EU]

Squamous: Scaly, or platelike. [EU]

Squamous cell carcinoma: Cancer that begins in squamous cells, which are thin, flat cells resembling fish scales. Squamous cells are found in the tissue that forms the surface of the skin, the lining of the hollow organs of the body, and the passages of the respiratory and digestive tracts. Also called epidermoid carcinoma. [NIH]

Squamous cell carcinoma: Cancer that begins in squamous cells, which are thin, flat cells resembling fish scales. Squamous cells are found in the tissue that forms the surface of the skin, the lining of the hollow organs of the body, and the passages of the respiratory and digestive tracts. Also called epidermoid carcinoma. [NIH]

Squamous cells: Flat cells that look like fish scales under a microscope. These cells cover internal and external surfaces of the body. [NIH]

Statistically significant: Describes a mathematical measure of difference between groups. The difference is said to be statistically significant if it is greater than what might be expected to happen by chance alone. [NIH]

Steel: A tough, malleable, iron-based alloy containing up to, but no more than, two percent carbon and often other metals. It is used in medicine and dentistry in implants and instrumentation. [NIH]

Stellate: Star shaped. [NIH]

Stem Cells: Relatively undifferentiated cells of the same lineage (family type) that retain the ability to divide and cycle throughout postnatal life to provide cells that can become specialized and take the place of those that die or are lost. [NIH]

Sterile: Unable to produce children. [NIH]

Sterility: 1. The inability to produce offspring, i.e., the inability to conceive (female s.) or to induce conception (male s.). 2. The state of being aseptic, or free from microorganisms. [EU]

Steroid: A group name for lipids that contain a hydrogenated cyclopentanoperhydrophenanthrene ring system. Some of the substances included in this group are progesterone, adrenocortical hormones, the gonadal hormones, cardiac aglycones, bile acids, sterols (such as cholesterol), toad poisons, saponins, and some of the carcinogenic hydrocarbons. [EU]

Stimulant: 1. Producing stimulation; especially producing stimulation by causing tension on muscle fibre through the nervous tissue. 2. An agent or remedy that produces stimulation. [EU]

Stimulus: That which can elicit or evoke action (response) in a muscle, nerve, gland or other excitable issue, or cause an augmenting action upon any function or metabolic process. [NIH]

Stomach: An organ of digestion situated in the left upper quadrant of the abdomen between the termination of the esophagus and the beginning of the duodenum. [NIH]

Stomatitis: Inflammation of the oral mucosa, due to local or systemic factors which may involve the buccal and labial mucosa, palate, tongue, floor of the mouth, and the gingivae. [EU]

Stool: The waste matter discharged in a bowel movement; feces. [NIH]

Stress: Forcibly exerted influence; pressure. Any condition or situation that causes strain or tension. Stress may be either physical or psychologic, or both. [NIH]

Stroke: Sudden loss of function of part of the brain because of loss of blood flow. Stroke may be caused by a clot (thrombosis) or rupture (hemorrhage) of a blood vessel to the brain. [NIH]

Stupor: Partial or nearly complete unconsciousness, manifested by the subject's responding only to vigorous stimulation. Also, in psychiatry, a disorder marked by reduced responsiveness. [EU]

Subacute: Somewhat acute; between acute and chronic. [EU]

Subclinical: Without clinical manifestations; said of the early stage(s) of an infection or other disease or abnormality before symptoms and signs become apparent or detectable by clinical examination or laboratory tests, or of a very mild form of an infection or other disease or abnormality. [EU]

Subcutaneous: Beneath the skin. [NIH]

Submaxillary: Four to six lymph glands, located between the lower jaw and the submandibular salivary gland. [NIH]

Subspecies: A category intermediate in rank between species and variety, based on a smaller number of correlated characters than are used to differentiate species and generally conditioned by geographical and/or ecological occurrence. [NIH]

Substance P: An eleven-amino acid neurotransmitter that appears in both the central and peripheral nervous systems. It is involved in transmission of pain, causes rapid contractions of the gastrointestinal smooth muscle, and modulates inflammatory and immune responses. [NIH]

Substrate: A substance upon which an enzyme acts. [EU]

Sulfur: An element that is a member of the chalcogen family. It has an atomic symbol S, atomic number 16, and atomic weight 32.066. It is found in the amino acids cysteine and methionine. [NIH]

Superantigens: Microbial antigens that have in common an extremely potent activating effect on T-cells that bear a specific variable region. Superantigens cross-link the variable region with class II MHC proteins regardless of the peptide binding in the T-cell receptor's pocket. The result is a transient expansion and subsequent death and anergy of the T-cells with the appropriate variable regions. [NIH]

Superoxide: Derivative of molecular oxygen that can damage cells. [NIH]

Supplementation: Adding nutrients to the diet. [NIH]

Suppression: A conscious exclusion of disapproved desire contrary with repression, in which the process of exclusion is not conscious. [NIH]

Survival Rate: The proportion of survivors in a group, e.g., of patients, studied and followed over a period, or the proportion of persons in a specified group alive at the beginning of a time interval who survive to the end of the interval. It is often studied using life table methods. [NIH]

Sympathetic Nervous System: The thoracolumbar division of the autonomic nervous system. Sympathetic preganglionic fibers originate in neurons of the intermediolateral column of the spinal cord and project to the paravertebral and prevertebral ganglia, which in turn project to target organs. The sympathetic nervous system mediates the body's response to stressful situations, i.e., the fight or flight reactions. It often acts reciprocally to the parasympathetic system. [NIH]

Sympathomimetic: 1. Mimicking the effects of impulses conveyed by adrenergic postganglionic fibres of the sympathetic nervous system. 2. An agent that produces effects similar to those of impulses conveyed by adrenergic postganglionic fibres of the sympathetic nervous system. Called also adrenergic. [EU]

Symphysis: A secondary cartilaginous joint. [NIH]

Symptomatic: Having to do with symptoms, which are signs of a condition or disease. [NIH]

Synapse: The region where the processes of two neurons come into close contiguity, and the nervous impulse passes from one to the other; the fibers of the two are intermeshed, but, according to the general view, there is no direct contiguity. [NIH]

Synaptic: Pertaining to or affecting a synapse (= site of functional apposition between neurons, at which an impulse is transmitted from one neuron to another by electrical or chemical means); pertaining to synapsis (= pairing off in point-for-point association of homologous chromosomes from the male and female pronuclei during the early prophase of meiosis). [EU]

Synergistic: Acting together; enhancing the effect of another force or agent. [EU]

Systemic: Affecting the entire body. [NIH]

Systemic lupus erythematosus: SLE. A chronic inflammatory connective tissue disease marked by skin rashes, joint pain and swelling, inflammation of the kidneys, inflammation of the fibrous tissue surrounding the heart (i.e., the pericardium), as well as other problems. Not all affected individuals display all of these problems. May be referred to as lupus. [NIH]

Systolic: Indicating the maximum arterial pressure during contraction of the left ventricle of the heart. [EU]

Tamoxifen: A first generation selective estrogen receptor modulator (SERM). It acts as an agonist for bone tissue and cholesterol metabolism but is an estrogen antagonist in mammary and uterine. [NIH]

Taste Buds: Small sensory organs which contain gustatory receptor cells, basal cells, and supporting cells. Taste buds in humans are found in the epithelia of the tongue, palate, and pharynx. They are innervated by the chorda tympani nerve (a branch of the facial nerve) and the glossopharyngeal nerve. [NIH]

Teratogenic: Tending to produce anomalies of formation, or teratism (= anomaly of formation or development : condition of a monster). [EU]

Testicular: Pertaining to a testis. [EU]

Testis: Either of the paired male reproductive glands that produce the male germ cells and the male hormones. [NIH]

Testosterone: A hormone that promotes the development and maintenance of male sex characteristics. [NIH]

Tetany: 1. Hyperexcitability of nerves and muscles due to decrease in concentration of extracellular ionized calcium, which may be associated with such conditions as parathyroid hypofunction, vitamin D deficiency, and alkalosis or result from ingestion of alkaline salts; it is characterized by carpopedal spasm, muscular twitching and cramps, laryngospasm with inspiratory stridor, hyperreflexia and choreiform movements. 2. Tetanus. [EU]

Tetrahydrocannabinol: A psychoactive compound extracted from the resin of Cannabis sativa (marihuana, hashish). The isomer delta-9-tetrahydrocannabinol (THC) is considered the most active form, producing characteristic mood and perceptual changes associated with this compound. Dronabinol is a synthetic form of delta-9-THC. [NIH]

Thalidomide: A pharmaceutical agent originally introduced as a non-barbiturate hypnotic, but withdrawn from the market because of its known tetratogenic effects. It has been reintroduced and used for a number of immunological and inflammatory disorders. Thalidomide displays immunosuppresive and anti-angiogenic activity. It inhibits release of tumor necrosis factor alpha from monocytes, and modulates other cytokine action. [NIH]

Therapeutics: The branch of medicine which is concerned with the treatment of diseases, palliative or curative. [NIH]

Thermogenesis: The generation of heat in order to maintain body temperature. The uncoupled oxidation of fatty acids contained within brown adipose tissue and shivering are examples of thermogenesis in mammals. [NIH]

Third Ventricle: A narrow cleft inferior to the corpus callosum, within the diencephalon, between the paired thalami. Its floor is formed by the hypothalamus, its anterior wall by the lamina terminalis, and its roof by ependyma. It communicates with the fourth ventricle by the cerebral aqueduct, and with the lateral ventricles by the interventricular foramina. [NIH]

Thoracic: Having to do with the chest. [NIH]

Threonine: An essential amino acid occurring naturally in the L-form, which is the active form. It is found in eggs, milk, gelatin, and other proteins. [NIH]

Threshold: For a specified sensory modality (e. g. light, sound, vibration), the lowest level (absolute threshold) or smallest difference (difference threshold, difference limen) or intensity of the stimulus discernible in prescribed conditions of stimulation. [NIH]

Thrombin: An enzyme formed from prothrombin that converts fibrinogen to fibrin. (Dorland, 27th ed) EC 3.4.21.5. [NIH]

Thrombocytopenia: A decrease in the number of blood platelets. [NIH]

Thrombomodulin: A cell surface glycoprotein of endothelial cells that binds thrombin and serves as a cofactor in the activation of protein C and its regulation of blood coagulation. [NIH]

Thrombosis: The formation or presence of a blood clot inside a blood vessel. [NIH]

Thromboxanes: Physiologically active compounds found in many organs of the body. They are formed in vivo from the prostaglandin endoperoxides and cause platelet aggregation, contraction of arteries, and other biological effects. Thromboxanes are important mediators of the actions of polyunsaturated fatty acids transformed by cyclooxygenase. [NIH]

Thymidine: A chemical compound found in DNA. Also used as treatment for mucositis. [NIH]

Thymidine Phosphorylase: The enzyme catalyzing the transfer of 2-deoxy-D-ribose from thymidine to orthophosphate, thereby liberating thymidine. EC 2.4.2.4. [NIH]

Thyroid: A gland located near the windpipe (trachea) that produces thyroid hormone, which helps regulate growth and metabolism. [NIH]

Thyroid Gland: A highly vascular endocrine gland consisting of two lobes, one on either side of the trachea, joined by a narrow isthmus; it produces the thyroid hormones which are concerned in regulating the metabolic rate of the body. [NIH]

Thyroxine: An amino acid of the thyroid gland which exerts a stimulating effect on thyroid metabolism. [NIH]

Tissue: A group or layer of cells that are alike in type and work together to perform a specific function. [NIH]

Tissue Culture: Maintaining or growing of tissue, organ primordia, or the whole or part of an organ in vitro so as to preserve its architecture and/or function (Dorland, 28th ed). Tissue culture includes both organ culture and cell culture. [NIH]

Tolerance: 1. The ability to endure unusually large doses of a drug or toxin. 2. Acquired drug tolerance; a decreasing response to repeated constant doses of a drug or the need for increasing doses to maintain a constant response. [EU]

Tooth Preparation: Procedures carried out with regard to the teeth or tooth structures preparatory to specified dental therapeutic and surgical measures. [NIH]

Topical: On the surface of the body. [NIH]

Toxic: Having to do with poison or something harmful to the body. Toxic substances usually cause unwanted side effects. [NIH]

Toxicity: The quality of being poisonous, especially the degree of virulence of a toxic microbe or of a poison. [EU]

Toxicology: The science concerned with the detection, chemical composition, and pharmacologic action of toxic substances or poisons and the treatment and prevention of toxic manifestations. [NIH]

Toxin: A poison; frequently used to refer specifically to a protein produced by some higher plants, certain animals, and pathogenic bacteria, which is highly toxic for other living organisms. Such substances are differentiated from the simple chemical poisons and the vegetable alkaloids by their high molecular weight and antigenicity. [EU]

Tracer: A substance (such as a radioisotope) used in imaging procedures. [NIH]

Trachea: The cartilaginous and membranous tube descending from the larynx and branching into the right and left main bronchi. [NIH]

Traction: The act of pulling. [NIH]

Transcriptase: An enzyme which catalyses the synthesis of a complementary mRNA molecule from a DNA template in the presence of a mixture of the four ribonucleotides (ATP, UTP, GTP and CTP). [NIH]

Transcription Factors: Endogenous substances, usually proteins, which are effective in the initiation, stimulation, or termination of the genetic transcription process. [NIH]

Transduction: The transfer of genes from one cell to another by means of a viral (in the case of bacteria, a bacteriophage) vector or a vector which is similar to a virus particle (pseudovirion). [NIH]

Transfection: The uptake of naked or purified DNA into cells, usually eukaryotic. It is analogous to bacterial transformation. [NIH]

Transforming Growth Factor alpha: Factor isolated in a variety of tissues including epithelium, and maternal decidua. It is closely related to epidermal growth factor and binds to the EGF receptor. TGF-alpha acts synergistically with TGF-beta in inducing phenotypic transformation, but its physiological role is unknown. [NIH]

Transforming Growth Factor beta: A factor synthesized in a wide variety of tissues. It acts synergistically with TGF-alpha in inducing phenotypic transformation and can also act as a negative autocrine growth factor. TGF-beta has a potential role in embryonal development, cellular differentiation, hormone secretion, and immune function. TGF-beta is found mostly as homodimer forms of separate gene products TGF-beta1, TGF-beta2 or TGF-beta3. Heterodimers composed of TGF-beta1 and 2 (TGF-beta1.2) or of TGF-beta2 and 3 (TGF-beta2.3) have been isolated. The TGF-beta proteins are synthesized as precursor proteins. [NIH]

Translation: The process whereby the genetic information present in the linear sequence of ribonucleotides in mRNA is converted into a corresponding sequence of amino acids in a protein. It occurs on the ribosome and is unidirectional. [NIH]

Translational: The cleavage of signal sequence that directs the passage of the protein through a cell or organelle membrane. [NIH]

Translocation: The movement of material in solution inside the body of the plant. [NIH]

Transmitter: A chemical substance which effects the passage of nerve impulses from one cell to the other at the synapse. [NIH]

Transplantation: Transference of a tissue or organ, alive or dead, within an individual, between individuals of the same species, or between individuals of different species. [NIH]

Trauma: Any injury, wound, or shock, must frequently physical or structural shock, producing a disturbance. [NIH]

Triad: Trivalent. [NIH]

Tricyclic: Containing three fused rings or closed chains in the molecular structure. [EU]

Trigeminal: Cranial nerve V. It is sensory for the eyeball, the conjunctiva, the eyebrow, the skin of face and scalp, the teeth, the mucous membranes in the mouth and nose, and is motor to the muscles of mastication. [NIH]

Trigeminal Nerve: The 5th and largest cranial nerve. The trigeminal nerve is a mixed motor and sensory nerve. The larger sensory part forms the ophthalmic, mandibular, and maxillary nerves which carry afferents sensitive to external or internal stimuli from the skin, muscles, and joints of the face and mouth and from the teeth. Most of these fibers originate from cells of the trigeminal ganglion and project to the trigeminal nucleus of the brain stem. The smaller motor part arises from the brain stem trigeminal motor nucleus and innervates the muscles of mastication. [NIH]

Triglyceride: A lipid carried through the blood stream to tissues. Most of the body's fat tissue is in the form of triglycerides, stored for use as energy. Triglycerides are obtained primarily from fat in foods. [NIH]

Tropomyosin: A protein found in the thin filaments of muscle fibers. It inhibits contraction of the muscle unless its position is modified by troponin. [NIH]

Troponin: One of the minor protein components of skeletal muscle. Its function is to serve as the calcium-binding component in the troponin-tropomyosin B-actin-myosin complex by conferring calcium sensitivity to the cross-linked actin and myosin filaments. [NIH]

Truncal: The bilateral dissection of the abdominal branches of the vagus nerve. [NIH]

Tryptophan: An essential amino acid that is necessary for normal growth in infants and for nitrogen balance in adults. It is a precursor serotonin and niacin. [NIH]

Tuberculosis: Any of the infectious diseases of man and other animals caused by species of Mycobacterium. [NIH]

Tumor marker: A substance sometimes found in an increased amount in the blood, other body fluids, or tissues and which may mean that a certain type of cancer is in the body. Examples of tumor markers include CA 125 (ovarian cancer), CA 15-3 (breast cancer), CEA (ovarian, lung, breast, pancreas, and gastrointestinal tract cancers), and PSA (prostate cancer). Also called biomarker. [NIH]

Tumor Necrosis Factor: Serum glycoprotein produced by activated macrophages and other mammalian mononuclear leukocytes which has necrotizing activity against tumor cell lines and increases ability to reject tumor transplants. It mimics the action of endotoxin but differs from it. It has a molecular weight of less than 70,000 kDa. [NIH]

Tumor-derived: Taken from an individual's own tumor tissue; may be used in the development of a vaccine that enhances the body's ability to build an immune response to the tumor. [NIH]

Tumour: 1. Swelling, one of the cardinal signs of inflammations; morbid enlargement. 2. A new growth of tissue in which the multiplication of cells is uncontrolled and progressive; called also neoplasm. [EU]

Tunica: A rather vague term to denote the lining coat of hollow organs, tubes, or cavities. [NIH]

Type 2 diabetes: Usually characterized by a gradual onset with minimal or no symptoms of metabolic disturbance and no requirement for exogenous insulin. The peak age of onset is 50 to 60 years. Obesity and possibly a genetic factor are usually present. [NIH]

Tyrosine: A non-essential amino acid. In animals it is synthesized from phenylalanine. It is also the precursor of epinephrine, thyroid hormones, and melanin. [NIH]

Ubiquitin: A highly conserved 76 amino acid-protein found in all eukaryotic cells. [NIH]

Ulcerative colitis: Chronic inflammation of the colon that produces ulcers in its lining. This condition is marked by abdominal pain, cramps, and loose discharges of pus, blood, and mucus from the bowel. [NIH]

Ultraviolet radiation: Invisible rays that are part of the energy that comes from the sun. UV radiation can damage the skin and cause melanoma and other types of skin cancer. UV radiation that reaches the earth's surface is made up of two types of rays, called UVA and UVB rays. UVB rays are more likely than UVA rays to cause sunburn, but UVA rays pass deeper into the skin. Scientists have long thought that UVB radiation can cause melanoma and other types of skin cancer. They now think that UVA radiation also may add to skin damage that can lead to skin cancer and cause premature aging. For this reason, skin specialists recommend that people use sunscreens that reflect, absorb, or scatter both kinds of UV radiation. [NIH]

Uncoupling Agents: Chemical agents that uncouple oxidation from phosphorylation in the metabolic cycle so that ATP synthesis does not occur. Included here are those ionophores that disrupt electron transfer by short-circuiting the proton gradient across mitochondrial membranes. [NIH]

Univalent: Pertaining to an unpaired chromosome during the zygotene stage of prophase to first metaphase in meiosis. [NIH]

Uraemia: 1. An excess in the blood of urea, creatinine, and other nitrogenous end products of protein and amino acids metabolism; more correctly referred to as azotemia. 2. In current usage the entire constellation of signs and symptoms of chronic renal failure, including nausea, vomiting anorexia, a metallic taste in the mouth, a uraemic odour of the breath, pruritus, uraemic frost on the skin, neuromuscular disorders, pain and twitching in the muscles, hypertension, edema, mental confusion, and acid-base and electrolyte imbalances. [EU]

Urea: A compound (CO(NH2)2), formed in the liver from ammonia produced by the deamination of amino acids. It is the principal end product of protein catabolism and constitutes about one half of the total urinary solids. [NIH]

Uremia: The illness associated with the buildup of urea in the blood because the kidneys are not working effectively. Symptoms include nausea, vomiting, loss of appetite, weakness, and mental confusion. [NIH]

Urethra: The tube through which urine leaves the body. It empties urine from the bladder. [NIH]

Urinary: Having to do with urine or the organs of the body that produce and get rid of urine. [NIH]

Urinary Retention: Inability to urinate. The etiology of this disorder includes obstructive, neurogenic, pharmacologic, and psychogenic causes. [NIH]

Urinate: To release urine from the bladder to the outside. [NIH]

Urine: Fluid containing water and waste products. Urine is made by the kidneys, stored in the bladder, and leaves the body through the urethra. [NIH]

Uterus: The small, hollow, pear-shaped organ in a woman's pelvis. This is the organ in which a fetus develops. Also called the womb. [NIH]

Vaccination: Administration of vaccines to stimulate the host's immune response. This includes any preparation intended for active immunological prophylaxis. [NIH]

Vaccine: A substance or group of substances meant to cause the immune system to respond to a tumor or to microorganisms, such as bacteria or viruses. [NIH]

Vacuoles: Any spaces or cavities within a cell. They may function in digestion, storage, secretion, or excretion. [NIH]

Vagina: The muscular canal extending from the uterus to the exterior of the body. Also called the birth canal. [NIH]

Vagus Nerve: The 10th cranial nerve. The vagus is a mixed nerve which contains somatic afferents (from skin in back of the ear and the external auditory meatus), visceral afferents (from the pharynx, larynx, thorax, and abdomen), parasympathetic efferents (to the thorax and abdomen), and efferents to striated muscle (of the larynx and pharynx). [NIH]

Valine: A branched-chain essential amino acid that has stimulant activity. It promotes muscle growth and tissue repair. It is a precursor in the penicillin biosynthetic pathway. [NIH]

Vascular: Pertaining to blood vessels or indicative of a copious blood supply. [EU]

Vasculitis: Inflammation of a blood vessel. [NIH]

Vasodilator: An agent that widens blood vessels. [NIH]

Vector: Plasmid or other self-replicating DNA molecule that transfers DNA between cells in nature or in recombinant DNA technology. [NIH]

Vein: Vessel-carrying blood from various parts of the body to the heart. [NIH]

Venous: Of or pertaining to the veins. [EU]

Ventral: 1. Pertaining to the belly or to any venter. 2. Denoting a position more toward the belly surface than some other object of reference; same as anterior in human anatomy. [EU]

Ventricle: One of the two pumping chambers of the heart. The right ventricle receives oxygen-poor blood from the right atrium and pumps it to the lungs through the pulmonary artery. The left ventricle receives oxygen-rich blood from the left atrium and pumps it to the body through the aorta. [NIH]

Ventricular: Pertaining to a ventricle. [EU]

Ventricular Dysfunction: A condition in which the ventricles of the heart exhibit a decreased functionality. [NIH]

Venules: The minute vessels that collect blood from the capillary plexuses and join together to form veins. [NIH]

Vertebrae: A bony unit of the segmented spinal column. [NIH]

Veterinary Medicine: The medical science concerned with the prevention, diagnosis, and treatment of diseases in animals. [NIH]

Viral: Pertaining to, caused by, or of the nature of virus. [EU]

Virulence: The degree of pathogenicity within a group or species of microorganisms or viruses as indicated by case fatality rates and/or the ability of the organism to invade the tissues of the host. [NIH]

Virus: Submicroscopic organism that causes infectious disease. In cancer therapy, some viruses may be made into vaccines that help the body build an immune response to, and kill, tumor cells. [NIH]

Viscera: Any of the large interior organs in any one of the three great cavities of the body, especially in the abdomen. [NIH]

Visceral: , from viscus a viscus) pertaining to a viscus. [EU]

Visceral Afferents: The sensory fibers innervating the viscera. [NIH]

Visceral fat: One of the three compartments of abdominal fat. Retroperitoneal and subcutaneous are the other two compartments. [NIH]

Viscosity: A physical property of fluids that determines the internal resistance to shear forces. [EU]

Vitreous: Glasslike or hyaline; often used alone to designate the vitreous body of the eye (corpus vitreum). [EU]

Vitreous Body: The transparent, semigelatinous substance that fills the cavity behind the crystalline lens of the eye and in front of the retina. It is contained in a thin hyoid membrane and forms about four fifths of the optic globe. [NIH]

Vitro: Descriptive of an event or enzyme reaction under experimental investigation occurring outside a living organism. Parts of an organism or microorganism are used together with artificial substrates and/or conditions. [NIH]

Vivo: Outside of or removed from the body of a living organism. [NIH]

Volition: Voluntary activity without external compulsion. [NIH]

Wakefulness: A state in which there is an enhanced potential for sensitivity and an efficient responsiveness to external stimuli. [NIH]

White blood cell: A type of cell in the immune system that helps the body fight infection and disease. White blood cells include lymphocytes, granulocytes, macrophages, and others. [NIH]

Windpipe: A rigid tube, 10 cm long, extending from the cricoid cartilage to the upper border of the fifth thoracic vertebra. [NIH]

Withdrawal: 1. A pathological retreat from interpersonal contact and social involvement, as may occur in schizophrenia, depression, or schizoid avoidant and schizotypal personality disorders. 2. (DSM III-R) A substance-specific organic brain syndrome that follows the cessation of use or reduction in intake of a psychoactive substance that had been regularly used to induce a state of intoxication. [EU]

Wound Healing: Restoration of integrity to traumatized tissue. [NIH]

Xenograft: The cells of one species transplanted to another species. [NIH]

X-ray: High-energy radiation used in low doses to diagnose diseases and in high doses to treat cancer. [NIH]

Yeasts: A general term for single-celled rounded fungi that reproduce by budding. Brewers' and bakers' yeasts are Saccharomyces cerevisiae; therapeutic dried yeast is dried yeast. [NIH]

Yolk Sac: An embryonic membrane formed from endoderm and mesoderm. In reptiles and birds it incorporates the yolk into the digestive tract for nourishing the embryo. In placental mammals its nutritional function is vestigial; however, it is the source of most of the intestinal mucosa and the site of formation of the germ cells. It is sometimes called the vitelline sac, which should not be confused with the vitelline membrane of the egg. [NIH]

Zygote: The fertilized ovum. [NIH]

Zymogen: Inactive form of an enzyme which can then be converted to the active form, usually by excision of a polypeptide, e. g. trypsinogen is the zymogen of trypsin. [NIH]

INDEX

5
5-Hydroxytryptophan, 109, 167
A
Abdomen, 167, 176, 191, 205, 208, 210, 212, 220, 221, 222, 236, 242, 243
Abdominal, 19, 48, 51, 132, 167, 168, 205, 208, 220, 222, 241, 243
Abdominal fat, 167, 243
Abdominal Pain, 48, 167, 241
Aberrant, 128, 132, 167
Ablation, 18, 167
Acceptor, 167, 208, 220
Accommodation, 167, 215
Acetylcarnitine, 116, 117, 167
Acetylcholine, 167, 180, 217
Acetylcysteine, 83, 167
Acquired Immunodeficiency Syndrome, 41, 118, 167
Actin, 32, 167, 215, 241
Activities of Daily Living, 14, 167
Acute renal, 167
Acute tubular, 28, 167
Adaptability, 167, 179
Adaptation, 28, 52, 168, 180, 204
Adenocarcinoma, 48, 168, 217
Adenosine, 53, 168, 223
Adipocytes, 91, 129, 168, 183, 207
Adipose Tissue, 17, 24, 49, 56, 63, 167, 168, 208, 238
Adjustment, 167, 168
Adjuvant, 6, 34, 94, 97, 168
Adrenal Cortex, 31, 168, 184, 226
Adrenal Glands, 168
Adrenal insufficiency, 74, 168
Adrenaline, 104, 168
Adrenergic, 79, 121, 168, 170, 188, 191, 237
Adverse Effect, 116, 168, 234
Aerobic, 19, 29, 46, 168, 213, 220
Aerobic Metabolism, 29, 168, 220
Aerobic Respiration, 168, 220
Aerosols, 36, 168
Afferent, 45, 168, 193, 207
Affinity, 168, 169, 173, 234
Agar, 169, 224
Age of Onset, 169, 241
Agonist, 36, 94, 121, 124, 133, 169, 188, 238
Albumin, 10, 12, 80, 86, 169, 224
Alendronate, 121, 169
Algorithms, 169, 176
Alimentary, 78, 169, 221
Alkaline, 169, 170, 177, 222, 238
Alkylating Agents, 169, 178, 180
Allantois, 169, 193
Allogeneic, 169, 198
Allograft, 169, 216
Allylamine, 169, 170
Alopecia, 169, 184
Alpha Particles, 170, 229
Alpha-1, 170, 223
Alpha-Linolenic Acid, 109, 170
Alternative medicine, 138, 170
Ameliorating, 115, 170
Amenorrhea, 170, 171, 225
Amine, 112, 170, 200
Amino Acid Sequence, 110, 170, 171, 195
Amino Acids, 5, 42, 56, 109, 170, 195, 216, 221, 225, 227, 232, 233, 237, 240, 242
Amitriptyline, 62, 170
Ammonia, 42, 170, 197, 242
Amnion, 170, 193
Amplification, 30, 170
Amyotrophy, 61, 170
Anabolic, 46, 59, 64, 68, 76, 170, 187, 194
Anaesthesia, 170, 171, 203
Analgesic, 170, 202, 213, 215
Analog, 171, 194
Analogous, 17, 171, 240
Anaplastic, 81, 171
Anatomical, 35, 171, 179, 202, 232
Androgens, 7, 168, 171, 211
Anemia, 16, 53, 123, 126, 130, 131, 171, 194, 210
Anergy, 171, 237
Anesthesia, 171, 205
Angina, 123, 171
Angina Pectoris, 123, 171
Animal model, 8, 24, 42, 65, 117, 120, 171
Anions, 122, 169, 171, 206
Anode, 171
Anorexia Nervosa, 21, 110, 112, 128, 133, 171
Anosmia, 45, 171
Anovulation, 171, 225
Antagonism, 23, 46, 57, 60, 171, 187
Anthropometry, 20, 171
Antiallergic, 171, 185

Antibiotic, 171, 185, 188, 221, 224
Antibodies, 110, 111, 112, 119, 125, 171, 172, 200, 213, 224, 229
Antibody, 11, 43, 89, 125, 127, 169, 172, 182, 200, 202, 203, 211, 213, 229, 235
Anticholinergic, 170, 172
Anticoagulant, 172, 227
Antidepressant, 167, 170, 172
Antiepileptic, 167, 172
Antigen, 169, 172, 182, 200, 201, 202, 203, 211
Anti-infective, 172, 201
Anti-inflammatory, 21, 115, 172, 187, 196, 202, 215
Anti-Inflammatory Agents, 115, 172
Antimetabolite, 172, 194
Antineoplastic, 73, 169, 172, 184, 188, 194, 195, 220, 224, 225
Antioxidant, 32, 109, 122, 172, 220
Antipruritic, 172, 185
Antipyretic, 172, 215
Antiviral, 32, 46, 167, 172, 195, 204, 221
Anuria, 172, 207
Anus, 172, 176, 182
Anxiety, 123, 172
Apnoea, 54, 172
Apolipoproteins, 172, 208
Apoptosis, 6, 21, 54, 60, 85, 172, 178
Aqueous, 173, 174, 185, 190, 201, 207
Arachidonic Acid, 173, 189, 207, 226
Arcuate Nucleus, 49, 173
Arginine, 173, 217
Argon, 64, 173
Arterial, 169, 173, 180, 201, 227, 238
Arteries, 173, 176, 184, 209, 214, 239
Arterioles, 173, 176, 177, 212, 215
Arteriovenous, 45, 173, 212
Artery, 13, 112, 128, 133, 173, 184, 215, 228, 231
Arthropathy, 117, 173
Articular, 173, 219
Asbestos, 173, 210, 212
Ascites, 8, 51, 63, 173
Assay, 29, 173
Asthenia, 53, 56, 109, 116, 117, 173
Astrocytes, 173, 199
Asymptomatic, 22, 31, 173, 220
Atrophy, 29, 39, 44, 129, 132, 173, 208, 216
Attenuated, 42, 174
Attenuation, 24, 103, 174
Autodigestion, 174, 220
Autoimmune disease, 111, 112, 116, 122, 174, 214
Autoimmunity, 27, 123, 174
Autonomic Nervous System, 49, 174, 222, 235, 237
Autopsy, 30, 174
Autosuggestion, 174, 202
Axons, 174, 205, 218, 219, 231

B

Bacteria, 127, 171, 172, 174, 183, 190, 192, 193, 198, 200, 212, 224, 228, 230, 233, 239, 240, 242
Bacterial Infections, 116, 174
Bacterial Physiology, 168, 174
Bacterium, 174, 183
Barbiturate, 174, 238
Basal cells, 174, 238
Basal Ganglia, 174, 195
Basal Ganglia Diseases, 174
Basal metabolic rate, 124, 174
Base, 14, 174, 186, 192, 195, 206, 207, 222, 225, 242
Basement Membrane, 119, 174, 192, 207
Basophil, 175, 200
Bed Rest, 132, 175
Benign, 72, 123, 175, 195, 212, 216, 229
Beta-Thromboglobulin, 175, 205
Bewilderment, 175, 183
Bilateral, 61, 175, 225, 241
Bile, 175, 194, 195, 199, 206, 208, 236
Bile Acids, 175, 195, 236
Biliary, 175, 199, 220
Biliary Tract, 175, 220
Bilirubin, 169, 175
Binding Sites, 128, 175
Bioassays, 26, 175
Bioavailability, 36, 175
Biochemical, 13, 23, 32, 63, 75, 102, 172, 175, 207, 219, 227, 233
Biogenesis, 38, 175
Biological response modifier, 175, 204
Biological therapy, 175, 198
Biomarkers, 40, 175
Biopsy, 44, 175
Biopterin, 176, 216
Biosynthesis, 12, 173, 176, 180, 216, 233
Biotechnology, 26, 50, 138, 149, 176
Bladder, 8, 176, 183, 214, 216, 227, 242
Blood Coagulation, 126, 176, 177, 194, 239
Blood Coagulation Factors, 176
Blood Glucose, 129, 176, 199, 201, 204
Blood Platelets, 176, 224, 233, 239

Blood pressure, 13, 167, 176, 178, 201, 202, 213, 234
Blood vessel, 169, 176, 178, 179, 180, 190, 196, 206, 209, 212, 222, 223, 234, 236, 239, 243
Blot, 33, 176
Body Composition, 19, 20, 40, 46, 66, 112, 176
Body Fluids, 175, 176, 194, 216, 218, 234, 241
Body Mass Index, 128, 133, 176, 220
Bone Marrow, 26, 115, 176, 195, 198, 209, 213, 214, 234
Bone Marrow Transplantation, 115, 176
Bowel, 108, 119, 123, 176, 187, 203, 205, 236, 241
Bowel Movement, 176, 187, 236
Brachytherapy, 176, 205, 229
Bradykinin, 176, 217, 224
Brain Stem, 177, 241
Breast Neoplasms, 177, 194
Bronchial, 177, 200
Bronchitis, 177, 180
Bronchodilator, 177, 181
Buccal, 177, 209, 236
Bulimia, 35, 45, 110, 112, 123, 128, 133, 177

C

Calcitonin, 121, 177
Calcium, 12, 32, 122, 173, 177, 182, 187, 201, 210, 215, 221, 223, 234, 238, 241
Caloric intake, 109, 177
Calpain, 32, 177
Cannabidiol, 177
Cannabinoids, 17, 94, 98, 177
Cannabinol, 177
Capillary, 71, 177, 196, 208, 243
Capsules, 104, 177, 196
Carbohydrate, 109, 177, 196, 197
Carbon Dioxide, 178, 185, 224, 231
Carcinogenic, 169, 178, 204, 226, 236
Carcinoma, 48, 65, 81, 90, 109, 178, 217
Cardiovascular, 13, 46, 78, 86, 94, 108, 123, 129, 178, 207, 233, 235
Cardiovascular disease, 13, 108, 123, 129, 178
Carmustine, 111, 178
Carnitine, 94, 117, 167, 178
Carotene, 109, 178, 231
Case report, 52, 64, 89, 178, 181
Case series, 178, 181
Caspase, 16, 178
Catabolism, 21, 32, 39, 45, 59, 80, 178
Cataract, 61, 178
Catecholamine, 178, 188
Caudal, 35, 178, 202, 225
Causal, 178, 233
Cause of Death, 36, 178
Cell Cycle, 6, 10, 24, 178, 181, 184, 192, 227
Cell Death, 26, 28, 39, 172, 179, 192, 216
Cell Differentiation, 124, 179, 234
Cell Division, 174, 178, 179, 185, 192, 198, 213, 224
Cell Fusion, 34, 179
Cell membrane, 179, 186, 189, 192, 223
Cell motility, 179, 199
Cell proliferation, 6, 44, 124, 179, 205, 234
Cell Respiration, 168, 179, 213, 220, 231
Cell Survival, 16, 179, 198
Central Nervous System, 45, 108, 119, 132, 167, 174, 179, 195, 197, 207, 213, 214, 219, 233
Ceramide, 16, 179
Cerebral, 108, 113, 174, 177, 179, 186, 191, 192, 210, 229, 238
Cerebrovascular, 174, 178, 179
Cerebrum, 179, 223
Cervical, 116, 117, 179
Cervix, 179
Character, 171, 179, 186
Chemoprevention, 11, 179
Chemotherapeutic agent, 12, 37, 111, 179
Chemotherapy, 6, 13, 36, 37, 48, 101, 109, 111, 114, 126, 154, 155, 179, 188
Chin, 179, 212
Chlorambucil, 111, 180
Chlorpromazine, 180, 194
Cholesterol, 60, 121, 175, 180, 184, 201, 208, 209, 211, 236, 238
Cholesterol Esters, 180, 208
Choline, 13, 180
Choline Kinase, 13, 180
Cholinergic, 170, 180
Chondrocytes, 180, 194
Chorda Tympani Nerve, 180, 238
Chorion, 180, 193
Choroid, 180, 231
Chromatin, 172, 180, 209, 217
Chromosomal, 170, 180, 224, 231
Chromosome, 29, 180, 183, 208, 242
Chronic Disease, 23, 44, 65, 123, 129, 133, 180, 182
Chronic Obstructive Pulmonary Disease, 39, 54, 180
Chronic renal, 108, 180, 225, 242

Chylomicrons, 180, 208
Cicatrix, 180, 181
Cicatrization, 116, 117, 181
Circadian, 39, 49, 181
Circadian Rhythm, 40, 181
Cirrhosis, 120, 181
CIS, 47, 181, 231
Cisplatin, 111, 181
Clamp, 38, 181
Clear cell carcinoma, 181, 186
Clenbuterol, 101, 181
Clinical Medicine, 181, 226
Clinical study, 104, 181
Clinical trial, 4, 25, 26, 36, 68, 112, 128, 149, 154, 181, 183, 188, 227, 229
Cloning, 23, 124, 176, 181, 208
Coagulation, 64, 118, 176, 181, 199, 224
Coenzyme, 117, 181
Cofactor, 132, 181, 227, 239
Colitis, 80, 181
Collagen, 47, 126, 175, 181, 182, 193, 194, 205, 210, 224, 226
Collagen disease, 126, 182
Collagenases, 119, 182
Colloidal, 169, 182, 189, 222
Colon, 86, 100, 105, 109, 181, 182, 203, 207, 241
Combination Therapy, 62, 87, 182
Complement, 182, 196, 213, 224
Complementary and alternative medicine, 97, 106, 182
Complementary medicine, 97, 182
Compliance, 13, 183
Computational Biology, 149, 183
Concomitant, 6, 45, 46, 78, 121, 183
Confusion, 85, 183, 187, 201, 242
Congestive heart failure, 18, 39, 54, 87, 119, 121, 183
Conjugated, 99, 183, 185
Conjugation, 28, 183
Conjunctiva, 183, 240
Connective Tissue, 119, 176, 181, 182, 183, 194, 195, 209, 212, 232, 237
Connective Tissue Cells, 183
Consciousness, 170, 183, 186, 188, 228
Constitutional, 183, 214
Contraceptive, 183, 211
Contraindications, ii, 183
Contralateral, 40, 183, 219
Control group, 45, 48, 183
Controlled study, 69, 89, 100, 183
Coordination, 183, 214
Cornea, 184
Corneal Ulcer, 120, 184
Coronary, 112, 128, 133, 171, 178, 184, 214
Coronary Circulation, 171, 184
Coronary heart disease, 178, 184
Coronary Thrombosis, 184, 214, 215
Corpus, 184, 223, 226, 238, 243
Corpus Luteum, 184, 226
Cortex, 184, 192, 229
Cortical, 13, 31, 184, 192, 233
Corticosteroids, 184, 196, 212
Cortisol, 7, 169, 184
Cortisone, 184, 187
Cranial, 180, 184, 193, 196, 211, 216, 218, 219, 222, 240, 242
Croton Oil, 184, 222
Curative, 126, 184, 217, 238
Cutaneous, 116, 117, 184, 207, 209
Cyclic, 53, 132, 177, 184, 198, 217, 223, 226
Cyclin, 16, 31, 69, 132, 184
Cyclophosphamide, 6, 184
Cyproheptadine, 51, 185
Cysteine, 4, 83, 84, 167, 177, 185, 237
Cystine, 185
Cytochrome, 185, 220
Cytogenetics, 11, 185
Cytopenia, 123, 185
Cytoplasm, 34, 172, 179, 185, 198, 209, 213, 215, 217, 232
Cytoskeletal Proteins, 177, 185, 189
Cytotoxic, 32, 111, 118, 126, 127, 185, 202, 229, 234
Cytotoxic chemotherapy, 111, 185
Cytotoxicity, 6, 169, 181, 185

D

Dactinomycin, 71, 185
Dantrolene, 33, 185
Daunorubicin, 185, 188
Deamination, 185, 242
Decarboxylation, 185, 200
Decidua, 186, 224, 240
Degenerative, 17, 116, 119, 186, 199, 210, 214, 219, 231
Dehydration, 111, 186
Dehydroepiandrosterone, 41, 186
Deletion, 172, 186
Delirium, 123, 186
Delivery of Health Care, 186, 198
Dementia, 14, 108, 123, 167, 186
Demyelinating Diseases, 120, 186
Dendrites, 186, 216, 218
Depolarization, 186, 234

Deprivation, 5, 27, 186
Dermatitis, 123, 186, 232
DES, 71, 186
Desensitization, 186, 202
Deuterium, 186, 201
Dexamethasone, 49, 82, 186
Diabetes Mellitus, 3, 28, 127, 132, 187, 196, 199
Diabetic Retinopathy, 120, 187, 223
Diagnostic procedure, 107, 138, 187
Dialyzer, 187, 199
Diarrhea, 34, 41, 53, 187
Diastolic, 187, 201
Dietary Fats, 187, 208
Digestion, 169, 175, 176, 187, 188, 205, 208, 236, 242
Digestive system, 187, 214
Digestive tract, 187, 234, 235, 244
Dihydrotestosterone, 187, 230
Diltiazem, 33, 187
Direct, iii, 6, 8, 41, 49, 111, 126, 141, 181, 187, 188, 230, 237
Discrete, 46, 187, 227
Disease Progression, 6, 14, 187
Disorientation, 183, 186, 187
Dissection, 187, 241
Dissociation, 169, 187, 206
Distal, 188, 195, 222, 228
Diuretic, 87, 188
Diverticulum, 64, 169, 188
Dopamine, 131, 132, 180, 188, 217, 222
Dose-dependent, 128, 188
Double-blind, 69, 79, 100, 188
Doxorubicin, 6, 111, 188
Drinking Behavior, 188, 217
Drive, ii, vi, 13, 24, 47, 93, 188, 207
Dronabinol, 36, 188, 238
Drug Interactions, 142, 188
Dumping Syndrome, 185, 188
Duodenum, 175, 188, 220, 236
Dura mater, 188, 211, 220
Dwarfism, 121, 188
Dysgeusia, 23, 30, 45, 188
Dyskinesia, 188
Dysmenorrhea, 188, 215
Dyspepsia, 35, 188
Dysphagia, 35, 53, 189
Dyspnea, 51, 85, 189
Dystrophin, 189, 214
Dystrophy, 12, 33, 189
E
Eating Disorders, 20, 154, 189
Edema, 126, 187, 189, 215, 242
Effector, 22, 167, 182, 189, 223
Efficacy, 6, 36, 117, 128, 189
Eicosanoids, 101, 189
Elasticity, 189, 234
Elastin, 182, 189, 193
Elective, 84, 189
Electrocoagulation, 181, 189
Electrolysis, 171, 189
Electrolyte, 131, 186, 189, 194, 207, 212, 218, 234, 242
Electrons, 172, 174, 189, 206, 220, 229
Electrophoresis, 71, 189
Electroporation, 130, 189
Emaciation, 167, 190
Embryo, 170, 179, 190, 193, 203, 244
Emesis, 74, 75, 190
Emetic, 36, 184, 190
Emollient, 190, 197
Emphysema, 180, 190
Emulsion, 105, 190
Enalapril, 87, 190
Endemic, 41, 190, 210, 235
Endocrine System, 190, 216
Endogenous, 18, 43, 50, 64, 111, 121, 122, 124, 176, 177, 188, 189, 190, 191, 240
Endorphins, 190, 217
Endothelial cell, 13, 190, 194, 205, 239
Endothelium, 190, 217
Endothelium-derived, 190, 217
Endotoxemia, 113, 190
Endotoxic, 113, 116, 127, 190
Endotoxin, 43, 116, 125, 190, 241
End-stage renal, 180, 190, 225
Energetic, 126, 191
Energy balance, 38, 88, 191, 207
Enhancer, 10, 19, 36, 191
Enkephalins, 191, 217
Environmental Exposure, 22, 191, 218
Environmental Health, 148, 150, 191
Enzymatic, 177, 178, 182, 191, 193, 200, 211, 231
Enzyme, 13, 21, 33, 39, 119, 132, 178, 180, 181, 189, 190, 191, 195, 197, 198, 208, 212, 215, 220, 223, 224, 227, 230, 234, 237, 239, 240, 243, 244
Ependyma, 173, 191, 238
Epidermal, 39, 191, 206, 211, 240
Epidermal Growth Factor, 39, 191, 240
Epidermis, 174, 191, 206
Epidermoid carcinoma, 191, 235
Epigastric, 191, 220

Epinephrine, 168, 188, 191, 217, 241
Epithelial, 80, 111, 168, 184, 186, 191, 199, 207
Epithelial Cells, 111, 191, 199, 207
Epithelium, 174, 190, 191, 218, 240
Erythrocytes, 171, 176, 177, 191, 230
Erythroid Progenitor Cells, 191, 214
Esophageal, 64, 78, 192
Esophagitis, 114, 192
Esophagus, 64, 187, 192, 195, 209, 222, 236
Estrogen, 14, 121, 192, 211, 233, 238
Etoposide, 111, 192
Eukaryotic Cells, 185, 192, 203, 219, 241
Evoke, 192, 236
Excipients, 36, 192
Excitation, 185, 192, 217
Excitatory, 5, 192, 197
Excrete, 172, 192, 206
Exhaustion, 126, 171, 192, 210
Exocrine, 192, 220
Exocytosis, 192, 200
Exogenous, 18, 121, 190, 192, 195, 241
Exotoxin, 126, 192
Expiration, 192, 231
Extensor, 192, 228
External-beam radiation, 192, 229
Extracellular, 18, 33, 47, 173, 183, 192, 193, 194, 210, 212, 234, 238
Extracellular Matrix, 18, 47, 183, 192, 194, 210
Extracellular Matrix Proteins, 47, 192, 210
Extracellular Space, 192, 193, 212
Extraction, 18, 193
Extrapyramidal, 14, 188, 193
Extremity, 46, 193
F
Facial, 180, 193, 235, 238
Facial Nerve, 193, 238
Failure to Thrive, 35, 129, 193
Family Planning, 149, 193
Fatigue, 66, 74, 129, 193, 198
Fatty acids, 101, 109, 117, 121, 167, 169, 189, 193, 197, 208, 226, 238
Feces, 193, 236
Feeding Behavior, 19, 23, 35, 124, 193
Fetal Membranes, 120, 193
Fetus, 193, 223, 242
Fibrin, 176, 193, 239
Fibrinogen, 86, 193, 224, 239
Fibrinolysis, 126, 193
Fibroblast Growth Factor, 33, 193
Fibroblasts, 30, 47, 183, 194, 205
Fibronectins, 193, 194
Fibrosarcoma, 21, 194
Fibrosis, 23, 85, 110, 112, 125, 128, 133, 169, 194, 232
Fluid Therapy, 194, 218
Fluorouracil, 111, 194
Fluoxymesterone, 82, 194
Fluphenazine, 62, 194
Folate, 22, 194
Folic Acid, 194
Follicles, 194, 204
Forearm, 176, 194
Free Radicals, 172, 187, 194, 215
Fumigation, 168, 194
G
Gallbladder, 167, 175, 187, 194
Gamma Rays, 194, 229
Gamma-interferon, 110, 194
Ganglia, 167, 174, 195, 216, 222, 237
Ganglion, 195, 219, 231, 241
Gas, 170, 173, 178, 194, 195, 201, 217
Gastrectomy, 185, 195
Gastric, 45, 174, 178, 191, 195, 200
Gastrin, 195, 200
Gastroesophageal Reflux, 35, 45, 195
Gastrointestinal Hemorrhage, 118, 195
Gastrointestinal tract, 7, 111, 195, 207, 233, 241
Gelatinases, 119, 195
Gemcitabine, 48, 195
Gene Expression, 10, 27, 28, 30, 47, 48, 111, 112, 127, 128, 195
Gene Targeting, 11, 195
Gene Therapy, 18, 33, 195
Genetic Code, 195, 218
Genetic Engineering, 176, 181, 196
Genetics, 11, 17, 44, 48, 183, 185, 196, 205, 213
Genotype, 129, 133, 196, 222
Geriatric, 63, 67, 69, 196
Germ Cells, 196, 219, 235, 238, 244
Germline mutation, 22, 196, 200
Ginseng, 6, 196
Gland, 39, 168, 184, 196, 209, 220, 221, 223, 227, 232, 236, 239
Glomerular, 12, 120, 196, 205, 207, 231
Glomerular Filtration Rate, 12, 196, 207
Glomerulus, 196
Glossopharyngeal Nerve, 196, 238
Glucocorticoid, 24, 32, 49, 187, 196
Gluconeogenesis, 109, 196
Glucose Intolerance, 109, 187, 196

Glucose tolerance, 132, 133, 196
Glucose Tolerance Test, 196, 197
Glucuronic Acid, 197, 199
Glutamate, 10, 197
Glutamic Acid, 194, 197, 217, 226
Glutamine, 4, 10, 31, 32, 73, 114, 197
Glutathione Peroxidase, 197, 233
Glycerol, 109, 197, 208, 223
Glycerophospholipids, 197, 223
Glycine, 197, 217, 233
Glycogen, 197, 223
Glycols, 197, 201
Glycoprotein, 71, 91, 193, 197, 198, 207, 214, 239, 241
Glycosaminoglycans, 193, 197
Glycosidic, 197, 223
Gonad, 197
Gonadal, 31, 197, 236
Gout, 197, 215
Governing Board, 198, 225
Gp120, 198, 221
Grade, 17, 26, 198
Graft, 108, 116, 119, 127, 198, 215
Graft Rejection, 108, 116, 119, 198
Grafting, 198, 203
Graft-versus-host disease, 127, 198
Gram-negative, 127, 190, 198
Granulocytes, 175, 198, 214, 234, 244
Granuloma, 43, 198
Granulosa Cells, 198, 204
Growth factors, 21, 33, 41, 117, 123, 198
Guanine, 22, 103, 198, 228
Guanylate Cyclase, 198, 217
H
Habituation, 24, 198
Haematemesis, 190, 198
Health Care Costs, 18, 198
Health Expenditures, 198
Heart attack, 178, 198
Heart failure, 45, 55, 59, 60, 64, 67, 68, 70, 72, 73, 79, 85, 87, 102, 119, 123, 198
Heart Transplantation, 55, 81, 199
Hematopoiesis, 111, 199
Hematopoietic Stem Cells, 199, 214
Hemodialysis, 63, 187, 199, 207
Hemoglobin, 12, 171, 191, 199, 206, 207
Hemoglobinopathies, 195, 199
Hemorrhage, 187, 189, 199, 215, 236
Hemostasis, 199, 233
Heparan Sulfate Proteoglycan, 19, 199
Heparin, 25, 199, 224
Hepatic, 47, 109, 116, 117, 118, 129, 169, 186, 196, 199, 208
Hepatitis, 115, 117, 122, 199
Hepatobiliary, 53, 199, 223
Hepatocyte, 10, 33, 118, 126, 199
Hepatocyte Growth Factor, 33, 126, 199
Hepatoma, 39, 199
Hepatorenal Syndrome, 118, 199
Hereditary, 196, 197, 199, 214, 216
Hereditary mutation, 196, 199
Heredity, 195, 196, 200
Hernia, 116, 117, 200
Histamine, 111, 185, 200
Histamine Release, 111, 200
Histidine, 200
Histology, 13, 200
Homeostasis, 38, 49, 121, 129, 200, 235
Homeotic, 11, 200
Homodimer, 200, 240
Homologous, 195, 200, 237
Hormonal, 6, 18, 41, 43, 68, 70, 173, 200
Hormonal therapy, 6, 200
Hormone Replacement Therapy, 200, 226
Hormone therapy, 13, 200, 211
Human growth hormone, 16, 200
Humoral, 198, 200
Hybrid, 200
Hybridization, 30, 179, 200, 213
Hybridomas, 190, 200, 205
Hydrazine sulfate, 154, 201
Hydrogen, 122, 167, 170, 174, 177, 186, 193, 197, 201, 208, 213, 217, 218, 220, 227
Hydrogen Peroxide, 122, 197, 201, 208
Hydrolysis, 181, 201, 208, 223, 225, 227
Hydrophobic, 197, 201, 208
Hydroxamic Acids, 119, 201
Hydroxides, 201
Hydroxyl Radical, 122, 201
Hydroxylysine, 182, 201
Hydroxyproline, 182, 201
Hypercalcemia, 65, 78, 89, 201, 224
Hyperlipidemia, 46, 109, 126, 128, 133, 201
Hyperlipoproteinemia, 201, 208
Hyperphagia, 112, 132, 201
Hyperplasia, 41, 44, 201
Hypersensitivity, 186, 201, 207, 232
Hypertension, 35, 45, 123, 128, 133, 178, 190, 201, 242
Hypertrophy, 18, 44, 123, 201
Hypnotic, 174, 201, 238
Hypoglycaemia, 186, 201
Hypoglycemic, 4, 201

Hypogonadism, 7, 194, 202
Hypotension, 123, 202
Hypothalamic, 19, 23, 49, 69, 72, 202
Hypothalamus, 35, 42, 49, 173, 174, 202, 223, 238
Hypoxia, 13, 186, 202
Hypoxic, 13, 202
I
Iatrogenic, 118, 202
Ibuprofen, 51, 202
Imaging procedures, 202, 239
Immune response, 41, 113, 168, 171, 172, 174, 184, 198, 202, 213, 237, 241, 242, 243
Immune system, 6, 41, 111, 113, 116, 174, 175, 202, 207, 209, 214, 216, 242, 244
Immunity, 50, 167, 202, 209, 218
Immunocompromised, 8, 202
Immunodeficiency, 6, 35, 41, 53, 65, 69, 123, 126, 128, 132, 167, 202
Immunologic, 39, 41, 69, 202, 229
Immunology, 9, 17, 81, 125, 168, 169, 202, 205
Immunosuppressant, 169, 194, 202
Immunosuppression, 41, 202, 209, 219
Immunosuppressive, 184, 196, 202
Immunosuppressive Agents, 202
Impairment, 22, 126, 175, 186, 188, 202, 212
Implant radiation, 203, 205, 229
Implantation, 25, 203
Impotence, 6, 203
In situ, 49, 203
In Situ Hybridization, 49, 203
In vitro, 6, 10, 11, 20, 21, 26, 30, 34, 36, 43, 49, 74, 78, 86, 101, 117, 179, 195, 203, 239
Incision, 203, 205
Incompetence, 195, 203
Incubated, 33, 203
Induction, 20, 26, 28, 34, 46, 49, 50, 70, 72, 81, 118, 126, 127, 171, 203
Infancy, 203
Infantile, 62, 203, 208
Infarction, 203, 231
Inflammatory bowel disease, 112, 119, 203
Infusion, 35, 42, 43, 113, 203, 215
Ingestion, 43, 197, 201, 203, 225, 238
Inhalation, 36, 168, 173, 203, 225
Inhibin, 31, 203
Initiation, 204, 240
Innervation, 193, 204, 228
Inorganic, 181, 201, 204, 214
Inotropic, 188, 204
Inpatients, 42, 204
Insight, 12, 17, 46, 49, 204
Institutionalization, 18, 204
Insulator, 204, 214
Insulin, 7, 16, 18, 19, 23, 33, 42, 46, 68, 71, 72, 90, 94, 98, 100, 101, 117, 119, 120, 122, 129, 132, 133, 196, 204, 206, 241
Insulin-dependent diabetes mellitus, 129, 204
Insulin-like, 18, 33, 90, 117, 204
Intensive Care, 66, 118, 204
Interferon, 73, 194, 204
Interferon-alpha, 73, 204
Interleukin-1, 71, 108, 110, 113, 204
Interleukin-2, 73, 204
Interleukin-6, 24, 86, 99, 113, 205
Interleukin-8, 113, 205
Interleukins, 65, 202, 205
Internal Medicine, 10, 32, 48, 60, 62, 90, 205, 211
Internal radiation, 205, 229
Interneurons, 5, 205
Interstitial, 47, 176, 193, 205, 231
Interstitial Collagenase, 47, 205
Intervertebral, 116, 117, 205
Intestinal, 6, 67, 116, 117, 178, 196, 205, 210, 244
Intestine, 176, 205, 207
Intoxication, 186, 205, 244
Intracellular, 22, 27, 29, 34, 47, 76, 123, 203, 205, 211, 217, 226, 230, 233, 234
Intramuscular, 205, 221
Intraperitoneal, 8, 205
Intravascular, 118, 205
Intravenous, 31, 131, 203, 205, 221
Intrinsic, 169, 175, 205
Inulin, 196, 205
Invasive, 116, 202, 205, 210
Investigative Techniques, 104, 205
Involuntary, 3, 174, 206, 215, 218, 233
Ionization, 71, 206
Ionizing, 170, 191, 206, 229
Ionophores, 122, 206, 242
Ions, 174, 187, 189, 201, 206
Ischemia, 173, 206, 215, 231
Isoleucine, 109, 206
J
Jaundice, 199, 206
K
Kb, 148, 206
Keratinocytes, 205, 206
Keratoconus, 120, 206

Ketoacidosis, 206
Ketone Bodies, 206
Ketosis, 98, 206
Kidney Disease, 29, 148, 206, 231
Kidney Failure, 130, 190, 206, 207
Kidney Failure, Acute, 207
Kidney Failure, Chronic, 207
Kinetics, 63, 72, 207
L
Laminin, 175, 193, 207
Large Intestine, 187, 205, 207, 230, 234
Latent, 12, 207, 226
Leishmaniasis, 90, 207
Lens, 178, 207, 243
Leptin, 43, 49, 50, 70, 72, 80, 120, 207
Lesion, 111, 126, 198, 207
Lethal, 114, 116, 207
Lethargy, 53, 129, 207
Leucine, 31, 45, 72, 109, 207
Leukemia, 11, 104, 109, 188, 195, 207
Leukocytosis, 65, 78, 207
Leukotrienes, 103, 173, 189, 207
Libido, 171, 207
Life Expectancy, 130, 208
Ligament, 208, 227
Ligands, 123, 208
Ligase, 33, 38, 208
Ligation, 33, 208
Linkages, 197, 199, 208
Lipase, 73, 208
Lipid, 24, 72, 81, 91, 94, 103, 122, 126, 172, 180, 197, 204, 206, 208, 214, 220, 241
Lipid Mobilization, 103, 208
Lipid Peroxidation, 208, 220
Lipodystrophy, 7, 46, 208
Lipolysis, 7, 82, 101, 109, 208
Lipopolysaccharide, 116, 127, 198, 208
Lipoprotein, 19, 72, 73, 86, 109, 198, 208, 209
Lipoprotein Lipase, 72, 86, 109, 208
Liposarcoma, 133, 208
Liver Cirrhosis, 57, 199, 208
Lobe, 200, 208
Localized, 57, 67, 189, 203, 207, 208, 209, 224
Loop, 37, 200, 209
Low-density lipoprotein, 208, 209
Lower Esophageal Sphincter, 195, 209
Lung Transplantation, 55, 89, 209
Lupus, 108, 209, 238
Lymph, 41, 179, 190, 209, 236
Lymph node, 179, 209
Lymphadenopathy, 41, 209
Lymphatic, 190, 203, 209, 212, 234
Lymphatic system, 209, 235
Lymphocyte Count, 167, 209
Lymphocyte Depletion, 202, 209
Lymphocytes, 32, 34, 113, 125, 167, 172, 194, 200, 204, 205, 209, 244
Lymphoid, 41, 172, 184, 209, 214
Lymphokines, 113, 209
Lymphoma, 11, 209
Lymphopenia, 41, 209
M
Macrophage, 21, 99, 126, 204, 209
Macula, 210
Macula Lutea, 210
Macular Degeneration, 120, 210
Magnetic Resonance Imaging, 20, 210
Malabsorption, 61, 66, 210
Malaise, 129, 210
Malaria, 108, 113, 115, 116, 127, 210
Malaria, Falciparum, 210
Malaria, Vivax, 210
Malformation, 19, 210
Malignancy, 21, 89, 98, 100, 109, 131, 210
Malignant, 13, 26, 55, 72, 73, 79, 109, 129, 167, 168, 172, 210, 212, 216, 229, 232
Malignant mesothelioma, 210, 212
Malnutrition, 23, 28, 37, 41, 43, 53, 102, 109, 124, 126, 129, 169, 173, 210
Mammary, 208, 210, 238
Mania, 210
Manic, 123, 210
Mastication, 210, 240, 241
Matrix metalloproteinase, 119, 210
Maxillary, 210, 211, 240
Maxillary Nerve, 211, 240
Mediate, 10, 17, 27, 34, 123, 188, 211
Mediator, 16, 27, 42, 72, 86, 116, 118, 123, 204, 211, 224, 233
Medical Oncology, 26, 68, 86, 211
MEDLINE, 149, 211
Medroxyprogesterone Acetate, 51, 211
Megestrol, 4, 51, 60, 68, 69, 73, 74, 75, 80, 81, 82, 84, 85, 86, 88, 89, 143, 211
Megestrol Acetate, 4, 51, 60, 68, 69, 73, 74, 80, 81, 82, 84, 85, 86, 88, 89, 211
Melanin, 211, 222, 241
Melanocytes, 211
Melanoma, 78, 83, 86, 211, 241
Membrane Lipids, 211, 223
Memory, 171, 186, 211
Meninges, 179, 188, 211

Meningitis, 115, 116, 211
Menstrual Cycle, 211, 226
Mental, iv, 4, 123, 148, 150, 179, 183, 186, 187, 193, 203, 210, 211, 212, 228, 232, 242
Mental Health, iv, 4, 148, 150, 212, 228
Mental Retardation, 123, 212
Mesenchymal, 191, 212
Mesothelioma, 71, 210, 212
Metabolic disorder, 10, 23, 30, 38, 43, 45, 120, 128, 132, 197, 212
Metabolite, 12, 20, 212
Metastasis, 13, 120, 130, 210, 212
Metastatic, 48, 81, 109, 212, 232
Metastatic cancer, 81, 212
Microbe, 212, 239
Microbiology, 9, 26, 168, 212
Microcirculation, 208, 212
Microdialysis, 5, 212
Micronutrients, 41, 212
Microorganism, 181, 212, 221, 244
Micro-organism, 116, 212, 233
Microscopy, 33, 175, 212
Microsporidiosis, 9, 212
Microtubules, 212, 220
Mineralocorticoids, 168, 212
Mitochondria, 29, 167, 213, 215, 219
Mitochondrial Swelling, 213, 216
Mitosis, 173, 213
Mitotic, 192, 213
Mobility, 121, 213
Mobilization, 10, 121, 208, 213
Modeling, 20, 213
Modification, 196, 213, 229
Molecular Probes, 189, 213
Monitor, 5, 15, 213, 217
Monoclonal, 200, 213, 229
Monocytes, 113, 125, 204, 205, 213, 214, 238
Monokines, 113, 126, 127, 213
Mononuclear, 48, 74, 75, 113, 116, 198, 213, 241
Morphine, 213, 215
Morphology, 178, 213
Motility, 213, 233
Motion Sickness, 214, 215
Movement Disorders, 214
Mucocutaneous, 207, 214
Mucolytic, 167, 214
Mucosa, 111, 209, 214, 236, 244
Mucositis, 111, 114, 214, 239
Mucus, 214, 241
Multiple Organ Failure, 115, 118, 214
Multiple sclerosis, 72, 115, 119, 214
Muscle Fibers, 214, 215, 241
Muscle Proteins, 29, 33, 59, 214
Muscle relaxant, 185, 214
Musculature, 85, 214
Myasthenia, 116, 117, 214
Myelin, 186, 214
Myeloid Cells, 214
Myeloid Progenitor Cells, 16, 214
Myelosuppression, 123, 214
Myocardial infarction, 123, 175, 184, 214, 215
Myocardial Ischemia, 171, 214
Myocardial Reperfusion, 215, 231
Myocardial Reperfusion Injury, 215, 231
Myocardium, 171, 214, 215
Myofibrils, 32, 177, 189, 215
Myopathy, 41, 215
Myopia, 120, 215, 216, 230
Myosin, 32, 45, 215, 241

N

Naproxen, 101, 215
Narcosis, 215
Narcotic, 111, 213, 215
Natural selection, 175, 215
Nausea, 36, 48, 74, 154, 155, 188, 206, 215, 242
NCI, 1, 147, 154, 181, 215
Nearsightedness, 215, 216
Necrosis, 17, 27, 28, 39, 47, 48, 50, 52, 64, 65, 66, 71, 83, 99, 108, 110, 113, 115, 116, 117, 125, 126, 131, 172, 184, 203, 214, 215, 216, 231, 238, 241
Neonatal, 73, 216
Neonatal period, 73, 216
Neoplasm, 216, 232, 241
Neopterin, 60, 80, 103, 216
Nephropathy, 3, 206, 216
Nephrosis, 199, 216
Nerve Growth Factor, 216, 217
Nervous System, 35, 119, 168, 174, 179, 211, 216, 217, 222, 237
Neural, 5, 35, 45, 168, 200, 216
Neuralgia, 116, 117, 216
Neurodegenerative Diseases, 131, 174, 216
Neuroendocrine, 7, 49, 124, 216
Neurogenic, 216, 242
Neurologic, 112, 216
Neuromuscular, 167, 185, 216, 242
Neuronal, 23, 117, 215, 216
Neurons, 10, 42, 49, 186, 192, 195, 205, 214, 216, 217, 218, 237

Neuropathy, 170, 216, 222
Neuropeptide, 13, 25, 76, 216
Neuropeptide Y, 25, 76, 216
Neurotoxicity, 116, 217
Neurotransmitter, 46, 167, 168, 177, 188, 197, 200, 217, 234, 237
Neurotrophins, 49, 217
Neutrons, 170, 217, 229
Neutropenia, 16, 123, 217
Neutrophils, 198, 205, 217
Niacin, 217, 241
Nitric Oxide, 32, 34, 76, 217
Nitrogen, 32, 42, 84, 98, 109, 129, 170, 171, 173, 184, 193, 197, 207, 217, 241
Non-small cell lung cancer, 11, 75, 217
Norepinephrine, 168, 170, 188, 217
Nuclear, 38, 39, 128, 133, 174, 183, 189, 192, 194, 195, 216, 217, 231
Nuclei, 170, 183, 189, 195, 196, 210, 213, 217, 219, 227
Nucleic acid, 111, 120, 124, 125, 127, 128, 130, 132, 195, 200, 203, 217, 218, 228, 229
Nucleic Acid Hybridization, 200, 218
Nutritional Status, 5, 7, 13, 41, 218
Nutritional Support, 62, 72, 81, 104, 154, 218
Nystagmus, 62, 218

O

Occult, 3, 218
Ocular, 120, 218
Odds Ratio, 218, 230
Olfactory Bulb, 218
Olfactory Nerve, 116, 117, 218
Oligo, 26, 218
Oligomenorrhea, 218, 225
Oliguria, 207, 218
Omega-3 fatty acid, 11, 102, 218
Oncogene, 199, 218
Oncologist, 54, 218
Oncology nurse, 15, 219
Oncolysis, 71, 219
Opacity, 178, 219
Ophthalmic, 219, 240
Opportunistic Infections, 7, 8, 35, 41, 167, 219
Optic Chiasm, 202, 219
Optic Disk, 187, 210, 219
Optic Nerve, 116, 117, 219, 220, 231
Organ Culture, 219, 239
Organelles, 29, 185, 211, 213, 219, 224
Osmotic, 169, 213, 219
Osteoarthritis, 108, 115, 119, 122, 123, 219
Osteoclasts, 177, 219
Osteoporosis, 108, 116, 117, 121, 123, 169, 219
Outpatient, 19, 219
Ovaries, 31, 219, 225, 233
Ovary, 184, 197, 219, 220
Overweight, 20, 95, 128, 132, 220
Ovulation, 171, 198, 211, 220
Ovum, 184, 186, 220, 226, 244
Oxidation, 31, 79, 109, 167, 172, 185, 197, 208, 220, 238, 242
Oxidative metabolism, 168, 207, 220
Oxidative Phosphorylation, 29, 220
Oxidative Stress, 10, 59, 76, 220
Oxygen Consumption, 220, 231
Oxygenase, 21, 220

P

Pachymeningitis, 211, 220
Paclitaxel, 6, 220
Palate, 196, 220, 236, 238
Palliative, 6, 52, 82, 94, 115, 211, 220, 238
Pancreas, 42, 65, 109, 167, 175, 187, 204, 208, 220, 241
Pancreatic, 22, 43, 48, 79, 84, 94, 99, 104, 105, 129, 178, 195, 220
Pancreatic cancer, 22, 43, 48, 79, 99, 104, 105, 220
Pancreatic Juice, 195, 220
Pancreatitis, 22, 118, 220
Paralysis, 116, 117, 220, 228
Paraneoplastic Syndromes, 65, 78, 131, 220
Parasite, 8, 43, 116, 221, 232
Parasitic, 43, 85, 221
Parathyroid, 12, 89, 131, 221, 238
Parathyroid Glands, 221
Parathyroid hormone, 12, 89, 131, 221
Parenteral, 56, 63, 75, 101, 111, 221
Parenteral Nutrition, 56, 63, 111, 221
Paroxysmal, 171, 221
Particle, 36, 221, 240
Pathogen, 127, 221
Pathologic, 173, 175, 184, 201, 221, 228
Pathologic Processes, 173, 221
Pathologies, 27, 35, 41, 113, 125, 221
Pathophysiology, 25, 79, 90, 102, 221
Patient Education, 154, 160, 162, 165, 221
Pelvic, 221, 227
Pelvis, 167, 219, 221, 242
Penicillin, 171, 221, 243
Peptide, 5, 12, 18, 26, 42, 177, 182, 193, 195, 207, 216, 221, 225, 227, 237

Peptide T, 42, 221
Perception, 30, 221, 232
Perfusion, 53, 202, 222
Pericardial Effusion, 51, 222
Pericardium, 222, 238
Periodontal disease, 120, 222
Peripheral blood, 48, 74, 75, 125, 204, 222
Peripheral Nervous System, 186, 191, 216, 217, 222, 237
Peripheral Neuropathy, 3, 29, 222
Peripheral stem cells, 198, 222
Peritoneal, 173, 205, 222
Peritoneal Cavity, 173, 205, 222
Peroxide, 122, 222
Petrolatum, 190, 222
Pharmacologic, 21, 39, 171, 184, 222, 239, 242
Pharynx, 195, 222, 238, 242
Phenolphthalein, 190, 222
Phenotype, 49, 120, 222
Phenylalanine, 222, 241
Phorbol, 10, 222
Phorbol Esters, 10, 222
Phosphodiesterase, 22, 223
Phospholipases, 223, 234
Phospholipids, 122, 193, 208, 211, 223
Phosphorus, 12, 177, 221, 223
Phosphorylase, 29, 177, 223
Phosphorylated, 16, 181, 223
Phosphorylates, 132, 223
Phosphorylation, 10, 27, 123, 132, 180, 223, 242
Phosphorylcholine, 180, 223
Photocoagulation, 181, 223
Physical Examination, 12, 223
Physiologic, 7, 169, 176, 205, 211, 212, 223, 226, 230, 233
Physiology, 6, 22, 29, 30, 35, 60, 67, 223
Pigment, 175, 211, 223
Pilot study, 11, 34, 51, 223
Pineal Body, 223
Pineal gland, 39, 223
Pituitary Gland, 193, 223
Pituitary Hormones, 217, 223
Placenta, 223, 226
Plants, 170, 178, 180, 196, 205, 213, 217, 224, 225, 232, 239
Plaque, 120, 224
Plasma cells, 172, 224
Plasma protein, 80, 169, 224
Plasmapheresis, 64, 224
Plasmid, 130, 224, 243
Plastids, 219, 224
Platelet Activation, 224, 234
Platelet Aggregation, 217, 224, 239
Platelet Factor 4, 205, 224
Platelets, 175, 177, 214, 217, 224
Plicamycin, 111, 224
Pneumonia, 34, 183, 224
Podophyllotoxin, 192, 225
Point Mutation, 29, 225
Poisoning, 186, 205, 215, 225
Polycystic, 132, 225
Polycystic Ovary Syndrome, 132, 225
Polyp, 54, 225
Polypeptide, 42, 49, 110, 123, 127, 128, 132, 170, 181, 191, 193, 200, 225, 227, 244
Polyunsaturated fat, 98, 103, 104, 225, 239
Port, 15, 225
Port-a-cath, 225
Posterior, 180, 196, 220, 223, 225
Postmenopausal, 169, 219, 225
Postnatal, 11, 225, 236
Postoperative, 65, 214, 225
Postprandial, 45, 225
Postsynaptic, 225, 234
Potentiates, 204, 225
Potentiating, 170, 225
Potentiation, 10, 225, 234
Practice Guidelines, 150, 225
Preclinical, 6, 225
Precursor, 119, 125, 167, 173, 180, 184, 188, 189, 190, 191, 216, 217, 222, 225, 240, 241, 243
Predisposition, 128, 226
Premarin, 121, 226
Preoperative, 55, 226
Presynaptic, 217, 226
Prevalence, 13, 22, 35, 110, 112, 218, 226
Probe, 30, 45, 212, 226
Progeny, 183, 226
Progesterone, 121, 211, 226, 236
Progression, 12, 13, 14, 24, 41, 48, 65, 82, 119, 130, 171, 226
Projection, 205, 217, 218, 219, 226
Proline, 182, 201, 226
Promoter, 10, 19, 127, 128, 226
Prophylaxis, 116, 117, 226, 242
Prostaglandin, 21, 113, 226, 239
Prostaglandins A, 226
Prostate, 65, 82, 100, 106, 109, 175, 227, 241
Protease, 46, 182, 227
Protein C, 26, 56, 103, 120, 121, 169, 170, 172, 208, 214, 227, 241, 242

Protein Conformation, 170, 227
Protein Folding, 29, 227
Protein S, 9, 16, 31, 32, 41, 60, 117, 123, 125, 129, 176, 195, 200, 224, 227, 232
Protein Subunits, 125, 227
Proteinuria, 13, 120, 227
Proteoglycans, 175, 193, 227
Proteolytic, 21, 48, 52, 170, 182, 193, 227
Protocol, 15, 227
Protons, 170, 201, 206, 227, 229
Proto-Oncogene Proteins, 220, 227
Proto-Oncogene Proteins c-mos, 220, 227
Protozoa, 183, 207, 212, 228
Protozoal, 228
Protozoan, 123, 210, 228
Proximal, 37, 188, 226, 228
Psoriasis, 108, 123, 228
Psychic, 207, 212, 228, 233
Psychoactive, 17, 228, 238, 244
Psychogenic, 228, 242
Psychotherapy, 228, 230
Ptosis, 29, 228
Puberty, 41, 194, 228
Public Health, 20, 24, 43, 150, 228
Public Policy, 149, 228
Publishing, 50, 228
Pulmonary, 77, 81, 86, 88, 113, 176, 207, 228, 243
Pulmonary Artery, 176, 228, 243
Pulmonary Edema, 207, 228
Pulse, 213, 228
Purines, 228, 233
Pyogenic, 229, 233
Pyramidal Tracts, 193, 229
Pyrimidines, 229, 233
Q
Quality of Life, 14, 16, 18, 23, 37, 40, 48, 83, 85, 229
Quaternary, 227, 229
Quiescent, 33, 229
R
Radiation, 13, 15, 37, 118, 171, 191, 192, 194, 202, 205, 206, 218, 229, 241, 244
Radiation oncologist, 218, 229
Radiation therapy, 15, 37, 192, 205, 229
Radioactive, 201, 203, 205, 206, 213, 217, 229
Radioimmunotherapy, 229
Radioisotope, 229, 239
Radiolabeled, 229
Radiotherapy, 101, 111, 114, 126, 176, 229
Randomized, 19, 48, 75, 79, 82, 189, 229
Randomized clinical trial, 48, 229
Reactive Oxygen Species, 38, 230
Reassurance, 4, 230
Receptors, Serotonin, 230, 233
Recombinant, 16, 47, 89, 108, 111, 112, 113, 123, 124, 127, 130, 230, 243
Recombination, 183, 195, 230
Rectum, 172, 176, 182, 187, 195, 203, 207, 227, 230
Recurrence, 13, 179, 181, 230
Red blood cells, 191, 214, 220, 230, 232
Reductase, 22, 230
Refer, 1, 177, 182, 190, 205, 210, 217, 229, 230, 239
Refraction, 215, 230
Refractive Power, 215, 230
Regeneration, 33, 116, 117, 194, 230
Regimen, 114, 189, 230
Regurgitation, 54, 195, 230
Reinfection, 42, 230
Relapse, 4, 230
Relative risk, 14, 230
Remission, 230
Renal cell carcinoma, 57, 231
Renal failure, 23, 28, 125, 129, 186, 199, 231
Renal Osteodystrophy, 13, 231
Reperfusion, 116, 117, 119, 215, 231
Reperfusion Injury, 119, 231
Reproductive cells, 196, 199, 231
Respiration, 38, 178, 193, 213, 231
Retina, 117, 180, 187, 207, 210, 215, 219, 231, 232, 243
Retinal, 187, 219, 231
Retinal Ganglion Cells, 219, 231
Retinopathy, 3, 120, 187, 231
Retrospective, 40, 231
Retroviral vector, 195, 231
Retrovirus, 113, 231
Rheumatoid, 23, 52, 57, 83, 108, 115, 116, 119, 122, 123, 125, 127, 128, 182, 215, 232
Rheumatoid arthritis, 23, 57, 83, 108, 115, 119, 122, 123, 125, 127, 128, 182, 215, 232
Ribose, 168, 232, 239
Ribosome, 232, 240
Risk factor, 12, 22, 55, 129, 230, 232
Rod, 174, 181, 190, 232
S
Salivary, 180, 187, 193, 220, 232, 236
Saponins, 232, 236
Sarcoma, 26, 109, 232, 234
Sarcomere, 33, 232
Satiation, 46, 232

Schistosome, 41, 43, 232
Schizoid, 232, 244
Schizophrenia, 123, 232, 244
Schizotypal Personality Disorder, 232, 244
Sclerosis, 108, 116, 117, 182, 214, 232
Screening, 22, 112, 122, 124, 181, 232
Secondary tumor, 212, 232
Secretory, 28, 232
Sedative, 170, 174, 233
Seizures, 186, 221, 233
Selective estrogen receptor modulator, 233, 238
Selenium, 109, 114, 233
Self Care, 167, 233
Semen, 227, 233
Seminiferous tubule, 203, 233
Semisynthetic, 192, 233
Senile, 108, 219, 233
Sepsis, 12, 32, 48, 108, 119, 127, 129, 132, 233
Septic, 12, 27, 28, 33, 48, 94, 115, 116, 119, 123, 128, 233
Septicaemia, 66, 233
Sequence Homology, 221, 233
Serine, 16, 123, 132, 227, 233
Serotonin, 74, 75, 167, 170, 185, 208, 217, 230, 233, 241
Serum, 6, 12, 18, 26, 32, 60, 94, 114, 117, 169, 182, 207, 209, 213, 233, 241
Sex Characteristics, 171, 228, 233, 238
Shivering, 233, 238
Shock, 12, 27, 94, 106, 113, 115, 116, 118, 119, 123, 126, 128, 190, 234, 240
Side effect, 6, 27, 36, 111, 114, 141, 143, 168, 175, 184, 214, 234, 239
Signal Transduction, 10, 40, 44, 47, 84, 123, 234
Signs and Symptoms, 230, 234, 242
Skeleton, 11, 167, 226, 234
Skin Aging, 120, 234
Small cell lung cancer, 234
Small intestine, 8, 180, 188, 200, 205, 234
Smooth muscle, 18, 169, 177, 183, 200, 213, 217, 234, 237
Social Environment, 229, 234
Sodium, 85, 197, 213, 215, 234
Soft tissue, 176, 194, 234
Soft tissue sarcoma, 194, 234
Solid tumor, 13, 120, 188, 234
Solitary Nucleus, 174, 235
Solvent, 197, 219, 235
Soma, 235
Somatic, 19, 35, 179, 196, 200, 213, 222, 235, 242
Somatic cells, 179, 213, 235
Soybean Oil, 225, 235
Spasticity, 185, 235
Specialist, 156, 235
Species, 9, 12, 113, 169, 191, 200, 207, 210, 213, 221, 230, 233, 235, 236, 240, 241, 243, 244
Specificity, 31, 169, 235
Spectroscopic, 13, 235
Sperm, 131, 171, 180, 196, 199, 231, 233, 235
Sperm Motility, 132, 235
Spermatozoon, 235
Spinal cord, 108, 173, 177, 179, 180, 188, 191, 195, 211, 216, 220, 222, 229, 235, 237
Sporadic, 216, 235
Squamous, 65, 78, 191, 217, 235
Squamous cell carcinoma, 78, 191, 217, 235
Squamous cells, 235
Statistically significant, 8, 236
Steel, 181, 236
Stellate, 47, 236
Stem Cells, 191, 214, 222, 236
Sterile, 221, 236
Sterility, 185, 236
Steroid, 115, 184, 194, 232, 236
Stimulant, 185, 200, 236, 242
Stimulus, 18, 108, 188, 192, 204, 205, 236, 239
Stomach, 31, 109, 167, 174, 187, 192, 195, 196, 200, 206, 209, 215, 222, 234, 236
Stomatitis, 114, 236
Stool, 8, 182, 207, 236
Stress, 10, 28, 122, 174, 178, 184, 215, 220, 226, 232, 236
Stroke, 27, 45, 108, 112, 128, 132, 133, 148, 178, 236
Stupor, 207, 215, 236
Subacute, 203, 236
Subclinical, 203, 233, 236
Subcutaneous, 25, 131, 168, 189, 208, 221, 236, 243
Submaxillary, 191, 236
Subspecies, 235, 236
Substance P, 212, 232, 237
Substrate, 16, 98, 237
Sulfur, 193, 237
Superantigens, 116, 237
Superoxide, 122, 237

Supplementation, 4, 37, 40, 98, 100, 101, 103, 114, 130, 237
Suppression, 39, 46, 86, 99, 237
Survival Rate, 118, 237
Sympathetic Nervous System, 174, 237
Sympathomimetic, 188, 191, 217, 237
Symphysis, 179, 227, 237
Symptomatic, 220, 237
Synapse, 168, 226, 237, 240
Synaptic, 217, 234, 237
Synergistic, 6, 18, 23, 43, 124, 237
Systemic lupus erythematosus, 115, 182, 237
Systolic, 201, 238

T

Tamoxifen, 6, 233, 238
Taste Buds, 30, 238
Teratogenic, 169, 187, 238
Testicular, 30, 123, 224, 238
Testis, 31, 238
Testosterone, 4, 7, 46, 230, 238
Tetany, 221, 238
Tetrahydrocannabinol, 17, 116, 177, 188, 238
Thalidomide, 78, 86, 238
Therapeutics, 11, 78, 142, 205, 238
Thermogenesis, 38, 63, 238
Third Ventricle, 173, 202, 223, 238
Thoracic, 78, 132, 209, 238, 244
Threonine, 123, 132, 221, 227, 233, 238
Threshold, 201, 238
Thrombin, 193, 224, 227, 239
Thrombocytopenia, 41, 239
Thrombomodulin, 227, 239
Thrombosis, 175, 227, 236, 239
Thromboxanes, 173, 189, 239
Thymidine, 22, 29, 239
Thymidine Phosphorylase, 29, 239
Thyroid, 52, 81, 177, 221, 239, 241
Thyroid Gland, 221, 239
Thyroxine, 169, 222, 239
Tissue Culture, 8, 239
Tolerance, 105, 167, 196, 239
Tooth Preparation, 168, 239
Topical, 201, 222, 239
Toxic, iv, 8, 25, 26, 36, 113, 169, 183, 185, 191, 192, 202, 216, 225, 233, 239
Toxicity, 6, 37, 116, 188, 239
Toxicology, 36, 150, 239
Toxin, 190, 239
Tracer, 45, 239
Trachea, 222, 239, 240
Traction, 181, 240
Transcriptase, 231, 240
Transcription Factors, 16, 27, 38, 48, 240
Transduction, 10, 23, 30, 123, 234, 240
Transfection, 176, 190, 195, 240
Transforming Growth Factor alpha, 111, 240
Transforming Growth Factor beta, 31, 47, 240
Translation, 28, 108, 127, 240
Translational, 11, 15, 108, 240
Translocation, 43, 123, 240
Transmitter, 167, 173, 188, 211, 217, 240
Transplantation, 81, 101, 180, 207, 209, 240
Trauma, 108, 116, 118, 174, 186, 192, 216, 220, 240
Triad, 129, 240
Tricyclic, 170, 224, 240
Trigeminal, 117, 211, 240
Trigeminal Nerve, 117, 240
Triglyceride, 94, 201, 208, 241
Tropomyosin, 214, 241
Troponin, 214, 241
Truncal, 46, 121, 241
Tryptophan, 12, 56, 60, 109, 182, 233, 241
Tuberculosis, 35, 116, 209, 241
Tumor marker, 175, 241
Tumor-derived, 24, 241
Tumour, 63, 64, 78, 84, 94, 100, 101, 104, 195, 241
Tunica, 214, 241
Type 2 diabetes, 38, 129, 133, 241
Tyrosine, 16, 33, 188, 241

U

Ubiquitin, 21, 25, 28, 32, 38, 39, 48, 52, 241
Ulcerative colitis, 115, 119, 203, 241
Ultraviolet radiation, 234, 241
Uncoupling Agents, 206, 242
Univalent, 201, 220, 242
Uraemia, 220, 242
Urea, 32, 42, 207, 242
Uremia, 207, 231, 242
Urethra, 227, 242
Urinary, 12, 20, 123, 218, 242
Urinary Retention, 123, 242
Urinate, 242
Urine, 26, 70, 172, 176, 188, 191, 206, 207, 218, 227, 242
Uterus, 179, 184, 186, 219, 226, 242

V

Vaccination, 34, 242
Vaccine, 42, 168, 227, 241, 242

Vacuoles, 219, 242
Vagina, 179, 186, 242
Vagus Nerve, 235, 241, 242
Valine, 109, 242
Vascular, 169, 180, 190, 203, 208, 212, 217, 223, 239, 243
Vasculitis, 220, 243
Vasodilator, 177, 188, 200, 215, 243
Vector, 25, 127, 240, 243
Vein, 173, 205, 217, 243
Venous, 44, 173, 175, 227, 243
Ventral, 173, 202, 243
Ventricle, 228, 238, 243
Ventricular, 13, 67, 215, 243
Ventricular Dysfunction, 67, 243
Venules, 176, 177, 212, 243
Vertebrae, 205, 235, 243
Veterinary Medicine, 149, 243
Viral, 7, 32, 113, 116, 123, 167, 184, 194, 216, 231, 240, 243
Virulence, 174, 239, 243
Virus, 6, 34, 41, 53, 65, 69, 117, 128, 167, 191, 196, 198, 204, 224, 231, 240, 243
Viscera, 235, 243
Visceral, 19, 35, 42, 45, 46, 63, 90, 174, 196, 207, 242, 243
Visceral Afferents, 174, 196, 242, 243
Visceral fat, 19, 243
Viscosity, 167, 243
Vitreous, 187, 207, 231, 243
Vitreous Body, 231, 243
Vitro, 6, 21, 26, 36, 43, 199, 243
Vivo, 6, 8, 11, 13, 17, 19, 21, 30, 31, 33, 39, 44, 49, 69, 78, 86, 101, 125, 130, 179, 195, 199, 203, 209, 212, 239, 244
Volition, 206, 244

W

Wakefulness, 186, 244
White blood cell, 172, 175, 203, 209, 214, 217, 224, 244
Windpipe, 222, 239, 244
Withdrawal, 55, 76, 186, 244
Wound Healing, 9, 47, 120, 121, 180, 194, 210, 244

X

Xenograft, 22, 71, 171, 244
X-ray, 20, 194, 217, 229, 244

Y

Yeasts, 222, 244
Yolk Sac, 193, 244

Z

Zygote, 183, 244
Zymogen, 227, 244

9 780497 001957

Printed in the United States
30322LVS00001B/176

9 780497 001957